Central Nervous System Tumors - Primary and Secondary

Edited by Feyzi Birol Sarica

Published in London, United Kingdom

Central Nervous System Tumors - Primary and Secondary
http://dx.doi.org/10.5772/intechopen.102249
Edited by Feyzi Birol Sarica

Contributors
José Luis Navarro-Olvera, Armando Armas-Salazar, Jesús Q. Beltrán, Gustavo Aguado-Carrillo, Fiacro Jiménez-Ponce, Edgar Abarca-Rojano, José Damián Carrillo-Ruiz, Edwina Ayaaba Ayabilah, Andrew Yaw Nyantakyi, Joseph Daniels, İsmail Kaya, Hüseyin Yakar, Nicollas Nunes Rabelo, Mateus Gonçalves de Sena Barbosa, G. Sethuram Rao, D. Vydeki, Raghunadharao Digumarti, Sujith Kumar Mullapally, Vidyasagar Dusi, Feyzi Birol Sarica, Gabriele Capo, Alberto Vandenbulcke, Cédric Yves Barrey, Ayfer Aslan, Gökhan Kurt, Mustafa Caglar Sahin, Nazmin Ahmed

First published in London, United Kingdom, 2023 by IntechOpen
IntechOpen is the global imprint of INTECHOPEN LIMITED, registered in England and Wales, registration number: 11086078, 5 Princes Gate Court, London, SW7 2QJ, United Kingdom

British Library Cataloguing-in-Publication Data
A catalogue record for this book is available from the British Library

Additional hard and PDF copies can be obtained from orders@intechopen.com

Central Nervous System Tumors - Primary and Secondary
Edited by Feyzi Birol Sarica
p. cm.
Print ISBN 978-1-80356-752-5
Online ISBN 978-1-80356-753-2
eBook (PDF) ISBN 978-1-80356-754-9

For EU product safety concerns:
IN TECH d.o.o., Prolaz Marije Krucifikse Kozulić 3, 51000 Rijeka, Croatia,
info@intechopen.com or visit our website at intechopen.com.

Meet the editor

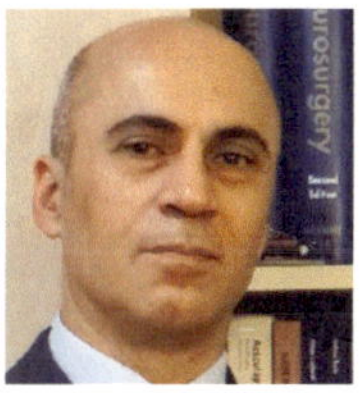

Feyzi Birol Sarica graduated in medicine from Ankara University in 1997. Following the presentation of his thesis, "Prognostic factors in Supratentorial Glial Tumors", at the Ankara Numune Education and Research Hospital, he was certified as a neurosurgeon. Between 2006 and 2015 he worked first as a neurosurgeon and then as a lecturer at Adana Education and Research Hospital, Baskent University. Further appointments were at Kudret International Hospital in Ankara, and the Department of Neurosurgery at Giresun University, where he became an associate professor in 2018. He is a member of the Turkish Neurosurgical Society and the Nervous System Surgery Association.

Contents

Preface

Tumors of the central nervous system (CNS), as described in the World Health Organization's 2021 *Classification of CNS Tumors*, may be of more than 100 types, originating from the brain, cerebellum, brain stem, spinal cord, and meninges. Thanks to advances in microsurgery and intraoperative assistive imaging technologies, total or gross-total resections of many CNS tumors can now be achieved. However, treatment of high-grade CNS tumors such as glioblastoma multiforme remains difficult. With adjuvant radiotherapy, chemotherapy (such as Temozolomide) and anti-angiogenic agents (such as Bevacizumab), partial increases in the life span of patients with these tumors have been observed. At the same time, due to advances in clinical and experimental studies, the genetic, molecular and immunological structures of many high-grade CNS tumors, as well as their interactions with the tumor microenvironment, are now better understood. Today, targeted therapies and vaccines developed with immunotherapy protocols are promising developments. This book is designed to increase understanding of the natural history of CNS tumors and to update knowledge on relevant treatment protocols.

Chapter 1 is the Introductory Chapter.

Chapter 2 focuses on histopathology, epidemiology, and multidisciplinary treatment protocols for intracranial meningiomas. Selective surgical approaches, depending on the location of these tumors, are explained in detail. The advantages of stereotactic radiosurgery (SRC), used in tumors that cannot be completely removed and whose residues are detected in the postoperative period, are discussed, and clinical studies are described in which therapeutically effective anti-angiogenic agents are used to target intracranial meningiomas. In Chapter 3 the role of radiotherapy and stereotactic radiosurgery in the treatment of residual or recurrent high-grade tumors is discussed. These techniques can be especially useful, with the MR-perfusion technique, or differentiating meningioma subtypes. A significant relationship has been established between MR elastography measurements and the intraoperative qualitative assessment of tumor consistency. The use of this technique is very useful in the gross-total removal of these tumors during surgery. Radiomics and artificial intelligence are described as potential methods for preoperative evaluation of high-grade meningiomas, prediction of recurrence and outcomes, and radiation therapy planning. Studies on smart drug molecules that can be developed in accordance with the molecular characteristics of high-grade meningiomas are also included.

Chapter 4 describes surgical and radiosurgical treatment (gamma-knife, etc.) options for pituitary neuroendocrine tumors. Surgical (transcranial and transsphenoidal) options for these tumors, and tumoral and hormonal control rates are also covered. It is reported that more than 90% of tumor control in non-functional adenomas is achieved with SRC, and the morbidity associated with radiosurgery is less than 1% in lesions invading the cavernous sinus. Chapter 5 discusses diagnostic methods, clinical findings and multidisciplinary treatment approaches to craniopharyngioma. Surgical and/or endoscopic approaches preferred for total or gross-total tumor resection, depending on craniopharyngioma classifications (including endoscopic ones), are explained.

Chapter 6 explores general metastatic pathways and pathobiological processes, with particular reference to tumors that metastasize to the brain. This study underlines the importance of radiotherapy (especially whole-brain radiotherapy) and SRC (gamma-knife, cyber-knife, etc.). Chapter 7 considers the incidence of pediatric CNS tumors in the world and specifically in India, with the different treatment protocols (such as surgery, WBRT, SRC, and proton therapy) and their contribution to patients' life expectancy. Attention is drawn to the lack of radiotherapy and oncology centers in India and other developing countries, and the consequent inadequacy of pediatric CNS tumor data reporting. It is especially important that guidelines containing treatment algorithms for pediatric CNS tumors should be established in developing countries.

Chapter 8 discusses brain tumor detection techniques based on MR images and using unconventional soft computing approaches. An extensive literature survey reveals that brain tumor detection and classification using artificial neural networks (ANN), self-organizing maps (SOM) and back propagation networks (BPN) is a promising research field. An automated tumor detection system using ANN is proposed to classify the images as metastasis, glioma, astrocytoma and meningioma. Analysis of a simulation using modified SOM and modified BPN techniques showed superior results for tumors of different sizes and shapes, compared to conventional MR imaging methods, with 96% accuracy in tumor classification and an average efficiency of 93% (improvements of 10% and 8%, respectively).

For optimal resection of brain tumors, intraoperative real-time 2D USG should be preferred by neurosurgeons to intraoperative neuro-navigation techniques because it is both cheaper and more accessible. Ultrasound is used during tumor resection for different purposes: tumor location and characterization, surgical planning, and evaluation of the extent of resection. Chapter 9 compares ultrasonography techniques for gross-total or total tumor resections.

The possible oncolytic effect of the Zika virus, especially in high-grade brain tumors, is explored in Chapter 10. Zika virus originates from non-structural protein 5 (NS5). In the future, there is the potential for Zika virus vaccines to be used as an adjuvant treatment in patients with glioblastoma multiforme tumors, whose life expectancy is quite short compared to other organ tumors. Tumor remission has been reported in mice inoculated with Zika virus-infected cells and in mice with diagnosed glioblastoma multiforme with intracranial injections of live attenuated Zika virus. These findings still need to be investigated in vivo, and there are currently no human studies to support the safety of CNS studies of the Zika virus.

Epidemiological, histopathological and genetic features of intradural intramedullary spinal tumors are described in Chapter 11. The relevant diagnostic imaging techniques are also indicated. Surgical and adjuvant radiotherapy protocols for these tumors are discussed. The pathogenesis, predisposing factors and clinical symptomatology of spinal meningiomas are reported in Chapter 12, together with appropriate surgical approaches, depending on the location and topography of the tumor, and factors affecting the prognosis of these patients.

Feyzi Birol Sarica
Associate Professor,
Department of Neurosurgery,
Giresun University Faculty of Medicine,
Giresun, Turkey

Section 1

Introduction

Chapter 1

Introductory Chapter: Significant Updates for Brain Tumors to the 2021 WHO Classification of the CNS Tumors (WHO CNS5) and Clinical Overview – Molecular Translation of the Brain Tumors

Feyzi Birol Sarica

1. Introduction

The incidence of the brain tumors is 14.8 per 100,000 people per year. An estimated 43,800 new brain tumors are diagnosed each year in the United States of America. It has been stated that 92.2% of these are observed in adults and over age groups, and 7.8% are observed in children and adolescents. About half of the brain tumors are histologically in benign character, and the most common histologically observed tumor type in this group is Meningioma. The primary brain tumors with the malignant character comprise 2% of all cancers. The primary brain tumors with the malignant character are in the 1st rank among the causes of death due to the solid tumors in children and in the 3rd rank among the causes of death due to the cancer in adolescents aged 15–34 and adults. The most common histologically observed tumor type in this group is glioblastoma [1].

2. Brain tumors

2.1 Clinical features

Depending on the histopathological structure of the brain tumors, they can only make external compression on the adjacent brain parenchyma or cause necrosis with different levels of the parenchymal infiltration. The most common symptom observed for the brain tumors is headache, which develops as a result of increased intracranial pressure. The epileptic seizures are frequently observed in the low-grade tumors. The focal neurological deficits, such as hemiparesis and hemihypoesthesia, are usually related to the localization of the tumor. The mental status changes that range from sleepiness to deep coma are observed in 15–20% of the patients with glioma [2].

2.2 Diagnostic techniques

The contrast-enhanced brain magnetic resonance imaging (MRI) is essential in the diagnosis of the primary brain tumors. Both the annular areas with the live tumor tissue with the contrast enhancement and the central necrotic areas can be displayed in more detail in the high-grade gliomas, especially like the glioblastoma by means of the contrast-enhanced brain MRI. The peritumoral vasogenic edema area is also evaluated on the MRI T2 sequences. The brain MR-spectroscopy, in which the metabolic activity of the relevant tumor is evaluated, is used especially in the diagnosis of the low-grade gliomas. The tumors such as medulloblastoma, which often spread to the leptomeninges *via* the subarachnoid space, are required to be scanned with the MRI in the spinal area along with the brain [2]. The definitive diagnosis of the brain tumors is made either by the surgical biopsy or by the histopathological examination of the tumoral tissue taken by the stereotaxic biopsy in the tumor localizations having a high risk of the surgical morbidity [3–5].

2.3 Treatment protocols

2.3.1 Surgery

In the benign brain tumors such as meningioma, the first treatment option is surgical tumor resection, and in most cases, total removal of the tumor is possible. Due to their infiltrative natural structure, there are difficulties encountered in total surgical removal of the high-grade brain tumors. However, since the level of surgical resection has been shown to have a positive effect on the prognosis of the malignant brain tumors, the radical tumor resection is recommended as much as possible without causing morbidity [3–5]. By means of the tumor cytoreduction, both the existing neurological conditions of the patients can be improved and the radiotherapy and/or chemotherapy protocols to be applied after the surgery can be applied more effectively. By means of the advances in the microsurgical techniques and surgical approaches, more radical resections of the brain tumors can be performed today. In addition, the development of auxiliary microsurgical techniques such as intraoperative neuronavigation, which allows real-time evaluation of the stereotaxic three-dimensional images during the surgery, greatly increases the success of microsurgical tumor resection. The cortical mapping of the brain and white matter pathways is used to prevent postoperative morbidity in the radical surgical resections of the tumors located near critical functional areas of the brain. In the tumors localized in the critical functional areas of the brain with an unacceptable high risk of the postoperative morbidity, the stereotaxic biopsy performed with the computed tomography is preferred for the histopathological diagnosis [2].

2.3.2 Radiotherapy, chemotherapy, and molecular targeted therapy

The radiotherapy has become the standard adjuvant treatment method, especially in the high-grade gliomas, after it was shown that the radiotherapy applied in the postsurgical period prolongs the median life span by 14–36 weeks [6]. For the brain tumors, the radiotherapy is used as adjuvant therapy in the postoperative period. By means of the calculated therapeutic rate by taking into account the radiosensitivity of the normal parenchymal tissue, currently, the fractionated radiotherapy protocols, in which the multiple small doses of the radiation are applied, have been developed for many infiltrative malignant brain tumors. In the non-infiltrative brain tumors such as brain metastases, meningiomas adjacent to the optic nerve, and residual vestibular schwannomas, the stereotaxic radiosurgery is preferred, in which a single fraction and high-dose radiotherapy can be applied to the tumor area [7]. The temozolomide is the most commonly used chemotherapeutic agent, with the proven usefulness as a postoperative adjuvant therapy for the high-grade gliomas. Currently, in the treatment of the glioblastoma, concomitant therapy protocol is used, which is planned to be continued with temozolomide for six more cycles after the temozolomide treatment used at the same time with radiotherapy. While the median life expectancy is 12.1 months in the patients who received only radiotherapy, this has been 14.6 months with this concomitant treatment with temozolomide [8]. Bevacizumab, which is a monoclonal antibody binding to the vascular endothelial growth factor, with its antiangiogenic effect, has increased progression-free survival rates in the patients with relapsed GBM following the concomitant treatment with temozolomide [9].

Especially in the treatment of high-grade brain tumors, by means of the positive developments observed in recent years, although the life span of the patients is partially prolonged, these treatment results are still not at an acceptable level today. Therefore, there is a need to develop new agents targeting the aberrant signaling pathways of the high-grade brain tumors. In this context, the World Health Organization's (WHO) Classification of Central Nervous System (CNS) Tumors for 2016, in which histology of the CNS tumors and molecular data were combined, was updated in 2021.

3. Significant updates for brain tumors to the 2021 WHO classification of CNS tumors

In the WHO 2021 classification of the CNS tumors (WHO CNS5), the natural course of the tumors as a result of their molecular and biological behavior was better characterized. In this classification, especially practical approaches obtained as a result of the molecular translation of the tumors occupy a place in the taxonomy of the CNS tumors [10]. The most important change in the WHO CNS5 updated classification is that the subtypes of the gliomas have been also stated by separating them as adult-type and pediatric-type gliomas by considering the deep-rooted molecular genetic differences. The data stated in this classification make important contributions both to the planning of optimal treatment specific to the tumor subtypes and to the development of new treatment protocols in this way. As a result, the prognosis of the homogeneous patient groups with the CNS tumors and subtypes will also be better understood [11].

When the adult-type gliomas were examined, the glioblastoma was divided into IDH-mutant type (10%) and IDH-wildtype (90%) tumors in the previous classifications. To eliminate the problems observed due to the very different biological behavior of these tumors, only IDH-wildtype tumors are included in glioblastoma in the WHO CNS5 classification. In addition, although it does not have the histological features of glioblastoma typical of adults, the IDH-wildtype diffuse astrocytic tumors with one or more of three genetic parameters have been included in the glioblastoma group. In these genetic parameters, there are TERT promoter mutation, EGFR gene amplification, or combined gain of entire chromosome 7 and loss of entire chromosome 10 (+7/−10). In the WHO CNS5 classification, all IDH-mutant diffuse astrocytic tumors have been classified separately and named as IDH-mutant astrocytoma.

The IDH-mutant astrocytomas have been graded as grades 2, 3, and 4. The tumors having the CDKN2A/B homozygous deletion have been classified as the WHO grade 4, and all IDH-mutant diffuse astrocytic tumors have been classified separately and named as IDH-mutant astrocytoma [11].

When the pediatric-type gliomas are examined, they have divided into two groups as pediatric-type diffuse low-grade glioma and pediatric-type diffuse high-grade glioma. There are four glioma subtypes that take place within these two tumor groups. The pediatric low-grade gliomas have been classified as tumors with the specific BRAF mutations and fusions, by taking into account the differences in the molecular structures. This situation is very important in terms of the current treatment protocols, especially in the pediatric patient groups having the low-grade glioma [12]. In addition, in the WHO CNS5 classification, as it is in the pilocytic astrocytomas having the complex histological features, in addition to the *BRAF* mutations and/or fusions having the prognostic significance for the high-grade astrocytomas with the piloid features, other accompanying mutations, such as CDKN2A/B and ATRX, have been stated [13]. In addition, the infant-type hemispheric gliomas associated with the NTRK family or other genetic abnormalities have been described in this classification. This situation is very important in the preparation of the current treatment plans for the patients having this group of tumors [11].

The modified ependymoma subtypes have been stated in the WHO CNS5 classification based on the histological and molecular features, as well as the anatomical locations of the ependymomas. In addition, it has been stated that the different predictive values are observed in these tumor subtypes as a result of the detection of the specific molecular changes such as loss of chromosome 6q in the ependymoma subtypes located in the posterior fossa [14]. For the medulloblastomas, the WHO CNS5 classification has been created based on the biological and clinical heterogeneity of the tumors generally used in the WHO 2016 classification [15]. In this classification, the non-WNT/non-SHH tumors appear to be the most common types of medulloblastoma. The SHH-associated tumors have been evaluated in two subgroups as TP53 wild-type and TP53-mutant type, due to the differences in their prognosis. In conclusion, 13 or more subgroups have been defined in the WHO CNS5 classification, by taking into account the molecular information of medulloblastoma tumors. Despite the surgical treatment, the local and craniospinal radiotherapy for the non-medulloblastoma embryonal tumors, except for the atypical teratoid/rhabdoid tumors, the prognosis is still poor in this patient group. For this reason, it is extremely important to develop molecular targeted therapy agents, as well as effective chemotherapeutic agents to be used in the treatment of the patients found in this group [11].

4. Conclusions

In addition to the genetic and molecular structures of the CNS tumors, which are tried to be described in detail in the WHO CNS5 classification, the interactions between the immunological aspects of the tumor and its microenvironment are better understood; various molecular targeted therapy protocols for these tumors will be able to be developed. In this context, the targeted therapies such as immunotherapy protocols currently being studied are promising developments today including vaccines. This book has been designed by many internationally respected authors in their field to understand the natural history and biological behavior of the CNS tumors and to update information on the treatment protocols.

Conflict of interest

The authors declare no conflict of interest.

Abbreviations

CNS	Central nervous system
MRI	magnetic resonance imaging
WHO	World Health Organization
WHO CNS5	2021 WHO classification of the CNS tumors

Author details

Feyzi Birol Sarica
Giresun University Faculty of Medicine, Department of Neurosurgery, Giresun Education and Research Hospital, Giresun, Turkey

*Address all correspondence to: saricafb@gmail.com

References

[1] Jemal A, Siegal R, Ward E, Murray T, Xu J, Thun MJ. Cancer statistics, 2007. CA: a Cancer Journal for Clinicians. 2007;**57**:43-66. DOI: 10.3322/canjckin.57.1.43

[2] Buckner JC, Brown PD, O'Neill BP, Meyer FB, Wetmore CJ, Uhm JH. Central nervous system tumors. Mayo Clinic Proceedings. 2007;**82**(10):1271-1286. DOI: 10.4065/82.10.1271

[3] Simpson JR, Horton J, Scott C, Curran WJ, Rubin P, Fischbach J, et al. Influence of location and extent of surgical resection on survival of patients with glioblastoma multiforme: Results of three consecutive radiation therapy oncology group (RTOG) clinical trials. International Journal of Radiation Oncology, Biology, Physics. 1993;**26**(2):239-244. DOI: 10.1016/0360-3016(93)90203-8

[4] Keles GE, Anderson B, Berger MS. The effect of extent of resection on time to tumor progression and survival in patients with glioblastoma multiforme of the cerebral hemisphere. Surgical Neurology. 1999;**52**(4):371-379. DOI: 10.1016/s0090-3019(99)00103-2

[5] Lacroix M, Abi-Said D, Fourney DR, Gokaslan ZL, Shi W, DeMonte F, et al. A multivariate analysis of 416 patients with glioblastoma multiforme: Prognosis, extent of resection, and survival. Journal of Neurosurgery. 2001;**95**(2):190-198. DOI: 10.3171/jns.2001.95.2.0190

[6] Stupp R, Tonn JC, Brada M, Pentheroudakis G. ESMO guidelines working group. High-grade malignant glioma: ESMO clinical practice guidelines for diagnosis, treatment and follow-up. Ann. Oncology. 2010;**21**(Suppl. 5):190-193. DOI: 10.1093/annonc/mdq187

[7] Souhami L, Seiferheld W, Brachman D, Poggorsak EB, Werner-Wasik M, Lustig R, et al. Randomized comparison of stereotactic radiosurgery followed by conventional radiotherapy with carmustine for patients with glioblastoma multiforme: Report of radiation therapy oncology group 39-05 protocol. International Journal of Radiation Oncology, Biology, Physics. 2004;**60**:853-860. DOI: 10.1016/j.ijrobp.2004.04.011

[8] Stupp R, Mason WP, Van Den Bent MJ, Weller M, Fisher B, Taphoorn MJB, et al. European Organisation for Research and Treatment of Cancer brain tumor and radiotherapy groups, National Cancer Institute of Canada clinical trials group. Radiotherapy plus concomitant and adjuvant temozolomide for glioblastoma. The New England Journal of Medicine. 2005;**352**:987-996. DOI: 10.1056/NEJMoa043330

[9] Friedman HS, Prados MD, Wen PY, Mikkelsen T, Schiff D, Abrey LE, et al. Bevacizumab alone and in combination with irinotecan in recurrent glioblastoma. Journal of Clinical Oncology. 2009;**27**:4733-4740. DOI: 10.1200/JCO.2008.19.8721

[10] Louis DN, Perry A, Wesseling P, Brat DJ, Cree IA, Figarella-Branger D, et al. The 2021 WHO classification of tumors of the central nervous system: A summary. Neuro-Oncology. 2021;**23**(8):1231-1251. DOI: 10.1093/neuonc/noab106

[11] Wen PY, Packer RJ. The 2021 WHO classification of tumors of the central nervous system: Clinical implications. Neuro-Oncology. 2021;**23**(8):1215-1217. DOI: 10.1093/neurooonc/noab120

[12] Jones DTW, Kieran MW, Bouffet E, Alexandrescu S, Bandopadhayay P, Bornhorst M, et al. Pediatric low-grade gliomas: Next biologically driven steps. Neuro-Oncology. 2018;**20**(2):160-173. DOI: 10.1093/neuonc/nox141

[13] Reinhardt A, Stichel D, Schrimpf D, Sahm F, Korshunov A, Reuss DE, et al. Anaplastic astrocytoma with piloid features, a novel molecular class of IDH wildtype glioma with recurrent MAPK pathway, CDKN2A/B and ATRX alterations. Acta Neuropathologica. 2018;**136**(2):273-291. DOI: 10.1007/s00401-018-1837-8

[14] Baroni L, Sundaresan L, Heled A, Coltin H, Pajtler KW, Lin T, et al. Ultra high-risk PFA ependymoma is characterized by loss of chromosome 6q. Neuro-Oncology. 2021;**23**(8):1372-1381. DOI: 10.1093/neuonc/noab034

[15] Hovestadt V, Ayrault O, Swartling FJ, Robinson GW, Pfister SM, Northcott PA. Medulloblastomics revisited: Biological and clinical insights from thousands of patients. Nature Reviews. Cancer. 2020;**20**(1):42-56. DOI: 10.1038/s41568-019-0223-8

Section 2

Intracranial Central Nervous System Tumors

Chapter 2

Meningiomas

İsmail Kaya and Hüseyin Yakar

Abstract

Meningiomas are among the most common central nervous system (CNS) tumors worldwide. These extra-axial lesions, which usually originate from neoplastic arachnoidal (meningothelial) cells, often appear in mid-late adulthood and are more common in women. Due to their heterogeneous morphology, the World Health Organization (WHO) divided meningiomas into three main groups, and these three main groups are divided into nine subgroups with histopathological differences according to their biological behavior. Clinical signs and symptoms, as in other central nervous system tumors, vary considerably depending on the compression or invasion of the neurovascular structures in the compartment where the meningioma is located. Meningiomas that are presented as benign lesions often have the potential to grow slowly, but could be associated with morbidity, such as poor quality of life, depending on the histopathological grade and localization of the lesion. Although fractionated radiotherapy or stereotactic radiosurgery is an alternative treatment option for meningiomas that cannot be completely removed (surgically inaccessible, or recurrent (atypical or anaplastic)) the primary treatment for these lesions is surgery. In this context, we have detailed meningiomas in this section.

Keywords: central nervous system tumors, intracranial meningioma, clinic, diagnosis, treatment

1. Introduction

Meningiomas, i.e., nonglial and extra-axial tumors of the central nervous system (CNS), are benign primary brain tumors that arise from neoplastic arachnoid (meningothelial) cells [1]. These epithelial cells, usually located in the arachnoid villi of the brain and spinal cord (rarely in the ventricles and extracranial area), are a component of the meninges that protect the brain [1]. Meningothelial cells, which form the interface between the parenchymal neurons and the cerebrospinal fluid (CSF), have an important barrier function for the CNS [1]. Thus, these cells are involved in removing waste products from the CSF with the protection of the optic nerve microenvironment and play a role in immunological processes through the secretion of proinflammatory cytokines in response to pathological stress conditions [2].

Felix Plater first defined meningioma in autopsy reports in 1614 as a roundish, fleshy, hard tumor with holes and the size of a medium-sized apple, covered with its membrane, and interspersed with venous lesions [3]. In the following years, different names were used for these pathological extra-axial structures, such as fungus durae matrix (Antoine Louis, 1774) and psammoma (Virchow, 1847), epithelioma

(Bouchard, 1864), endothelioma (Golgi1869) [4–7]. In 1922, Harvey Cushing's current definition of "meningiomas" prevailed in the literature to eliminate the diversity and confusion of this definition and to group many different pathologic tumor types arising from the meninges [6].

Meningiomas are common tumors, accounting for approximately 36% of all CNS tumors and 53% of non-malignant CNS tumors [8].

While meningiomas present as benign lesions they are often associated with treatable focal neurologic deficits and epileptic seizures, they may rarely be associated with morbidity, such as poor quality of life, depending on the histopathologic grade and location of the lesion [8].

Although the treatment principles are almost the same, spinal meningiomas and meningiomas of childhood are not discussed in this section to maintain the integrity of the topic. In this section, we aimed to give basic information about meningiomas, the importance of which we briefly mentioned.

2. Epidemiology, incidence, and prevalence

The incidence of meningiomas is based on hospital- or population-based information [8]. In parallel with developments in neuroradiology and increasing accuracy of disease reporting, the incidence has gradually increased over the years [9]. Hospital-based brain tumor series reported approximately 20% of all intracranial tumors, whereas autopsy studies found an overall incidence of almost 30% [10]. Meningiomas have the highest incidence rate among CNS tumors [10, 11]. They account for 38% of all intracranial tumors in women and 20% in men [10, 11]. Population-based studies have found an overall annual incidence of 6/100,000 [10, 11]. The incidence increases significantly with age. It is considered an age-related incidence, being 0.3/at 100,000 in childhood and 8.4/100,000 in the elderly [12, 13]. Intracranial meningiomas are most common in adults between the fourth and sixth decade [13]. While the incidence increases in patients with breast tumors and after head trauma, it reaches the highest rates after 50 years [9, 14, 15]. Although intracranial tumors have an overall higher prevalence in men than in women, the situation is reversed for meningiomas (women/men: 2/1) [9]. It is suggested that this increase is due to steroid receptors activating tumor growth [9]. However, female dominance of meningiomas, which is reported to be more common in Black people, has not been demonstrated in Black people [9]. Prevalence rates vary from 50.4/100,000 to 70.7/100,000 [16, 17]. Asymptomatic meningiomas are estimated to be discovered incidentally in 2–3% of the population and more than one in 8% of these cases [17]. Interestingly, non-malignant meningiomas are predominantly female, whereas atypical and anaplastic meningiomas are more common in men [18].

3. Neuropathological features and classification

Meningiomas are neoplastic changes of meningothelial cells tasked with barrier-like functions [2]. They originate from any region where the dura mater is located, often from the skull base and rarely from the extensions of the dura mater such as falx cerebri, tentorium cerebelli, and rarely from the optic nerve sheath and internal choroid plexuses in the ventricles [1]. Meningiomas, an extra-axial lesion, have a slow growth character, and macroscopically, a CSF cleft may be present adjacent to the

WHO grade 1	WHO grade 2	WHO grade 3
Meningothelial	Chordoid	Papillary
Fibrous	Clear cell	Rhabdoid
Transitional	Atypical	Anaplastic (malignant)
Angiomatous		
Psammomatous		
Microcystic		
Secretory		
Lymphoplasmacyte-rich		
Metaplastic		

Table 1.
WHO classification of meningiomas.

tumor, facilitating dissection between neuronal tissues at surgery [19]. These masses often present as a single, lobulated, and solitary extra-axial lesion [19]. Multiple lesions defined as "meningiomatosis" in syndromic patients, such as neurofibromatosis type 2 (NF2), can be seen [19].

Meningiomas can be classified according to their dural site of origin, involvement of adjacent tissues (e.g., bone, venous sinus, nerves, and brain), and histologic grading [20]. According to the World Health Organization (WHO), meningiomas are classified into three main groups based on their heterogeneous morphology: WHO Grade 1 (80% most common), WHO Grade 2 (10–18%), WHO Grade 3 (2–4% most aggressive) [20]. These three main groups were also subdivided into subgroups with histopathological differences [20]. This classification is based on pathologic criteria and is used to estimate the tumor progress (**Table 1**) [19, 20]. WHO Grading depends on brain invasion, specific histological features, or mitotic rate [21]. Although grade 1 meningiomas are designated as benign histopathologically, and they have a low recurrence rate of 5 years after surgery, the lifetime recurrence rate is approximately 30% [22]. In contrast, the 5-year recurrence rate for atypical (WHO 2) and anaplastic (WHO 3) meningiomas can be as high as 50% and 80% [21, 22]. The increase in recurrence rate after surgery is related to factors such as high-grade meningioma, brain or bone involvement, and a high proliferation index [23, 24]. However, it is impossible to determine which tumors will recur, based on the histologic criteria alone [20]. In addition, grade I and grade II meningiomas can progress to grade III by malignant transformation, but it is still unclear in which cases such progression occurs [20]. To this end, molecular characterization of meningiomas has defined several genetic biomarkers that can hopefully predict tumor behavior, and clinical trials are underway to address genetic subtypes [20]. These include BAP1 (rhabdoid and papillary subtype), SMARCE1 (clear cell subtype), TERT promoter mutation, and/or homozygous deletion of CDKN2A/B (CNS WHO grade 3), H3K27me3 loss of nuclear expression (potentially worse prognosis), KLF4/TRAF7 (secretory subtype) mutations, and methylome profiling (prognostic subtyping) [20].

3.1 WHO classification

3.1.1 WHO grade 1 (benign)

The most common meningiomas are classified into nine subgroups (**Table 1**). WHO grade 1 meningiomas generally have a good clinical course and a low risk of recurrence [20]. They rarely present with a histopathologic feature characterized by the presence of mitotic figures with pleomorphic nuclei [20, 25, 26].

3.1.2 WHO grade 2 (atypical)

WHO grade II meningiomas, referred to as the atypical group, have increased mitotic activity and a recurrence rate of up to 40% in 5 years [20, 25, 26].

3.1.3 WHO grade 3 (anaplastic)

This group represents malignant tumors with a very high recurrence rate as well as high mortality and morbidity. The 5-year progression-free survival for anaplastic variants is only 10% [20, 25, 26].

As mentioned before, CNS meningiomas are also named after the regions from which they arise. There are several classifications on this subject, but one of the most important is the one established by Yaşargil in 1966 [27]. According to Yaşargil, they are divided into six main groups (**Table 2**) [27].

3.2 Meningiomas, according to their localization

3.2.1 Olfactory groove meningiomas

This meningioma develops from arachnoid cap cells around the cribriform plate and crista galli [28, 29]. They may occur unilaterally or bilaterally [29]. Olfactory

A. Basal meningiomas		
1. Median	2. Paramedian	3. Lateral
Olfactory groove Tuberculum sella Dorsum sella Clivus Foramen magnum	Orbital ceiling Inner sphenoid wing Intracavernous Cavum Meckel Cerebellopontine	Outer sphenoid wing Sphenoorbital Sphenetemporal Sphenofrontal Sphenosilvian
B. Fissural meningiomas		
Falsin Tentorial Falkotentorial Silvian		
C. Dorsal meningiomas		
1. Supratentorial		2. Infratentorial
A. Parasagittal	B. Paramedian	Median Paramedian Lateral
Frontal Central Parietal Occipital	Frontal Central Parietal Occipital Temporal	
D. Intraventricular	**E. Orbital**	**F. Calvarial**
Lateral ventricles Third ventricle Fourth ventricle	Foraminal Canalicular Infraorbital	

Table 2.
Yaşargil meningioma classification.

groove meningiomas generally cause compression of the olfactory nerve and grow into the hemispheres [29]. Larger ones grow in the epidural plane and invade the ethmoid and sphenoid sinuses [29]. The most common findings in these cases are headache, personality changes, epilepsy, memory visual, and olfactory disturbances [28–30]. The arterial supply is usually through the ethmoid, meningeal, and ophthalmic arteries [29]. For this reason, central enucleation of the tumor should be performed after occluding the dural arterial supplies during surgery [27]. When removing the tumor, attention should be paid to the optic nerve and the anterior communicating arterial complex [27]. The operation is performed in two ways. One is the unilateral pterional transsylvian approach, and the other is bifrontal craniotomy [29, 31]. In the bifrontal craniotomy approach, less frontal lobe retraction and direct tumor intervention are easily possible, but more scar tissue is formed [29, 31]. With the pterional approach, although it provides relatively minor surgery, frontal lobe resection may sometimes be required [27, 30, 32]. To prevent CSF leakage from the cribriform plate after surgery, it should be covered with a pericranial flap, and fibrin glue should be used if necessary [27]. Postoperative CSF fistula may still occur [31]. It is recommended that lumbar drainage be attempted first, and if this attempt fails, radical dural repair is recommended [31].

3.2.2 Tuberculum sella meningiomas

These meningiomas arise from the tuberculum sellae, limbus sphenoidale, chiasmatic sulcus, and planum sphenoidale [33]. They account for 3% of all intracranial meningiomas [33]. Tuberculum sellae meningiomas most commonly originate from the optic nerves and chiasm [33]. Tuberculum sella meningiomas push the optic nerves upward and sideways [33]. The tumor grows posteriorly and superiorly, compressing the anterior cerebral artery and the anterior communicating artery complex [33]. Again, because of its growth, the tumor may invade the optic canal and frontobasal interhemispheric fissure [33]. When they reach a larger volume, they can compress the hypothalamus and cause an upward displacement of the third ventricle [33]. Very rarely, they can cause carotid artery dislocation [33]. In their clinic, they most commonly cause asymmetric vision loss [27]. In such cases, unilateral optic atrophy is noted [27]. This situation is in itself an indication of surgery [27]. Depending on the size and direction of the tumor, subfrontal, unilateral, supraorbital, or pterional transsylvian surgery may be performed [27, 33–36]. In the postoperative period, a 42–64% improvement in vision is observed [27, 30, 37, 38]. Vision impairment is observed in 10–20% of cases [27, 30, 37, 38]. The duration of visual impairment before surgery, tumor size, extent of visual loss, and advanced optic atrophy are key factors in postoperative recovery [9, 30, 37, 38]. In recent series, recurrence rates are less than 3% [39–44].

3.2.3 Sphenoid wing meningiomas

According to Al-Mefty, meningiomas of the sphenoid and parasellar regions are classified into five regions, including:

1. optic nerve, orbit, anterior visual pathways.

2. tuberculum sella.

3. clinoidal.

4. cavernous sinus

5. middle and outer wing meningiomas [33].

All of these have been mentioned in the classification of Yaşargil later on.

3.2.4 Clinoidal meningiomas

They are also meningiomas of the internal or medial sphenoid wing and arise from the anterior sphenoid process and the periphery of the lesser sphenoid wing [45]. As tumors grow, they compress the optic nerve, internal carotid artery, and branches, causing displacement [45]. Sometimes they can encircle these entities. Al-Mefty divided this group of meningiomas into three groups [45].

Group 1: These tumors originate on the underside of the anterior clinoid process and mainly involve the adventitia of the carotid artery [45]. For this reason, it may not be possible to distinguish this group of tumors from the branches of the carotid and middle cerebral arteries [45].

Group 2: These tumors originate at the superior or lateral projection of the anterior clinoid process [45]. The arachnoid of the carotid cistern separates it from the tumor adventitia [45]. Therefore, it is easy to separate the tumor from the carotid artery [45].

Group 3: The origin of these tumors is the optic foramen, so it grows toward the tip of the optic canal and anterior clinoid process [45]. These are relatively small tumors [46]. They are more easily scraped from the carotid arteries [45]. Clinically, unilateral optic atrophy is the most important finding [46–48]. In some cases, papilledema (Foster-Kennedy syndrome) may be observed on the opposite side of the eye [28, 49]. Depending on the size and orientation of the tumor, mental changes, hemiparesis, anosmia, and epileptic seizures may be observed [46–48]. It is more common in women and may enlarge during pregnancy [49]. The headache often manifests as orbital pain [49].

Pterional craniotomy is often preferred in treating this tumor group [50]. With advancing surgical techniques, vascular structures can be scraped microsurgically, and cranial nerves can be preserved safely, as with cavernous intrasinusal spread [50–52]. Despite all these options, the surgical cure of meningiomas of the middle sphenoid wing is still problematic [53, 54]. Radical resection is difficult despite all the developments [27, 31, 36, 45, 53, 54]. In Al-Mefty's series, it was reported that complete resection was not possible in group 1 cases, while group 2 and 3 cases could be treated without problems [45].

3.2.5 Lateral and middle sphenoid wing meningiomas

Rosal et al. divided this group of meningiomas into seven groups by extending the classification of Brotchi and Bonnal (**Figure 1**) [53].

Brotchi and Bonnal classification modified by Rosal et al.: Group 1: Medial sphenoid wing no cavernous sinus infiltration; Group 2: Medial sphenoid wing with cavernous sinus infiltration; Group 3: Middle sphenoid wing; Group 4: Lateral sphenoid wing; Group 5: En-plaque no cavernous sinus infiltration (first third and fourth areas combined); Group 6: En-plaque with cavernous sinus infiltration (first second third and fourth areas combined); Group 7: Pure intraosseous tumor infiltration.

They form clinics according to their location. While the second group tends to cause exophthalmos, the third and fourth groups cause hemiparesis and epilepsy [53]. In the

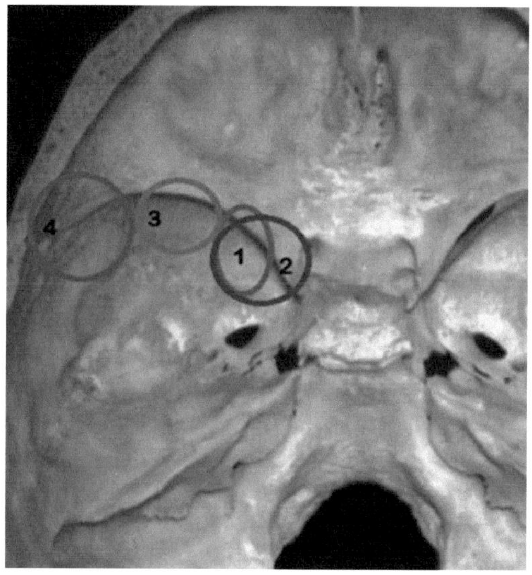

Figure 1.
Lateral and middle sphenoid wing meningiomas classification.

fifth group, there is localized and prolonged pain due to the spread of the plaques [53]. This sometimes occurs with the orbit and sphenoid bone invasion without mass effect [53]. In the case of invasion of the cavernous sinus, paralysis of the third, fourth, and sixth nerves may be observed [53]. When meningiomas in either group grow into the Sylvian fissure, they may encircle the middle cerebral artery [53]. In this case, differentiation from important structures is difficult. It is necessary to leave some tumor tissue [27]. Bone resection may be required to achieve a complete cure, especially because of bone invasion in groups 5, 6, and 7 [27]. The most appropriate surgical approach is the pterional approach [27]. The lateral sphenoid wing should be straightened to obtain an optimal field of view of this area [27].

3.2.6 Cavernous sinus meningiomas

While cavernous meningiomas can arise outside the cavernous sinus and invade it, they can also arise primarily from the cavernous sinus and invade externally [54]. The cavernous sinus is frequently invaded by meningiomas located in the orbital apex, internal sphenoid wing, middle fossa, tentorium, and superior clival region [54]. The reverse is also true [54]. Cavernous meningiomas were classified into five groups by Sekhar [55]. This classification was based on the location of the tumor in the sinus and the condition of the cavernous portion of the internal carotid artery [55]. Clinical findings refer to 3, 4, first and second branches of 5, and 6 nerves [55]. Therefore, diplopia and ophthalmoplegia can be seen [55]. The disease generally progresses slowly and worsens over time [55]. Angiography should be performed in all cases [55]. Patients should undergo a balloon occlusion test to determine collateral circulation [55]. After this test, cases are classified into low, intermediate, and high risk [55]. Because of the high likelihood of potential morbidities, adequate information and appropriate patient selection are important [55]. The main indication of surgery is a progressive deterioration of neurologic findings and evidence of radiographic growth [55]. While the indication for surgery is straightforward in large tumors and young patients, the decision to operate should be cautioned in elderly and high-risk patients with balloon occlusion tests [55]. Parkinson first performed surgery in 1965 [55]. Many authors have reported new surgical approaches and techniques [51, 52, 55–57]. Frontotemporal craniotomy and orbitozygomatic osteotomy are mostly used in surgery [51, 52, 55–57]. If the tumor infiltrates Meckel's cavity, tumor dissection should be performed [50, 56, 57].

3.2.7 Foramen magnum meningiomas

They are studied in two groups. The craniospinal ones arise from the basal groove in the lower part of the ⅓-clivus and extend from anteriorly and anterolaterally of the medulla to the foramen magnum [58]. The spinocranial, on the other hand, begins in the upper cervical region and extends upward from the posterior and postero-lateral aspect of the medulla to the cerebellomedullary cistern [58]. The most common finding is neck pain that is unilateral and occurs primarily with coughing, Lhermitte's phenomenon, cold dysesthesia due to the eleventh nerve compression, progressive sensorineural and motor deficits that begin in one arm and spread to the other extremities, and atrophy of intrinsic limb muscles [58–60]. Lower cranial nerve palsies, Horner syndrome, respiratory problems, sphincter disturbances, nystagmus, and papilledema are observed less frequently [58–60]. To reach foramen magnum meningiomas, there are four main entry sites [44, 61–67]. These are posterior, postero-lateral, anterior, and transcervical approaches [44, 61–67]. The most commonly used approaches are posterior ones and among them, transcondylar and inferior suboccipital approaches are widespread [44, 61–67]. Most lesions can be resected simply with the inferior suboccipital approach [44, 61–67]. The most important factor to complicate the approach is the venous plexus [44, 61–67]. For those originating from the anterior aspect of foramen magnum, the postero-lateral (far lateral) approach is beneficial, especially when the tumor is large, opening a corridor to the anterior aspect of the brain stem and upper spinal cord [44, 61–67]. The transcondylar approach is associated with a higher morbidity rate than the far lateral approach [44, 61–67]. But it gives a wider viewing angle and accesses hard-to-reach areas [44, 61–67]. It should be applied if the benefit of the transcondylar approach is greater when weighed against the risks associated with CN XI dissection, VA transposition, and condyle drilling [44, 61–67].

3.2.8 Cerebellopontine angle meningiomas

Cerebellopontine angle meningiomas, which arise from the dorsal part of the petrous bone, are divided into two parts according to their location [67, 68]. These are antero-medial angle meningiomas and postero-lateral angle meningiomas [67, 68]. While the first group originates from the anteromedial side of the internal meatus acousticus, the tumors of the second group originate from the postero-lateral side [68]. These tumors spread toward the jugular foramen and hypoglossal foramen [68]. These can cause compression of the cerebellar hemispheres and pons, which results in their displacement [68]. Cerebellopontine angle meningiomas may cause erosions in the petrous bone [68]. About half of all meningiomas of the posterior fossa consist of cerebellopontine angle meningiomas [67]. While their incidence peaks in the fifth decade cerebellopontine angle meningiomas are 2–4 times more common in women than men [68]. Symptoms it causes include hearing loss, tinnitus, vertigo, headache, trigeminal neuralgia, long-track findings, and increased cerebral pressure (ICP) [68].

Meningiomas of this region invade the fifth and seventh nerves more frequently than acoustic neuromas [68]. Lower cranial nerve findings are also seen in large lesions [68]. It is difficult to differentiate meningiomas in this region from acoustic neuromas [42, 68]. In the differential diagnosis, subarachnoid hemorrhage, which Yaşargil noted at a rate of 6%, may be a clue to angle meningiomas [67–70]. Another distinguishing feature for meningiomas could be the dural tail [68–70]. Angiographic staining is common in meningiomas but not in acoustic neuromas [68–70]. While intracanalicular tumors are rare in meningiomas, they are always found in acoustic neuromas [68–70]. As well as there is no hyperostosis in acoustic neuromas, it is found in meningiomas [68–70]. Additionally, the internal auditory canal is enlarged in acoustic neuromas, it is normal in meningiomas [68–70]. Despite these differences, diagnosing is not always easy [68–70]. While the facial nerve is anterior or anterosuperior to the tumor in acoustic neuromas, it can be located anywhere in the tumor in meningiomas [68–70]. For this reason, it is relatively easy to preserve hearing in meningiomas, but this is often impossible in acoustic neuromas [69, 70]. To reach these tumors, petrosal procedures in the anteromedial location of the tumor and retrosigmoid suboccipital procedures in the cerebellopontine angle location are used [70]. The surgeon's choice of surgical approach mainly depends on the characteristics of the tumor and the surgeon's personal preferences and the patient's clinic [70]. Most neurosurgeons prefer a single approach, while others use combinations. However, there are some points that need to be mentioned [70]. Petrosal procedures should be performed in patients with hearing loss because hearing preservation is not possible with this technique [70]. Retrosigmoid suboccipital procedures can be used in lesions that have serviceable hearing and can be resected posteriorly [70]. However, in the retrosigmoid approach, it is relatively more difficult to protect the adjacent cranial nerves [70].

3.2.9 Petroclival meningiomas

Petroclival meningiomas arise from the upper part of the ⅔ clivus and petrous region medial to the fifth nerve [71]. The brainstem and basilar artery complex are typically pushed to the opposite side [71]. Clival meningiomas originate in the superior part of the clivus ⅔ and midline [71]. They cause backward displacement of the brainstem and basilar artery complex [72–74]. Another group is the sphenopetroclival meningiomas defined by Yaşargil [71]. This type occurs when Meckel's cave is invaded by petroclival meningiomas [71]. In addition to the features of petroclival meningiomas, they invade the lateral wall of the cavernous sinus [71–75]. In the typical clinic of these tumors, headache and ataxia are observed with a frequency of 70%, while spastic paraparesis and somatosensory deficits are less common [71–75]. In these tumors, the fifth and eighth nerves are involved in ⅔ of the cases, the seventh nerve in half of the cases, and inferior cranial nerves in ⅓ of the cases [67, 72, 76]. Commonly used approaches for resection of these tumors are petrosal procedures, mid-fossa base procedures, or extended petrosal procedures that combine these two procedures [72, 76, 77].

3.2.10 Falx meningiomas

They can originate from any part of the falx [78]. Depending on their location, they are examined in three sections called anterior, middle, and posterior [78].

Anterior falx meningiomas are found in the part of the falx between the crista galli and the coronal suture [78]. Meningiomas of this region show an insidious course clinically and become noticeable only when they have reached a large size [78]. Common findings include headaches, visual disturbances, personality changes, and dementia [78]. Seizures are observed less frequently than in other regions [78].

Meningiomas of the middle falx arise in the falx region between the coronal suture and the lambdoid suture [78]. This region's most common clinical finding is focal motor or Jacksonian spasms [78]. Similarly, motor deficits may be seen [78].

Posterior falx meningiomas are meningiomas consisting of the falx portion between the lambdoid suture and the torcula [78]. They most commonly present with headaches [78]. Visual hallucinations and homonymous hemianopsia may occur in these patients [78].

For the resection of these tumors, various approaches can be used depending on the site of onset [27, 78].

3.2.11 Parasagittal meningiomas

These tumors are meningiomas that infiltrate the sagittal sinus, surrounding convex dura, and falx [79]. Bone involvement may also occur. According to the classification system of Sindou and Alvernia, sinus invasion is studied in six types (**Figure 2**) [79].

Type I: Lesion attachment to the outer surface of the sinus wall.

Type II: Tumor fragment inside the lateral recess.

Type III: Invasion of the ipsilateral wall.

Type IV: Invasion of the lateral wall and roof.

Types V and VI: Complete sinus occlusion with or without one wall free, respectively [79].

As with falx meningiomas, they are studied as anterior, middle, and posterior. Again, the symptoms and findings are the same as in Falx tumors [78, 79].

The most important question in surgical treatment is the condition of the sinuses [27, 78, 79]. Anterior meningiomas can be resected even if the sinus is open, but excision cannot be performed in intermediate and posterior tumors without complete closure of the sinus [27, 78, 79]. In such cases, subtotal resection (STR) is performed [27, 78, 79].

Surgical intervention for these lesions can be performed in various ways, depending on the location of the tumor [27, 78, 79]. All surgical methods used in other meningioma lesions can be used singly or in combination [27, 78, 79].

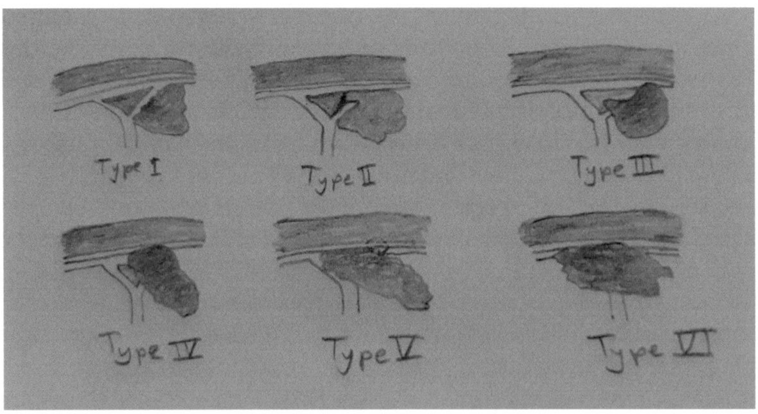

Figure 2.
Sindou and Alvernia classification.

3.2.12 Convexity meningiomas

Convexity meningiomas are meningiomas that are not associated with the dura of the skull base and do not invade the dural venous sinuses [80, 81]. They account for 15% of all meningiomas [80, 81]. They have been classified into precoronal, coronal, postcoronal, paracentral, parietal, occipital, and temporal subgroups by Cushing and Eisenhardt [28]. Clinically, the main findings are headache, mental symptoms, visual disturbances, and epilepsy [80, 81]. The surgical approach differs depending on the origin of the lesion [35, 82, 83]. Complete excision is simple compared with other groups, and mortality is negligible [35, 82, 83].

3.2.13 Tentorial meningiomas

Tentorial meningiomas are divided into three groups as medial, lateral, and falcotentorial meningiomas [84]. Tentorial meningiomas grow below or above the tentorium [84]. In most cases, the tumor grows infratentorial and typically causes headaches and ataxia [84].

The subtemporal approach is recommended for medial and lateral tentorial meningiomas [84]. An interhemispheric or supratentorial approach is recommended for posterior tentorial and falcotentorial meningiomas, and a combined supratentorial approach is recommended for the infratentorial portion of lateral tentorial meningiomas [27, 84].

3.2.14 Intraventricular meningiomas

Intraventricular meningiomas account for 5% of all meningiomas [85]. They originate from the tela choroidea or the choroid plexus, and 80% are in the lateral ventricle, 15% in the third ventricle, and 5% in the fourth ventricle [85]. Most of the meningiomas in the lateral ventricle are located in the trigone region [85]. Headache, vomiting, speech disorders, homonymous hemianopsia, and sensorimotor hemiparesis are observed in meningiomas at the trigonal region [85]. Papilledema, vomiting, and hypothalamic disturbances are common in third ventricular meningiomas [85]. Obstructive hydrocephalus findings occur in the fourth ventricle meningiomas [85]. Intraventricular meningiomas are supplied by the choroidal arteries and their venous drainage is through the ependymal veins [85]. They are often of the fibroblastic type [85]. Since 90% of intraventricular meningiomas are WHO grade I, the prognosis is favorable [85]. Surgery is considered curative if gross total resection is possible [85]. However, 10% of patients have intraventricular meningiomas WHO grades II and III and may require additional radiosurgery [85]. According to the WHO grading for all types of meningiomas, survival rates are valid for intraventricular meningiomas, but the recurrence and mortality rates are lower due to their generally lower grade and a better rate of complete surgical resection [85].

Transcortical interventions (middle frontal gyrus, posterior-middle temporal gyrus, superior parieto-occipital fissure) and interhemispheric transcallosal approaches are used in the surgery of meningiomas located in the lateral ventricle [44]. While the interforniceal approach is preferred for meningiomas in the third ventricle, the suboccipital route is preferred for meningiomas in the fourth ventricle [44].

3.2.15 Orbital meningiomas

Meningiomas in orbit are divided into primary and secondary meningiomas [49]. Whereas primary orbital meningiomas arise from the optic nerve sheath and are located throughout the orbit, secondary tumors arise from the dura around the orbit and grow into the orbit [49]. Orbital meningiomas account for 9% of all orbital tumors [49]. They commonly occur in childhood [49]. Loss of vision is the most important symptom [49]. In addition, optic disk changes, visual field loss, proptosis, and pain may also occur [49]. The recurrence rate ranges from about 17–42% [86]. The recurrence rate is lower in patients receiving postoperative radiation therapy, depending on the WHO grade [86]. Surgical interventions include transorbital and transcranial procedures [86].

3.2.16 Calvarial meningiomas

This group is a rare tumor that arises from the calvarium [27]. They do not have intradural components [27]. Cases have been reported in the scalp, temporal bone, jugular foramen, orbit, paranasal sinuses, infratemporal fossa, and parotid gland [27]. They are more common in childhood and among the elderly [27].

4. Etiology

Compared with malignant glial tumors, there are fewer studies on the etiologic risk factors for meningiomas. Although the exact etiology of meningiomas is still unknown, some recognized risk factors are present.

4.1 Molecular etiology (genetic)

Although meningiomas have benign pathophysiology, they are thought to arise from clonal growth from a single cell, which is a characteristic of carcinomas [87, 88]. Sporadic meningiomas are generally associated with one or more focal chromosomal deletion(s) [87, 88]. In contrast, atypical and malignant meningiomas usually have more than one chromosomal replica number change [89]. It is now known that the complexity of genetic abnormalities also leads to an increase in tumor grade in meningiomas [90]. The most common genetic disorder associated with an increased risk of meningiomas is NF2 [91]. These patients are more likely to develop second- and third-grade meningiomas or multiple meningiomas [91]. Gorlin, von Hippel-Lindau, Li-Fraumeni, multiple endocrine neoplasia (MEN), and Cowden disease are also syndromes that predispose to the development of meningiomas [92].

4.2 Ionizing radiation

Exposure to ionizing radiation is the most important risk factor for developing meningiomas [92, 93]. It has been found that there is an increased risk for the development of meningiomas when ionizing radiation is used in the context of indications for the treatment of various diseases (e.g., cranial irradiation for tinea capitis, dental radiography) [93]. This risk is increased not only in patients who have been exposed to ionizing radiation for treatment but also in people who have been exposed to the effects of the atomic bomb [93]. Ionizing radiation is a risk factor for the predisposition of meningiomas, with a six- to tenfold relative risk after a delay and without a dose relationship [93]. Based on this risk, ionizing radiation of radiographic examinations was recalculated and reduced [93].

4.3 Hormone

Because of the high incidence of meningiomas in women of reproductive age and women with breast cancer as well as the changes in meningioma size found in studies during pregnancy, the menstrual cycle, and menopause, it has been suggested that the increased risk for meningiomas may be related to hormones [94]. However, no association has been found between the use of oral contraceptives and the development of meningiomas [95, 96]. In addition, some other studies find no association between meningioma development and hormonal factors [95, 96].

Among the etiologically explained risk factors, head trauma, the presence of breast cancer, smoking, and cell phone use are mentioned. However, the causal relationship between these factors and meningioma development has not been established. For this reason, future studies will clarify these issues and uncover new developmental/acquired etiologic factors.

5. Diagnosis

These dural-based tumors are routinely discovered incidentally by neurologists, neurosurgeons, and other clinicians because of the wider use of computed tomography (CT) and magnetic resonance imaging (MRI) [97]. Nowadays, radiologic imaging with contrast-enhanced cranial CT or MRI provides very useful information not only in the diagnosis of meningiomas but also in monitoring asymptomatic cases, deciding on surgical/systemic treatment, and distinguishing between tumor recurrence and radiologic changes [97]. Histopathologic analysis by biopsy or resection is required for definitive diagnosis. However, thanks to evolving neuroradiology, MRI results have become the standard method for radiologic diagnosis and follow-up of meningiomas [97]. Contrast-enhanced CT can be performed in patients whose MRI is contraindicated for patient-related reasons (e.g., pacemakers, in-body metallic implants, claustrophobia) [97]. In addition, CT is superior to MRI in radiologic diagnosis by revealing the chronic effects of the tumor such as intra-tumoral calcification (25% of cases seen) and changes in the bone structure such as hyperostosis and interosseous bone growth [97]. However, the simultaneous use of both diagnostic tools provides more detailed information before and after surgery in most cases [97]. When imaging findings suggest meningioma, a biopsy is not required in these patients [97].

Benign meningiomas are usually isointense or mildly hypointense on T1-weighted brain imaging and hyperintense on T2-weighted/FLAIR sequences of MRI [97]. They have a characteristic thickened, contrast-enhancing dural tail (60%), and contain a CSF cleft [97]. Additionally, they have clearly defined margins and homogeneous enhancement (95%) [97]. Meningiomas displace the brain away from the overlying dura [97]. The dural tail is a useful radiologic finding at diagnosis to distinguish meningiomas from other lesions such as schwannomas [97]. However, the dural tail is not pathognomonic for meningiomas and may also be seen in metastases or hemangiopericytomas [97]. Again, it should be remembered that approximately 10–15% of meningiomas may have an atypical appearance on MRI images that mimics metastases or malignant gliomas [98]. Central necrosis, which is specific for malignant gliomas (hypointense, non-enhancing central necrotic area in the lesion at the T1-weighted images), can interestingly be found in both benign and malignant variants of meningiomas [98]. A cystic appearance is a rare radiologic finding for this tumor [98]. Although uncertain, peritumoral edema can be seen on T2-weighted and FLAIR images [98]. Peritumoral edema is attributed to more aggressive meningiomas invading the brain [98]. In particular, significant peritumoral edema may be present in secretory meningiomas [98].

MRI spectroscopy (MRIs) can be used for differential diagnosis of meningiomas [99]. This modality can be particularly beneficial in patients who cannot undergo surgery [99]. Compared with normal brain tissue, MRIs usually reveal decreased N-acetyl-aspartate and creatinine peaks and increased choline and alanine peaks. In contrast, atypical meningiomas may have an increased lactate peak caused by necrotic tumor tissue [99, 100]. Buhl et al. reported a characteristic lactate peak in more than 63% of patients with atypical meningiomas on preoperative MRIs [100].

Depending on radiology, WHO grading degrees may be suspected [101]. However, there are currently no imaging criteria for preoperative differentiation of the various WHO grades of intracranial meningiomas [101]. Therefore, there is still uncertainty about which patients should be followed up or operated on early [102]. Although it is not possible today to determine the variants of meningiomas radiologically, invasion of the adjacent brain parenchyma and bone tissue in its location, heterogeneous contrast enhancement, intense peritumoral edema, seen in T2-weighted and FLAIR sequences, and central necrosis seen as hypointense in the T1-weighted sequence (non-enhancing tumor area) are also considered indicative of high-grade meningiomas [102, 103]. In addition, meningiomas with calcifications on cranial CT (hyperdense) and T2-weighted MRI imaging (hypointense) have been associated with a slower growth rate [104, 105].

Recently, the role of radiomics has been investigated in meningiomas. Radiomics consists of the correlation of quantitative radiological features with pathological and molecular features of the tumor [106]. This novel method has the potential to increase knowledge of the tumor, which is beneficial given the tumor's hard-to-access location [106]. Several studies showed a potential role of radiomics in predicting the pathological grade and subtypes of meningiomas [106–109]. However, it is not currently in standard clinical use.

Because meningiomas easily invade the cerebral veins and cerebral venous sinuses, the MRI venogram is useful to visualize the relationship of the tumor to the lateral or superior sagittal sinus (direct invasion or compression) to determine the degree of tumor invasion and to reveal collateral venous outflow [107].

Conventional angiography no longer has a place in diagnosing meningiomas [110]. However, this technique can be used for intravascular embolization or to clarify the diagnosis when the appearance on CT or MRI remains unclear [110]. Angiographic findings suggest that meningioma includes dural arteries supplying the central tumor and pial arteries supplying the tumor periphery and bilateral vasculature [110].

Although positron emission tomography (PET) is not routinely used in clinical practice, it can be useful for meningiomas at the skull base, which are often difficult to detect with standard imaging modalities CT and MRI [111, 112]. Furthermore, PET(68-Ga-DOTATATE) can aid in the diagnosis during follow-up of recurrent meningiomas in cases where biopsy specimens cannot be obtained easily or undecided ones [111, 112].

6. Clinic

We have briefly mentioned above the clinical appearance caused by meningioma subgroups specifically. In general, clinical findings in meningiomas result from the tumor tissue compressing adjacent neural, vascular structures or occluding CSF flow pathways, cortical veins, and venous sinuses, depending on the compartment in which meningioma originated [113, 114]. Symptoms and signs of ICP such as papilledema, headache, nausea, and vomiting can occur not only in anterior skull base meningiomas that reach giant sizes (6 cm in diameter) but also in small tumors that cause severe reactive vasogenic edema [113, 114]. Although not common, they may present with clinical signs of transient ischemic attack or intracranial hemorrhage [113, 114]. Usually, meningiomas commonly cause peritumoral edema and epileptic seizures episodes (27–67%), which are thought to be site-dependent and may be partial (37%), complex partial (8%), generalized (60%), or a combination thereof [115, 116].

7. Treatment

The treatment of meningiomas varies widely and depends on patient-related factors such as age, performance status, concomitant medical conditions, and the targeted treatment modality (observation, symptomatic treatment, surgical treatment). Currently, the main treatment modality is observation with intermittent radiologic imaging for asymptomatic meningiomas, whereas complete surgical resection is sought for meningiomas that progress or cause symptoms (**Table 3**) [117].

7.1 Observation

Because the tumor growth rate for asymptomatic intracranial meningiomas is 2–4 mm/year, they can be treated conservatively. However, close surveillance is required clinically and radiologically, especially in young patients, because they can grow rapidly [117]. When a patient with a meningioma is planned for follow-up, the gold standard for it is intermittent MRI [117]. Contrast-enhanced T1-weighted sequences provide images suitable for evaluating volume increases in tumor mass [117]. In a study to determine tumor growth behavior in 64 patients with asymptomatic meningiomas, no patient had tumor-related symptoms in a 5-year follow-up [117]. During this 5-year follow-up period, 48 (75%) of the 64 patients experienced an increase in tumor size of 15% or more [117]. Therefore, serial imaging can follow asymptomatic meningiomas until permanent tumor growth is detected radiologically or symptoms develop [117]. However, even if an increase in tumor size is detected on serial volume measurements in the follow-up, the decision to proceed

Grade 1: Complete tumor resection, including dura and ingrown bone
Grade 2: Gross total resection (dura coagulation is present)
Grade 3: Macroscopic resection (no dural excision or coagulation)
Grade 4: Subtotal resection
Grade 5: Biopsy only [121]

Table 3.
SIMPSON grade.

with surgery still depends on the patient's age, symptomatology, and comorbidities [118, 119]. This is because the morbidity rate in surgically treated asymptomatic meningiomas is not negligible, especially in patients older than 70 [118, 119]. Therefore, the natural history of incidentally discovered tumors remains a concern for physicians and patients.

7.2 Surgery

Surgery is the primary treatment for meningiomas with volume increase on symptomatic or neuroradiologic follow-up [117–120]. The main goal of surgery is:

1. Preservation of existing neurological functions.

2. Elimination of neurological symptoms caused by the mass effect.

3. Prevention of recurrence with low morbidity (the recurrence rate is inversely proportional to the width of the resection); there should be maximal resection of the tumor, including all relevant dural and bony structures [120].

The basic principles of surgical treatment are central debulking and peripheral dissection, which facilitates resection in hard and calcified tumors, with good control of bleeding during surgery [27, 119]. Often, an arachnoid plane allowing reliable differentiation of the tumor from normal structures is discovered during surgery [27]. If this arachnoid plane is preserved, bleeding and injury to neurovascular structures are largely avoided [27].

As with other CNS tumors, the primary goal of surgical treatment for meningiomas is complete resection of the pathologic tissue [120]. However, several patient-related factors, such as tumor location, invasion of adjacent brain parenchyma, venous sinuses, encasement of arteries and cranial nerves by tumor tissue, or age and cardiovascular disease, may prevent complete resection from achieving good outcomes [27, 119, 120]. Therefore, complete resection is impossible without compromising functional outcomes for meningiomas in near-critical neurologic structures or surrounding neurovascular structures in some patients [27, 119, 120]. While resection for convexity meningiomas is relatively simple, resection for parasagittal tumors is more complicated because they often invade the sagittal sinus [120]. In cases where the tumor invades the sinus and venous flow persists, the portion of the tumor within the sinus should not be resected because of the risk of air embolism, hemorrhage, and acute sinus thrombosis [120]. Skull base meningiomas in the tuberculum sella, sphenoid wing, cerebellopontine angle, olfactory groove, or petroclival region require advanced surgical techniques [120]. Endoscopic endonasal procedures have been described that allow safe access without retraction of the parenchyma, especially for tumors located in the anterior midline region of the skull base [120]. Where necessary, an attempt should be made to achieve gross total resection (GTR) using all available modalities.

As with other intracranial tumors, it is possible to assess the success of the surgical resection with contrast-enhanced CT or MRI in the first 72 h after surgery [121]. In addition, neuro-radiologic imaging forms the basis for the Simpson grading system, which can predict recurrence after surgery [121]. According to Simpson's criteria, the extent of resection is considered a factor for progression-free and disease-free survival [121]. As the grade increases from Simpson grade 1 to grade 5, recurrence rates also increase (**Table 4**) [121]. Another factor affecting recurrence rates is the histopathologic grading of meningiomas [122, 123]. The 5-year recurrence rate after total gross resection of WHO grade I meningiomas was 7–23%, whereas WHO grade 2 meningiomas were 50–55%, and WHO grade 3 was 72–78% [122, 123]. However, the 15-year recurrence rate in patients who underwent GTR for all types of meningiomas was 24–60%, whereas this rate was over 70% in patients who underwent STR [124]. Other factors affecting survival include patient age and tumor location.

Preoperative embolization may be performed before surgery in very large or difficult-to-remove tumors with complex vascular feeding [125, 126]. However, because of cardiovascular complications, preoperative embolization is not a routine procedure and is not recommended in every case [125, 126]. In addition to shortening the operative

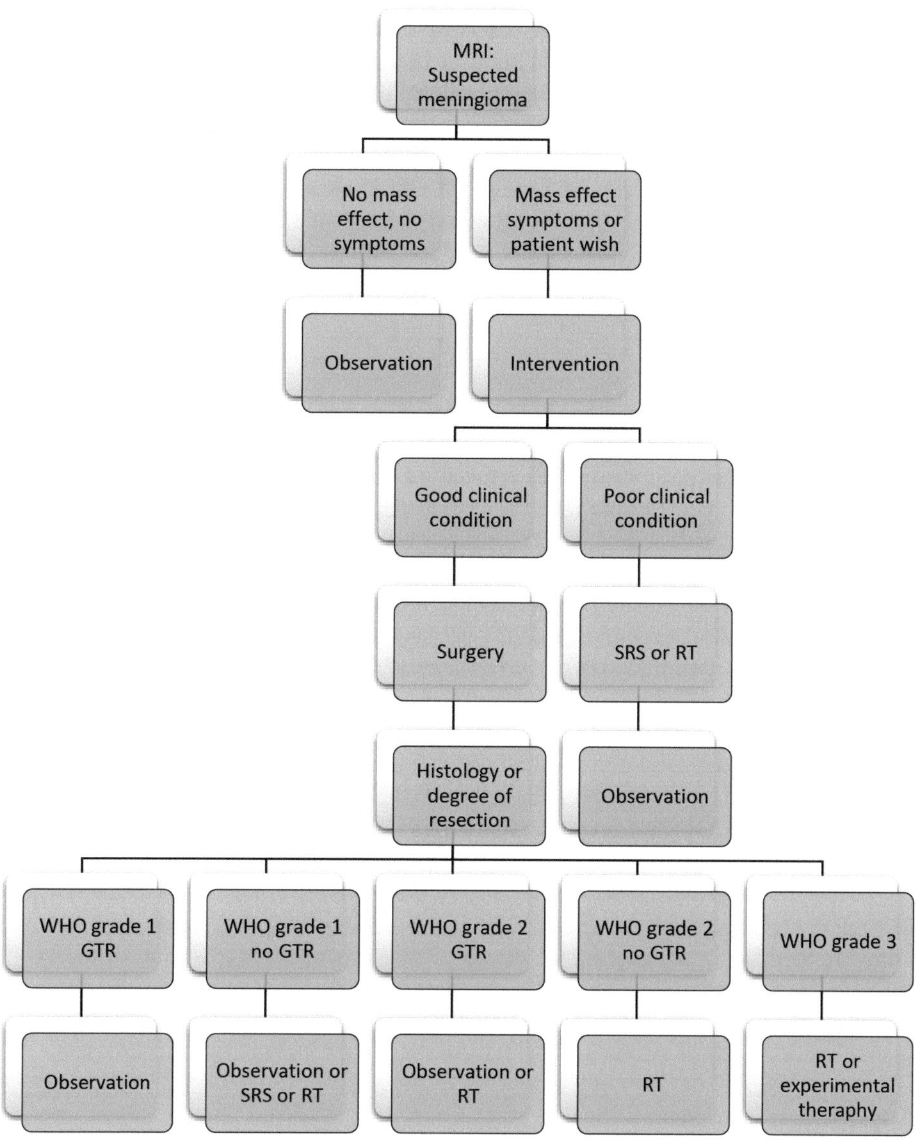

Table 4.
Overall evidence-based treatment algorithm.

time, preoperative embolization may be beneficial in cases where it is difficult to reach the feeding arteries, such as petroclival meningiomas [125, 126]. Therefore, the surgical team should evaluate the decision individually in each case [125, 126].

7.3 Endovascular treatment

The increase in interventional neuroradiologic applications and developments in microvascular catheters have also raised hopes for endovascular treatment of meningioma, which is a vascular tumor [127]. Some studies on this topic have found that the benefits of endovascular therapy are uncertain [128]. Therefore, significant obstacles remain to accepting endovascular intervention as a treatment modality. Selective microcatheter embolization of the meningeal arterial supply with various agents can be remarkably effective in the devascularization of the tumor, and preoperative embolization reduces perioperative bleeding [129]. However, there is still uncertainty about when preoperative embolization before resection is appropriate [129]. Furthermore, because atypical histopathologic features are more common in patients undergoing endovascular embolization, embolization could induce atypical histologic changes associated with benign (WHO 1) meningiomas [130, 131]. For the above reasons, endovascular embolization may be considered an alternative treatment option for managing meningiomas, but only for patients in whom surgical intervention is not feasible. It is not a stand-alone treatment modality.

7.4 Radiotherapy

Although radiation therapy has been used to treat tumors for many years, there are not as much clinical studies on treating meningiomas with radiation therapy as other pathologies. While radiotherapy (RT) is usually a secondary treatment modality to surgical resection to prevent higher-grade progression of meningiomas and reduce the recurrence rate, it may be considered a primary treatment option in a well-defined, inoperable small group of patients [132]. For this purpose, both fractionated external beam radiation therapy (EBRT) and stereotactic single-fraction radiation therapy (SRS) are used as adjuvant treatment tools [132]. SRS is increasingly used for lesions and may better protect the surrounding brain parenchyma from potential radiation toxicity [132]. Single-fraction SRS is usually limited to tumors <30 mm diameter and for meningiomas not directly adjacent to (or compressing) sensitive structures such as the hypothalamus [132]. Multifractional SRS can be used for bigger tumors [132]. Local control of meningiomas of a diameter of 3 cm or less after SRS was the effect of Simpson Grade I resection [133]. Two retrospective series found that a reduction of tumor size after SRS or EBRT provided tumor control after 5 and 10 years [134, 135]. The 10-year recurrence-free follow-up is 93.4% and 95.7%, respectively [135]. WHO grade II and III meningiomas are aggressive tumors [135]. The 1- and 4-year progression-free survival of these lesions after the first SRS is 92% and 31%, respectively [135]. Radiosurgery may be an important adjuvant and salvage therapy for lesions that will likely require more than one treatment [135]. Although discussions continue, combined treatment approaches that include surgery and fractionated RT are increasingly preferred.

7.5 Systemic treatments

There is no effective medical treatment for meningiomas because the beneficial effects of systemic agents have not been fully demonstrated in clinical trials.

Currently, conventional cytotoxic agents are not thought to have a beneficial effect on the tumor. Data about that subject are generally based on observational or retrospective data from a small group of patients rather than prospective studies.

Systemic therapy is currently an alternative treatment option for a small group of patients with recurrent/progressive diseases who cannot be treated with RT or for whom further surgical resection is not possible. Thus, systemic treatment is not the initial treatment for meningiomas but the final treatment step. These can be studied as follows.

7.5.1 Hormone therapy

Knowing that 70% of meningiomas have progesterone receptors, 60% have prolactin receptors, 30% have estrogen receptors, and female predominance suggests the growth of such tumors may be hormone-dependent [136–139]. Knowledge of the presence of hormone receptors has led to the idea that hormone antagonists can also be used in treating meningiomas. To this end, Koide et al. used mifepristone (progesterone antagonist) at 200 or 400 mg daily doses [140]. Although they reported improvement in 25% of the patients included in the study, they noted a decrease in tumor size in 35% of fourteen patients using the same hormone antagonist at similar doses [140]. Grunberg et al. used similar doses of mifepristone and had five out of 14 patients show a meaningful decrease in tumor size [141]. However, continuing studies with larger patient groups failed to achieve the cure mentioned above rates [140–142]. The trial with tamoxifen, an estrogen receptor modulator, conducted with 19 patients also failed to provide positive results [142].

7.5.2 Chemotherapy

Hydroxyurea, a drug commonly used in cancers, inhibits proliferation by inhibiting the S phase of replication [143, 144]. Swinnen et al. reported a decrease in tumor size in three of four patients in their study with hydroxyurea [143]. However, these responses could not be replicated in phase II clinical trials, and Chamberlain's study also failed to demonstrate efficacy [143, 144]. Currently, there is no routine clinical use.

7.5.3 Somatostatin analogs

Somatostatin receptors were found to be expressed in approximately 90% of meningiomas using single-photon emission computed tomography (SPECT) scanning [145]. Although 44% of 16 patients treated with a somatostatin agonist with a high affinity for somatostatin receptors (Sandostatin LAR) had positive results in terms of progression-free survival at 6 months, this agonist was found to have no effect in recurrent high-grade meningiomas [146]. In a study conducted with pasireotide, another agonist with higher receptor affinity than Sandostatin, no improvement in progression-free survival (PFS) at 6 months was observed [147]. The studies remain controversial, with no consensus. Currently, there is no routine clinical use.

7.5.4 Targeted agents

In recent studies, bevacizumab, an antibody against vascular endothelial growth factor (VEGF), has been shown to inhibit growth in meningiomas [148, 149]. Bevacizumab shows this effect possibly by blocking angiogenesis [148, 149]. Overall, bevacizumab appears to be an effective therapeutic approach for patients with atypical and anaplastic meningiomas who have exhausted surgical and radiation therapy options [148, 149]. Also because of the programmed death receptor (PDL1) in solid organ tumors outside the CNS, immunotherapeutics such as nivolumab and ipilimumab are quite effective [150]. After Du et al. presented evidence of PDL1 receptors in meningiomas, the use of nivolumab in recurrent meningiomas and pembrolizumab in atypical and anaplastic meningiomas paved the way for promising clinical trials [151]. There is currently an intense debate on the subject [151]. There is still no opinion due to the studies concluded in both directions [151]. Currently, there is no routine clinical use.

8. Conclusion

Within the framework of the rules of the book, we have tried to write this section without going into unnecessary detail. We hope it is useful for the reader.

Acknowledgements

We would like to thank our devoted families, whom we would not be able to reach without their support and sacrifice, and Operator Doctor Engin ELMACI for his support in our clinic.

Conflict of interest

The authors declare that they have no known competing financial interests or personal relationships between any person/persons or institution/institutions and the authors that could have appeared to influence the work reported in this paper.

Other declarations

Finally, we dedicate it to the great Türk nation, which sheds light on our future with its thousands of years of history.

Appendices and nomenclature

CNS	central nervous system
CSF	cerebrospinal fluid
CT	computed tomography
EBRT	external beam radiation therapy
GTR	gross total resection
ICP	increased cerebral pressure
MEN	multiple endocrine neoplasia
MRI	magnetic resonance imaging
MRIs	magnetic resonance imaging spectroscopy
NF2	neurofibromatosis type 2

PET	positron emission tomography
PDL1	programmed death receptor 1
RT	radiotherapy
SPECT	single-photon emission computed tomography
SRS	stereotactic radiosurgery
STR	subtotal resection
VEGF	vascular endothelial growth factor
WHO	World Health Organization

Author details

İsmail Kaya* and Hüseyin Yakar
Faculty of Medicine, Department of Neurosurgery, Niğde Ömer Halisdemir University, Niğde, Turkey

*Address all correspondence to: hekimikaya@gmail.com

References

[1] Del Maestro R. Al-Mefty's Meningiomas. Second Edition. 2011. Edited by Franco DeMonte, Michael W. McDermott, Ossama Al-Mefty. Published by Thieme Medical Publishers, Inc. 432pages. C$210 approx. Canadian Journal of Neurological Sciences/Journal Canadien Des Sciences Neurologiques. 2013;**40**(1):131-132. DOI: 10.1017/S0317167100017455

[2] Li J, Fang L, Killer H, Flammer J, Meyer P, Neutzner A. Meningothelial cells as part of the central nervous system host defence. Biology of the Cell. 2013;**105**(7):304-315. DOI: 10.1111/boc.201300013

[3] Bir S, Maiti T, Bollam P, Nanda A. Felix platter and a historical perspective of the meningioma. Clinical Neurology and Neurosurgery. 2015;**134**:75-78. DOI: 10.1016/j.clineuro.2015.02.018. Epub 2015 Apr 17

[4] Louis A. Memoire sur les Tumeurs Fongueuses de la Dure-Mere. Mémoires. Académie de chirurgie. 1774;**5**:1-59

[5] Plater F. Observationum in Hominis Affectibus Plerisque Corpori et Amino, Funtionum Laesione, Dolore Aliave molestiaet Vitio Incommendantibus. Libri Tres, Basileae: Impensis Ludivici Konig; 1614

[6] Cushing H. Themeningiomas (dural endotheliomas): Their source, and favoured seats of origin. Brain. 1992;**45**:282-316

[7] Drummond K, Zhu J, Black P. Meningiomas: Updating basic science, management, and outcome. The Neurologist. 2004;**10**(3):113-130. DOI: 10.1097/01.nrl.0000126588.14216.f3

[8] Gittleman H, Ostrom Q, Rouse C, Dowling J, de Blank P, Kruchko C, et al. Trends in central nervous system tumor incidence relative to other common cancers in adults, adolescents, and children in the United States, 2000 to 2010. Cancer. 2014;**121**(1):102-112. DOI: 10.1002/cncr.29015. Epub 25 Aug 2014

[9] Longstreth W, Dennis L, McGuire V, Drangsholt M, Koepsell T. Epidemiology of intracranial meningioma. Cancer. 1993;**72**(3):639-648. DOI: 10.1002/1097-0142(19930801)72:3<639::aid-cncr2820720304>3.0.co;2-p

[10] Bondy M, Lee LB. Epidemiology and etiology of intracranial meningiomas: A review. Journal of Neuro-Oncology. 1996;**29**(3):197-205. DOI: 10.1007/BF00165649

[11] De Monte F. Current management of meningiomas. Oncology (Williston Park). 1995;**9**(1):83-91, 96; discussion 96, 99-101

[12] Baumgartner J, Sorenson J. Meningioma in the pediatric population. Journal of Neuro-Oncology. 1996;**29**(3):223-228

[13] Blumenthal D, Berho M, Bloomfield S, Schochet S, Kaufman H. Childhood meningioma associated with meningioangiomatosis. Journal of Neurosurgery. 1993;**78**(2):287-289. DOI: 10.3171/jns.1993.78.2.0287

[14] Watkins D, Rouleau GA. Genetics, prognosis and therapy of central nervous system tumors. Cancer Detection and Prevention. 1994;**18**(2):139-144

[15] Preston-Martin S. Descriptive epidemiology of primary tumors of the brain, cranial nerves and cranial

meninges in Los Angeles County. Neuroepidemiology. 1989;**8**(6):283-295. DOI: 10.1159/000110196

[16] Davis FG, Kupelian V, Freels S, McCarthy B, Surawicz T. Prevalence estimates for primary brain tumors in the United States by behavior and major histology groups. Neuro-Oncology. 2001;**3**(3):152-158. DOI: 10.1093/neuonc/3.3.152

[17] Baldi I, Engelhardt J, Bonnet C, Bauchet L, Berteaud E, Grüber A, et al. Epidemiology of meningiomas. Neuro-Chirurgie. 2018;**64**(1):5-14. DOI: 10.1016/j.neuchi.2014.05.006. Epub 2014 Sep 22

[18] Mahmood A, Caccamo DV, Tomecek FJ, Malik GM. Atypical and malignant meningiomas: A clinicopathological review. Neurosurgery. 1993;**33**(6):955-963. DOI:10.1227/00006123-199312000-00001

[19] Backer-Grøndahl T, Moen BH, Torp SH. The histopathological spectrum of human meningiomas. International Journal of Clinical and Experimental Pathology. 2012;**5**(3):231-242. Epub 2012 Mar 25

[20] Chhabda S, Carney O, D'Arco F, Jacques TS, Mankad K. The 2016 World Health Organization classification of tumours of the central nervous system: What the paediatric neuroradiologist needs to know. Quantitative Imaging in Medicine and Surgery. 2016;**6**(5):486-489. DOI: 10.21037/qims.2016.10.01

[21] Adegbite AB, Khan MI, Paine KW, Tan LK. The recurrence of intracranial meningiomas after surgical treatment. Journal of Neurosurgery. 1983;**58**(1):51-56. DOI: 10.3171/jns.1983.58.1.0051

[22] de Almeida AN, Pereira BJA, Pires Aguiar PH, Paiva WS, Cabrera HN, da Silva CC, et al. Clinical outcome, tumor recurrence, and causes of death: A long-term follow-up of surgically treated meningiomas. World Neurosurgery. 2017;**102**:139-143. DOI: 10.1016/j.wneu.2017.03.009. Epub 2017 Mar 12

[23] Kim D, Niemierko A, Hwang WL, Stemmer-Rachamimov AO, Curry WT, Barker FG, et al. Histopathological prognostic factors of recurrence following definitive therapy for atypical and malignant meningiomas. Journal of Neurosurgery. 2018;**128**(4):1123-1132. DOI: 10.3171/2016.11.JNS16913. Epub 2017 Jun 16

[24] Adeberg S, Hartmann C, Welzel T, Rieken S, Habermehl D, von Deimling A, et al. Long-term outcome after radiotherapy in patients with atypical and malignant meningiomas—Clinical results in 85 patients treated in a single institution leading to optimized guidelines for early radiation therapy. International Journal of Radiation Oncology, Biology, Physics. 2012;**83**(3):859-864. DOI: 10.1016/j.ijrobp.2011.08.010. Epub 2011 Dec 2

[25] Buerki RA, Horbinski CM, Kruser T, Horowitz PM, James CD, Lukas RV. An overview of meningiomas. Future Oncology. 2018;**14**(21):2161-2177. DOI: 10.2217/fon-2018-0006. Epub 2018 Aug 7

[26] Mawrin C, Perry A. Pathological classification and molecular genetics of menin-giomas. Journal of Neuro-Oncology. 2010;**99**:379-391

[27] Yaşargil MG. In: Yaşargil MG, editor. Microneurosurgery IV B: Microneurosurgery of CNS Tumors. Georg Thieme Verlag: Stuttgart, New York; 1995

[28] Meningiomas. Their classification, regional behaviour, life history, and surgical end results. Bulletin

of the Medical Library Association. 1938;**27**(2):185

[29] Ojemann RG. Olfactory groove meningiomas. In: Al-Mefty O, editor. Meningioma. New York: Raven Press; 1991. pp. 383-393

[30] Solero CL, Giombini S, Morello G. Suprasellar and olfactory meningiomas. Report on a series of 153 personal cases. Acta Neurochirurgica. 1983;**67**(3-4):181-194. DOI: 10.1007/BF01401420

[31] Guthrie BL, Ebersold MJ, Scheithauer BW. Neoplasms of intra-cranial meninges. In: Youmans JR, editor. Neurological Surgery. III ed. Vol. 5. Philadelphia: WB Saunders; 1990. pp. 32-53

[32] Hassler W, Zentner J. Pterional approach for surgical treatment of olfactory groove meningiomas. Neurosurgery. 1989;**25**(6):942-945; discussion 945-7

[33] Al-Mefty O, Smith R. Tuberculum sellae meningiomas. New York: Raven Press; 1991. pp. 311-395

[34] Ojemann R. Meningiomas of the basal parapituitary region: Technical considerations. Clinical Neurosurgery. 1980;**27**(CN_suppl_1):233-262

[35] Ojemann RG. Meningiornas: Clinical features and surgical management. In: Wilkens R, Rengachary S, editors. Neurosurgery. New York: McGraw-Hill; 1985. pp. 635-654

[36] Ojemann RG. Surgical management of cranial and spinal meningiomas. Clinical Neurosurgery. 1993;**40**:321-383

[37] Kadis GN, Mount LA, Ganti SR. The importance of early diagnosis and treatment of the meningiomas of the planum sphenoidale and tuberculum sellae: A retrospective study of 105 cases. Surgical Neurology. 1979;**12**(5):367-371

[38] Symon L, Rosenstein J. Surgical management of suprasellar meningioma. Part 1: The influence of tumor size, duration of symptoms, and microsurgery on surgical outcome in 101 consecutive cases. Journal of Neurosurgery. 1984;**61**(4):633-641. DOI: 10.3171/jns.1984.61.4.0633

[39] Grisoli F, Diaz-Vasquez P, Riss M, Vincentelli F, Leclercq TA, Hassoun J, et al. Microsurgical management of tuberculum sellae meningiomas. Results in 28 consecutive cases. Surgical Neurology. 1986;**26**(1):37-44. DOI: 10.1016/0090-3019(86)90061-3

[40] Al-Mefty O, Holoubi A, Rifai A, Fox JL. Microsurgical removal of suprasellar meningiomas. Neurosurgery. 1985;**16**(3):364-372. DOI:10.1227/00006123-198503000-00014

[41] Philippon J, Cornu P. The recurrence of meningiomas. In: Al-Mefty O, editor. Meningiomas. New York: Raven Press; 1991. pp. 87-105

[42] Granick MS, Martuza RL, Parker SW, Ojemann RG, Montgomery WW. Cerebellopontine angle meningiomas: Clinical manifestations and diagnosis. The Annals of Otology, Rhinology, and Laryngology. 1985;**94**(1 Pt 1):34-38. DOI: 10.1177/000348948509400108

[43] Guidetti B, Ciappetta P, Domenicucci M. Tentorial meningiomas: Surgical experience with 61 cases and long-term results. Journal of Neurosurgery. 1988;**69**(2):183-187. DOI: 10.3171/jns.1988.69.2.0183

[44] Guidetti B, Delfini R. Lateral and fourth ventricle meningiomas. In: Al-Mefty O, editor. Meningiomas. New York: Raven Press; 1991. pp. 569-587

[45] Al-Mefty O. Clinoidal meningiomas. Journal of Neurosurgery.

1990;**73**(6):840-849. DOI: 10.3171/jns.1990.73.6.0840

[46] Uihlein A, Weyand RD. Meningiomas of anterior clinoid process as a cause of unilateral loss of vision; surgical considerations. A.M.A. Archives of Ophthalmology. 1953;**49**(3):261-270. DOI: 10.1001/archopht.1953.00920020270003

[47] Bonnal J, Thibaut A, Brotchi J, Born J. Invading meningiomas of the sphenoid ridge. Journal of Neurosurgery. 1980;**53**(5):587-599. DOI: 10.3171/jns.1980.53.5.0587

[48] Newell FW, Beaman TC. Ocular signs of meningioma. Transactions of the American Ophthalmological Society. 1957-1958;**55**:297-312; discussion 312-6

[49] Henderson JW, Campbell RJ, Farrow GM, et al. Orbital tumors. In: Metastatic Carcinomas. 3rd ed. New York, NY: Raven Press; 1994. pp. 361-376

[50] Sekhar LN, Sen CN, Jho HD, Janecka IP. Surgical treatment of intracavernous neoplasms: A four-year experience. Neurosurgery. 1989;**24**(1):18-30. DOI: 10.1227/00006123-198901000-00004

[51] Dolenc VV. Anatomy of the cavernous sinus. In: Anatomy and Surgery of the Cavernous Sinus. Vienna: Springer; 1989. DOI: 10.1007/978-3-7091-6942-1_2

[52] Al-Mefty O, Smith RR. Surgery of tumors invading the cavernous sinus. Surgical Neurology. 1988;**30**(5):370-381. DOI: 10.1016/0090-3019(88)90200-5

[53] Brotchi J, Bonnal JP. Lateral and middle sphenoid wing meningiomas. In: Al-Mefty O, editor. Meningiomas. New York: Raven Press; 1991. pp. 413-425

[54] Basso AJ, Carrizo A. Sphenoid ridge meningiomas. In: Schmidek HH, editor. Meningiomas and Their Surgical Management. Philadelphia: WB Saunders; 1991. pp. 242-259

[55] Sekhar LN, Altschuler EM. Meningiomas of the cavernous sinus. In: Al-Mefty O, editor. Meningiomas. New York: Raven Press; 1991. pp. 445-460

[56] Parkinson D. A surgical approach to the cavernous portion of the carotid artery. Anatomical studies and case report. Journal of Neurosurgery. 1965;**23**(5):474-483. DOI: 10.3171/jns.1965.23.5.0474

[57] van Loveren HR, Keller JT, el-Kalliny M, Scodary DJ, Tew JM Jr. The Dolenc technique for cavernous sinus exploration (cadaveric prosection). Technical note. Journal of Neurosurgery. 1991;**74**(5):837-844. DOI: 10.3171/jns.1991.74.5.0837

[58] Bruneau M, George B. Foramen magnum meningiomas: Detailed surgical approaches and technical aspects at Lariboisière Hospital and review of the literature. Neurosurgical Review. 2008;**31**(1):19-32; discussion 32-3. DOI: 10.1007/s10143-007-0097-1. Epub 2007 Sep 20

[59] Yasuoka S, Okazaki H, Daube JR, MacCarty CS. Foramen magnum tumors. Analysis of 57 cases of benign extramedullary tumors. Journal of Neurosurgery. 1978;**49**(6):828-838. DOI: 10.3171/jns.1978.49.6.0828

[60] Meyer FB, Ebersold MJ, Reese DF. Benign tumors of the foramen magnum. Journal of Neurosurgery. 1984;**61**(1):136-142. DOI: 10.3171/jns.1984.61.1.0136

[61] al-Mefty O, Borba LA, Aoki N, Angtuaco E, Pait TG. The transcondylar approach to extradural nonneoplastic lesions of the craniovertebral junction. Journal of Neurosurgery. 1996;**84**(1):1-6. DOI: 10.3171/jns.1996.84.1.0001

[62] George B, Lot G. Anterolateral and posterolateral approaches to the foramen magnum: Technical description and experience from 97 cases. Skull Base Surgery. 1995;**5**(1):9-19. DOI: 10.1055/s-2008-1058945

[63] Welling B, Al-Mefty O. Foramen magnum tumors. In: Cohen AR, editor. Surgical Disorders of the Fourth Ventricle. Cambridge: Blackwell Science; 1996. pp. 251-261

[64] Baldwin HZ, Spetzler RF, Wascher TM, Daspit CP. The far lateral-combined supra- and infratentorial approach: Clinical experience. Acta Neurochirurgica. 1995;**134**(3-4):155-158. DOI: 10.1007/BF01417683

[65] Sen CN, Sekhar LN. An extreme lateral approach to intradural lesions of the cervical spine and foramen magnum. Neurosurgery. 1990;**27**(2):197-204. DOI: 10.1097/00006123-199008000-00004

[66] Samii M, Klekamp J, Carvalho G. Surgical results for meningiomas of the craniocervical junction. Neurosurgery. 1996;**39**(6):1086-1094; discussion 1094-5. DOI: 10.1097/00006123-199612000-00003

[67] Yaşargil M, Mortara R, Curcic M. Meningiomas of basal posterior cranial fossa. In: Advances and Technical Standards in Neurosurgery, Advances and Technical Standards in Neurosurgery. Vol. 7. Vienna: Springer; 1980. pp. 3-115. DOI: 10.1007/978-3-7091-7051-9_1

[68] 11.Tekkök I, Süzer T, Erbengi A. Non-acoustic tumors of the cerebellopontine angle. Neurosurgical Review. 1992;**15**(2):117-123. DOI: 10.1007/BF00313506

[69] Nassif PS, Shelton C, Arriaga M. Hearing preservation following surgical removal of meningiomas affecting the temporal bone. The Laryngoscope. 1992;**102**(12 Pt 1):1357-1362. DOI: 10.1288/00005537-199212000-00009

[70] Arnautovic KI, Al-Mefty O. Cerebellopontine angle meningiomas. In: Kaye AH, Black PM, editors. Operative Neurosurgery. Vol. 1. London, England: Churchill Livingstone; 2000. pp. 545-558

[71] Mayberg MR, Symon L. Meningiomas of the clivus and apical petrous bone. Report of 35 cases. Journal of Neurosurgery. 1986;**65**(2):160-167. DOI: 10.3171/jns.1986.65.2.0160

[72] Hakuba A, Nishimura S, Tanaka K, Kishi H, Nakamura T. Clivus meningioma: Six cases of total removal. Neurologia Medico-Chirurgica (Tokyo). 1977;**17**(1 Pt 1):63-77. DOI: 10.2176/nmc.17pt1.63

[73] Samii M, Ammirati M, Mahran A, Bini W, Sepehrnia A. Surgery of petroclival meningiomas: Report of 24 cases. Neurosurgery. 1989;**24**(1):12-17. DOI: 10.1227/00006123-198901000-00003

[74] Zentner J, Meyer B, Vieweg U, Herberhold C, Schramm J. Petroclival meningiomas: Is radical resection always the best option? Journal of Neurology, Neurosurgery, and Psychiatry. 1997;**62**(4):341-345. DOI: 10.1136/jnnp.62.4.341

[75] Sekhar LN, Jannetta PJ, Burkhart LE, Janosky JE. Meningiomas involving the clivus: A six-year experience with 41 patients. Neurosurgery. 1990;**27**(5):764-781; discussion 781

[76] Al-Mefty O, Fox JL, Smith RR. Petrosal approach for petroclival meningiomas. Neurosurgery. 1988;**22**(3):510-517. DOI: 10.1227/00006123-198803000-00010

[77] Morrison AW, King TT. Experiences with a translabyrinthine-transtentorial approach to the cerebellopontine angle. Technical note. Journal of Neurosurgery. 1973;**38**(3):382-390. DOI: 10.3171/jns.1973.38.3.0382

[78] Mooney MA, Abolfotoh M, Bi WL, Tavanaiepour D, Almefty RO, Bassiouni H, et al. Is falcine meningioma a diffuse disease of the falx? Case series and analysis of a "grade zero" resection. Neurosurgery. 2020;**87**(5):900-909. DOI: 10.1093/neuros/nyaa038

[79] Sindou MP, Alvernia JE. Results of attempted radical tumor removal and venous repair in 100 consecutive meningiomas involving the major dural sinuses. Journal of Neurosurgery. 2006;**105**(4):514-525. DOI: 10.3171/jns.2006.105.4.514

[80] Giombini S, Solero CL, Lasio G, Morello G. Immediate and late outcome of operations for parasagittal and falx meningiomas. Report of 342 cases. Surgical Neurology. 1984;**21**(5):427-435. DOI: 10.1016/0090-3019(84)90446-4

[81] Marks SM, Whitwell HL, Lye RH. Recurrence of meningiomas after operation. Surgical Neurology. 1986;**25**(5):436-440. DOI: 10.1016/0090-3019(86)90081-9

[82] Chan RC, Thompson GB. Morbidity, mortality, and quality of life following surgery for intracranial meningiomas. A retrospective study in 257 cases. Journal of Neurosurgery. 1984;**60**(1):52-60. DOI: 10.3171/jns.1984.60.1.0052

[83] Giombini S, Solero CL, Morello G. Late outcome of operations for supratentorial convexity meningiomas. Report on 207 cases. Surgical Neurology. 1984;**22**(6):588-594. DOI: 10.1016/0090-3019(84)90436-1

[84] Kenichiro S, Yushio S. Tentorial meningiomas. In: AlMefty O, editor. Meningiomas. New York: Raven Press; 1991. pp. 357-361

[85] Fornari M, Savoiardo M, Morello G, Solero CL. Meningiomas of the lateral ventricles. Neuroradiological and surgical considerations in 18 cases. Journal of Neurosurgery. 1981;**54**(1):64-74. DOI: 10.3171/jns.1981.54.1.0064

[86] Newman SA, Jane JA. Meningiomas of the optic nerve, orbit, and anterior visual pathways. In: Al-Mefty O, editor. Meningiomas. New York: Raven Press; 1991. pp. 461-494

[87] Al Saadi A, Latimer F, Madercic M, Robbins T. Cytogenetic studies of human brain tumors and their clinical significance. II. Meningioma. Cancer Genetics and Cytogenetics. 1987;**26**(1):127-141. DOI: 10.1016/0165-4608(87)90140-3

[88] Hansson CM, Buckley PG, Grigelioniene G, Piotrowski A, Hellström AR, Mantripragada K, et al. Comprehensive genetic and epigenetic analysis of sporadic meningioma for macro-mutations on 22q and micro-mutations within the NF2 locus. BMC Genomics. 2007;**8**:16. DOI: 10.1186/1471-2164-8-16

[89] Shen Y, Nunes F, Stemmer-Rachamimov A, James M, Mohapatra G, Plotkin S, et al. Genomic profiling distinguishes familial multiple and sporadic multiple meningiomas. BMC Medical Genomics. 2009;**2**:42. DOI: 10.1186/1755-8794-2-42

[90] Riemenschneider MJ, Perry A, Reifenberger G. Histological classification and molecular genetics of meningiomas. Lancet Neurology. 2006;**5**(12):1045-1054. DOI: 10.1016/S1474-4422(06)70625-1. Erratum in: Lancet Neurology 2007 Feb;6(2):105

[91] Abi Jaoude S, Peyre M, Degos V, Goutagny S, Parfait B, Kalamarides M. Validation of a scoring system to evaluate the risk of rapid growth of intracranial meningiomas in neurofibromatosis type 2 patients. Journal of Neurosurgery. 2020;**134**(5):1377-1385. DOI: 10.3171/2020.3.JNS192382

[92] Chamberlain MC. Meningiomas. In: Norden AD, Reardon DA, Wen PCY, editors. Primary Central Nervous System Tumors: Pathogenesis and Therapy. NJ, USA: Humana Press; 2011. pp. 355-375

[93] Brenner AV, Sugiyama H, Preston DL, Sakata R, French B, Sadakane A, et al. Radiation risk of central nervous system tumors in the Life Span Study of atomic bomb survivors, 1958-2009. European Journal of Epidemiology. 2020;**35**(6):591-600. DOI: 10.1007/s10654-019-00599-y. Epub 2020 Jan 25

[94] Supartoto A, Sasongko MB, Respatika D, Mahayana IT, Pawiroranu S, Kusnanto H, et al. Relationships between neurofibromatosis-2, progesterone receptor expression, the use of exogenous progesterone, and risk of orbitocranial meningioma in females. Frontiers in Oncology. 2019;**8**:651. DOI: 10.3389/fonc.2018.00651

[95] Claus EB, Black PM, Bondy ML, Calvocoressi L, Schildkraut JM, Wiemels JL, et al. Exogenous hormone use and meningioma risk: What do we tell our patients? Cancer. 2007;**110**(3):471-476. DOI: 10.1002/cncr.22783

[96] Hatch EE, Linet MS, Zhang J, Fine HA, Shapiro WR, Selker RG, et al. Reproductive and hormonal factors and risk of brain tumors in adult females. International Journal of Cancer. 2005;**114**(5):797-805. DOI: 10.1002/ijc.20776

[97] Watts J, Box G, Galvin A, Brotchie P, Trost N, Sutherland T. Magnetic resonance imaging of meningiomas: A pictorial review. Insights Imaging. 2014;**5**(1):113-122. DOI: 10.1007/s13244-013-0302-4. Epub 2014 Jan 8

[98] Buetow MP, Buetow PC, Smirniotopoulos JG. Typical, atypical, and misleading features in meningioma. Radiographics. 1991;**11**(6):1087-1106. DOI: 10.1148/radiographics.11.6.1749851

[99] Harting I, Hartmann M, Bonsanto MM, Sommer C, Sartor K. Characterization of necrotic meningioma using diffusion MRI, perfusion MRI, and MR spectroscopy: Case report and review of the literature. Neuroradiology. 2004;**46**(3):189-193. DOI: 10.1007/s00234-003-1144-4. Epub 2004 Feb 4

[100] Buhl R, Nabavi A, Wolff S, Hugo HH, Alfke K, Jansen O, et al. MR spectroscopy in patients with intracranial meningiomas. Neurological Research. 2007;**29**(1):43-46. DOI: 10.1179/174313206X153824

[101] Spille DC, Adeli A, Sporns PB, Heß K, Streckert EMS, Brokinkel C, et al. Predicting the risk of postoperative recurrence and high-grade histology in patients with intracranial meningiomas using routine preoperative MRI. Neurosurgical Review. 2021;**44**(2):1109-1117. DOI: 10.1007/s10143-020-01301-7. Epub 2020 Apr 23. Erratum in: Neurosurg Rev. 2022 Apr;45(2):1815

[102] Hale AT, Wang L, Strother MK, Chambless LB. Differentiating meningioma grade by imaging features on magnetic resonance imaging. Journal of Clinical Neuroscience. 2018;**48**:71-75. DOI: 10.1016/j.jocn.2017.11.013. Epub 2017 Nov 22

[103] Nowak A, Dziedzic T, Krych P, Czernicki T, Kunert P, Marchel A. Benign versus atypical meningiomas: Risk

factors predicting recurrence. Neurologia i Neurochirurgia Polska. 2015;**49**(1):1-10. DOI: 10.1016/j.pjnns.2014.11.003. Epub 2014 Nov 28

[104] Nakamura M, Roser F, Michel J, Jacobs C, Samii M. The natural history of incidental meningiomas. Neurosurgery. 2003;**53**(1):62-70; discussion 70-1. DOI: 10.1227/01.neu.0000068730.76856.58

[105] Kuratsu J, Kochi M, Ushio Y. Incidence and clinical features of asymptomatic meningiomas. Journal of Neurosurgery. 2000;**92**(5):766-770. DOI: 10.3171/jns.2000.92.5.0766

[106] Niu L, Zhou X, Duan C, Zhao J, Sui Q, Liu X, et al. Differentiation researches on the meningioma subtypes by radiomics from contrast-enhanced magnetic resonance imaging: A preliminary study. World Neurosurgery. 2019;**126**:e646-e652. DOI: 10.1016/j.wneu.2019.02.109. Epub 2019 Mar 1

[107] Li X, Lu Y, Xiong J, Wang D, She D, Kuai X, et al. Presurgical differentiation between malignant haemangiopericytoma and angiomatous meningioma by a radiomics approach based on texture analysis. Journal of Neuroradiology. 2019;**46**(5):281-287. DOI: 10.1016/j.neurad.2019.05.013. Epub 2019 Jun 18

[108] Zhang Y, Chen JH, Chen TY, Lim SW, Wu TC, Kuo YT, et al. Radiomics approach for prediction of recurrence in skull base meningiomas. Neuroradiology. 2019;**61**(12):1355-1364. DOI: 10.1007/s00234-019-02259-0. Epub 2019 Jul 19

[109] Zhang J, Yao K, Liu P, Liu Z, Han T, Zhao Z, et al. A radiomics model for preoperative prediction of brain invasion in meningioma non-invasively based on MRI: A multicentre study. EBioMedicine. 2020;**58**:102933. DOI: 10.1016/j.ebiom.2020.102933. Epub 2020 Jul 30

[110] Sindou MP, Alaywan M. Most intracranial meningiomas are not cleavable tumors: Anatomic-surgical evidence and angiographic predictibility. Neurosurgery. 1998;**42**(3):476-480. DOI: 10.1097/00006123-199803000-00007

[111] Rachinger W, Stoecklein VM, Terpolilli NA, Haug AR, Ertl L, Pöschl J, et al. Increased 68Ga-DOTATATE uptake in PET imaging discriminates meningioma and tumor-free tissue. Journal of Nuclear Medicine. 2015;**56**(3):347-353. DOI: 10.2967/jnumed.114.149120. Epub 2015 Jan 29

[112] Afshar-Oromieh A, Wolf MB, Kratochwil C, Giesel FL, Combs SE, Dimitrakopoulou-Strauss A, et al. Comparison of ^{68}Ga-DOTATOC-PET/CT and PET/MRI hybrid systems in patients with cranial meningioma: Initial results. Neuro-Oncology. 2015;**17**(2):312-319. DOI: 10.1093/neuonc/nou131. Epub 2014 Jul 9

[113] Cameron EW. Transient ischaemic attacks due to meningioma—Report of 4 cases. Clinical Radiology. 1994;**49**(6):416-418. DOI: 10.1016/s0009-9260(05)81829-x

[114] Roux-Vaillard S, Mercier P, Fournier HD, Hayek G, Menei P, Guy G. Méningiomes intracrâniens révélés par une hémorragie [Intracranial meningiomas revealed by hemorrhage. Report of three cases and literature review]. Neurochirurgie. 1999;**45**(5):407-412. French

[115] Lieu AS, Howng SL. Intracranial meningiomas and epilepsy: Incidence, prognosis and influencing factors. Epilepsy Research. 2000;**38**(1):45-52. DOI: 10.1016/s0920-1211(99)00066-2

[116] Chozick BS, Reinert SE, Greenblatt SH. Incidence of seizures after surgery for supratentorial meningiomas: A modern analysis. Journal of Neurosurgery. 1996;**84**(3):382-386. DOI: 10.3171/jns.1996.84.3.0382

[117] Behbahani M, Skeie GO, Eide GE, Hausken A, Lund-Johansen M, Skeie BS. A prospective study of the natural history of incidental meningioma-Hold your horses! Neuro-Oncology Practice. 2019;**6**(6):438-450. DOI: 10.1093/nop/npz011. Epub 2019 Apr 17

[118] Zeidman LA, Ankenbrandt WJ, Du H, Paleologos N, Vick NA. Growth rate of non-operated meningiomas. Journal of Neurology. 2008;**255**(6):891-895. DOI: 10.1007/s00415-008-0801-2. Epub 2008 Mar 20

[119] Yano S, Kuratsu J. Kumamoto brain tumor research group. Indications for surgery in patients with asymptomatic meningiomas based on an extensive experience. Journal of Neurosurgery. 2006;**105**(4):538-543. DOI: 10.3171/jns.2006.105.4.538

[120] Zada G, Baskaya MK, Shah MV. Introduction: Surgical management of skull base meningiomas. Neurosurgical Focus. 2017;**43**(videosuppl2):Intro

[121] Simpson D. The recurrence of intracranial meningiomas after surgical treatment. Journal of Neurology, Neurosurgery, and Psychiatry. 1957;**20**(1):22-39. DOI: 10.1136/jnnp.20.1.22

[122] Ostrom QT, Gittleman H, Xu J, Kromer C, Wolinsky Y, Kruchko C, et al. CBTRUS statistical report: Primary brain and other central nervous system tumors diagnosed in the United States in 2009-2013. Neuro-Oncology. 2016;**18**(suppl_5):v1-v75. DOI: 10.1093/neuonc/now207

[123] Rogers L, Barani I, Chamberlain M, Kaley TJ, McDermott M, Raizer J, et al. Meningiomas: Knowledge base, treatment outcomes, and uncertainties. A RANO review. Journal of Neurosurgery. 2015;**122**(1):4-23. DOI: 10.3171/2014.7.JNS131644

[124] Kaley T, Barani I, Chamberlain M, McDermott M, Panageas K, Raizer J, et al. Historical benchmarks for medical therapy trials in surgery- and radiation-refractory meningioma: A RANO review. Neuro-Oncology. 2014;**16**(6):829-840. DOI: 10.1093/neuonc/not330. Epub 2014 Feb 4

[125] Wirsching HG, Richter JK, Sahm F, Morel C, Krayenbuehl N, Rushing EJ, et al. Post-operative cardiovascular complications and time to recurrence in meningioma patients treated with versus without pre-operative embolization: A retrospective cohort study of 741 patients. Journal of Neuro-Oncology. 2018;**140**(3):659-667. DOI: 10.1007/s11060-018-2996-0. Epub 2018 Sep 8

[126] Iacobucci M, Danieli L, Visconti E, Maresca M, Anile C, Colosimo C, et al. Preoperative embolization of meningiomas with polyvinyl alcohol particles: The benefits are not outweighed by risks. Diagnostic and Interventional Imaging. 2017;**98**(4):307-314. DOI: 10.1016/j.diii.2016.08.006. Epub 2016 Sep 24

[127] Gruber A, Killer M, Mazal P, Bavinzski G, Richling B. Preoperative embolization of intracranial meningiomas: A 17-years single center experience. Minimally Invasive Neurosurgery. 2000;**43**(1):18-29. DOI: 10.1055/s-2000-8812

[128] Bendszus M, Rao G, Burger R, Schaller C, Scheinemann K, Warmuth-Metz M, et al. Is there a benefit of preoperative meningioma

embolization? Neurosurgery. 2000;**47**(6):1306-1311; discussion 1311-2

[129] Rosen CL, Ammerman JM, Sekhar LN, Bank WO. Outcome analysis of preoperative embolization in cranial base surgery. Acta Neurochirurgica. 2002;**144**(11):1157-1164. DOI: 10.1007/s00701-002-0965-y

[130] Ng HK, Poon WS, Goh K, Chan MS. Histopathology of post-embolized meningiomas. The American Journal of Surgical Pathology. 1996;**20**(10):1224-1230. DOI: 10.1097/00000478-199610000-00008

[131] Perry A, Chicoine MR, Filiput E, Miller JP, Cross DT. Clinicopathologic assessment and grading of embolized meningiomas: A correlative study of 64 patients. Cancer. 2001;**92**(3):701-711. DOI: 10.1002/1097-0142(20010801)92:3<701::aid-cncr1373>3.0.co;2-7

[132] Vera E, Iorgulescu JB, Raper DM, Madhavan K, Lally BE, Morcos J, et al. A review of stereotactic radiosurgery practice in the management of skull base meningiomas. Journal of Neurological Surgery Part B: Skull Base. 2014;**75**(3):152-158. DOI: 10.1055/s-0033-1354747. Epub 2014 Mar 12

[133] Bir SC, Patra DP, Maiti TK, Bollam P, Minagar A, Nanda A. Direct comparison of gamma knife radiosurgery and microsurgery for small size meningiomas. World Neurosurgery. 2017;**101**:170-179. DOI: 10.1016/j.wneu.2017.01.105. Epub 2017 Feb 6

[134] Patibandla MR, Lee CC, Tata A, Addagada GC, Sheehan JP. Stereotactic radiosurgery for WHO grade I posterior fossa meningiomas: Long-term outcomes with volumetric evaluation. Journal of Neurosurgery. 2018;**129**(5):1249-1259. DOI: 10.3171/2017.6.JNS17993

[135] Cohen-Inbar O, Tata A, Moosa S, Lee CC, Sheehan JP. Stereotactic radiosurgery in the treatment of parasellar meningiomas: Long-term volumetric evaluation. Journal of Neurosurgery. 2018;**128**(2):362-372. DOI: 10.3171/2016.11.JNS161402. Epub 2017 Mar 24

[136] Jhawar BS, Fuchs CS, Colditz GA, Stampfer MJ. Sex steroid hormone exposures and risk for meningioma. Journal of Neurosurgery. 2003;**99**(5):848-853. DOI: 10.3171/jns.2003.99.5.0848

[137] Sanson M, Cornu P. Biology of meningiomas. Acta Neurochirurgica. 2000;**142**(5):493-505. DOI: 10.1007/s007010050462

[138] Muccioli G, Ghè C, Faccani G, Lanotte M, Forni M, Ciccarelli E. Prolactin receptors in human meningiomas: Characterization and biological role. The Journal of Endocrinology. 1997;**153**(3):365-371. DOI: 10.1677/joe.0.1530365

[139] Jimenez-Hakim E, el-Azouzi M, Black PM. The effect of prolactin and bombesin on the growth of meningioma-derived cells in monolayer culture. Journal of Neuro-Oncology. 1993;**16**(3):185-190. DOI: 10.1007/BF01057032

[140] Koide SS. Mifepristone. Auxiliary therapeutic use in cancer and related disorders. The Journal of Reproductive Medicine. 1998;**43**(7):551-560

[141] Grunberg SM, Weiss MH, Spitz IM, Ahmadi J, Sadun A, Russell CA, et al. Treatment of unresectable meningiomas with the antiprogesterone agent mifepristone. Journal of Neurosurgery. 1991;**74**(6):861-866. DOI: 10.3171/jns.1991.74.6.0861

[142] Goodwin JW, Crowley J, Eyre HJ, Stafford B, Jaeckle KA, Townsend JJ.

A phase II evaluation of tamoxifen in unresectable or refractory meningiomas: A southwest oncology group study. Journal of Neuro-Oncology. 1993;**15**(1):75-77. DOI: 10.1007/BF01050266

[143] Swinnen LJ, Rankin C, Rushing EJ, Laura HF, Damek DM, Barger GR. Phase II study of hydroxyurea for unresectable meningioma (Southwest Oncology Group S9811). Journal of Clinical Oncology. 2009;**27**(15_suppl):2063-2063

[144] Chamberlain MC, Johnston SK. Hydroxyurea for recurrent surgery and radiation refractory meningioma: A retrospective case series. Journal of Neuro-Oncology. 2011;**104**(3):765-771. DOI: 10.1007/s11060-011-0541-5. Epub 2011 Feb 13

[145] Simó M, Argyriou AA, Macià M, Plans G, Majós C, Vidal N, et al. Recurrent high-grade meningioma: A phase II trial with somatostatin analogue therapy. Cancer Chemotherapy and Pharmacology. 2014;**73**(5):919-923. DOI: 10.1007/s00280-014-2422-z. Epub 2014 Mar 12

[146] Chamberlain MC, Glantz MJ, Fadul CE. Recurrent meningioma: Salvage therapy with long-acting somatostatin analogue. Neurology. 2007;**69**(10):969-973. DOI: 10.1212/01.wnl.0000271382.62776.b7. Erratum in: Neurology 2008 Jan 22;70(4):325

[147] Norden AD, Ligon KL, Hammond SN, Muzikansky A, Reardon DA, Kaley TJ, et al. Phase II study of monthly pasireotide LAR (SOM230C) for recurrent or progressive meningioma. Neurology. 2015;**84**(3):280-286. DOI: 10.1212/WNL.0000000000001153. Epub 2014 Dec 19

[148] Pistolesi S, Boldrini L, Gisfredi S, De Ieso K, Camacci T, Caniglia M, et al. Angiogenesis in intracranial meningiomas: Immunohistochemical and molecular study. Neuropathology and Applied Neurobiology. 2004;**30**(2):118-125. DOI: 10.1046/j.0305-1846.2003.00516.x

[149] Nayak L, Iwamoto FM, Rudnick JD, Norden AD, Lee EQ, Drappatz J, et al. Atypical and anaplastic meningiomas treated with bevacizumab. Journal of Neuro-Oncology. 2012;**109**(1):187-193. DOI: 10.1007/s11060-012-0886-4. Epub 2012 Apr 29

[150] Gubin MM, Schreiber RD. Cancer. The odds of immunotherapy success. Science. 2015;**350**(6257):158-159. DOI: 10.1126/science.aad4140

[151] Du Z, Abedalthagafi M, Aizer AA, McHenry AR, Sun HH, Bray MA, et al. Increased expression of the immune modulatory molecule PD-L1 (CD274) in anaplastic meningioma. Oncotarget. 2015;**6**(7):4704-4716. DOI: 10.18632/oncotarget.3082

Chapter 3

Management of High-Grade Meningioma: Present, Past and Promising Future

Nazmin Ahmed

Abstract

High-grade meningiomas have a persistent therapeutic challenge, which the World Health Organization (WHO) categorizes as grade II and III lesions, represent 10–20% and 5% of individuals with meningiomas, respectively. Although grade I meningiomas can be completely surgically removed and have long-term progression-free survival, higher grade meningiomas are more likely to return aggressively and to be resistant to conventional treatments. Recently, stereotactic radiosurgery (SRS) has offered promise for the treatment of localized tumors. The era of molecular targeted treatment is now upon us. Patients are being enrolled in clinical trials with a variety of innovative medications that target driver mutations, and these trials might result in more effective treatment plans. Alpha-interferon, vascular endothelial growth factor inhibitors, and somatostatin receptor agonists are among the medications that are advised for the medical treatment of meningiomas in addition to radiation and surgical excision. For the treatment of meningioma, efforts to find novel informative mutations and protein biomarkers have advanced. Several patient populations have shown promise for improved outcomes with EZH2 inhibition. Overall, it is hoped that targeted research and the application of those strategies, such as PRRT and TTF devices, would lead to better results in future. This chapter aims to discuss the neuro-imaging features of high grade meningiomas, diagnostic and therapeutic implications of recently discovered genetic alterations and outcome. There will be a brief review focusing on ongoing clinical trials of novel therapeutic agents and future research scope in this arena.

Keywords: meningioma, molecular targeted therapy, surgery

1. Introduction

The majority of primary central nervous system (CNS) tumors (37% of cases) are meningiomas. The prognosis for low grade (I) meningiomas is generally good, with a 20-year recurrence rate of 20%. Grade II meningiomas is difficult to cure and have a high chance of coming back after treatment. However, the prognosis for anaplastic meningiomas is dismal, with a median overall survival of only 1.5 years [1–3]. Additionally, clinical professionals frequently have to make tough treatment choices in instances with complicated morphology or localization, close to important brain structures like the optic nerve, or when incidental cancers are present. Here, we have discussed the epidemiology, natural history and cytogenetics of high grade meningioma. Moreover, we have discussed current theories of diagnosis, therapy, molecular biology. Additionally, improvements in imaging, particularly positron emission tomography (PET) and molecular profiling, are likely to soon have an influence on current clinical practice and be included into existing guidelines [4–6].

2. Epidemiology

Around 70% of cases are classified as WHO grade I meningiomas, 28% as WHO grade II meningiomas, and just around 3% as WHO grade III meningiomas. Meningiomas of grades II and III are more prevalent in males than in girls, according to various studies, however some also found different findings [7]. Research among participants in USA found that the age-adjusted incidence rate for WHO grade II meningiomas is 0.26/100,000 in the male population and 0.30/100,000 in the female population. On the other hand, age-adjusted incidence rates for meningiomas of WHO grade III are 0.08 per 100,000 for men and 0.09 per 100,000 for women [8]. Black individuals are more likely than white people, Asian-Pacific Islanders, and then white people to have high grade meningiomas. With aging comes an increased chance of developing these meningiomas, which often affect adults around the age of 60 [9].

Around 90% of WHO grade II meningiomas survive after five years. The number of tissue and cell abnormalities is increased in atypical meningiomas (WHO grade II). These tumors have a larger chance of recurrence than benign meningiomas, develop more quickly than benign meningiomas, and frequently invade the brain (WHO grade I). In comparison to benign and atypical meningiomas, malignant meningiomas (WHO grade III) have more cellular abnormalities and progress more quickly. The two kinds of malignant meningiomas return more frequently than the other two and are more likely to penetrate the brain. 1.7% of meningiomas with tissue confirmation

Characteristics	Grade-I	Grade-II & Grade-III
Somatic mutation [12–16]	Relatively low somatic mutation burden. *TRAF7*, *KLF4*, *AKT1*, *SMO*, *PIK3CA*, and RNA polymerase II subunit A (*POLR2A*) typically seen in grade-1 meningiomas and mostly do not coexist with *NF2* mutations	High-grade meningiomas exhibit a relatively high somatic mutation burden. The mutations tended to be C > T transitions. a higher expression of miR-21 is found in WHO grade II or III meningioma.
Genomic profile [12, 13, 15]	Alterations in NF2 is less common in low-grade meningiomas	Alterations in *NF2* or chromosome 22 occurred significantly more frequently in high-grade (80%) than low-grade meningiomas
Copy number alterations [13, 16]	Less frequent copy number alterations	High-grade meningiomas demonstrate frequent copy number alterations
Genomic disruption [17]	3%	19%
Loss of chromosome 22 [18]	More frequently (87%)	Less frequently (58%)

Characteristics		Grade-I	Grade-II & Grade-III
Gene Mutation [11, 19]	NF2	Yes	Yes & Yes
	TRAF7	Yes	Yes & Yes
	TERT	Yes	Yes & Yes
	SMARCB1	Yes	No & No
	PIK3CA	Yes	Yes & Yes
	POLR2A	Yes	No & No
	KLF4	Yes	No & No
	AKTI	Yes	No & No
	SMO	Yes	No & No
	SMARCEL	No	Yes & No
	BAPI	No	No & Yes
Chromosomal Alterations [19]		Loss: 22q	Grade II: Loss: 1p, 6q, 10, 14q, 18q; Gain: 1q, 9q, 12q, 15q, 17q, 20q Grade III: Loss: 9p Amplification: 17q

Table 1.
Cytogenetic variation of Grade-I, Grade-II and Grade-III meningioma.

are malignant, making up the bulk of meningiomas (WHO grade III) [8, 10]. After age 65, the chance of high grade meningiomas dramatically increases with age. The least at risk age group is 0 to 14 year olds. In comparison to other ethnic groups in the United States, African Americans have been found to have greater incidence of high grade meningioma [8]. High levels of ionizing radiation exposure have been linked to an increased risk of high grade meningiomas. Additionally, there is evidence between low radiation exposures to meningiomas. The most frequent source of ionizing radiation exposure in the US is dental X-rays. Numerous studies have connected a higher risk of meningioma to the frequency of full mouth dental radiographs. It is thought that individuals with the genetic condition Neurofibromatosis type 2 (NF2) have an increased chance of developing meningioma. Additionally, meningiomas that are malignant or numerous may be more common in NF2 patients [10]. While post-menopausal women without these traits are more likely to have Grade I meningiomas, meningioma patients with past CVA and those with grade 4/4 vascularity are more likely to develop WHO Grade II-III tumors [11] (**Table 1**).

3. Natural history of high-grade meningioma

The natural history of high-grade meningioma remains largely unknown. Based on the natural history of patients younger than 60 to 70 years of age and those with meningiomas characterized by surrounding brain hyperintensity on T2-weighted MRI, absence of calcification, and tumor diameter > 25–30 mm exhibit a higher risk for early recurrence [20–23]. For patients with NF2 linked malignancies, which typically exhibit a saltatory growth pattern, it is extremely important to be aware of and take

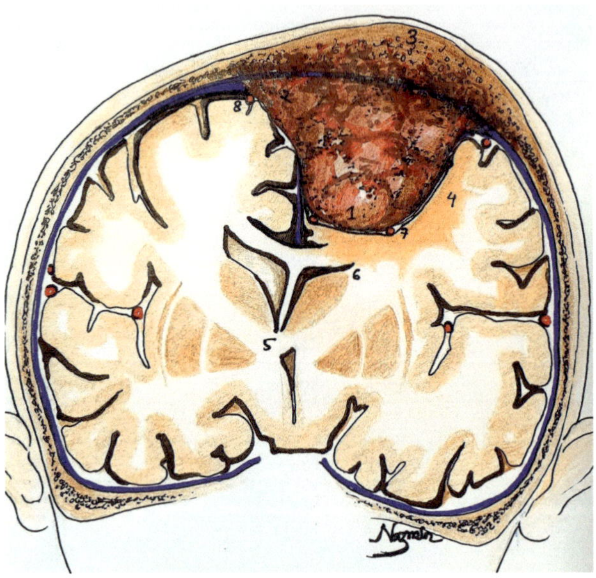

Figure 1.
Schematic picture demonstrated the natural history of an untreated high grade parasagittal meningioma. With the course of time, progressive invasion of SSS and overlying hyperostosis and/or, osteolysis occur. Later on, pial invasion and aquisition of pial feeders give to peritumoral edema, compression/effacement of ventricles and midline shifting. (1) parasagittal meningioma, (2) invasion of superior sagittal sinus, (3) hyperostosis of overlying bone, (4) peritumoral edema, (5) midline shifting, (6) effacement of lateral ventricle, (7&8) acquisition of pial feeders.

appropriate action in response to genetic abnormalities [24]. Because new tumors can develop in NF2 patients over their lifetime and because radiographic and symptomatic progression are unpredictable, resection may be best reserved for symptom-producing tumors, de novo, and brain edema-associated meningiomas in NF2 patients [24, 25]. Numerous investigations revealed that a number of chromosomal changes were linked to the development of cancer, and these changes may also be indicators of cancerous potential that affect tumor recurrence and a bad prognosis. Young age, lack of calcification, peritumoral edema, and high-intensity signal on T2WI were associated with clinical progression, according to Kim et al. [26] (**Figure 1**).

4. Diagnostic neuroimaging

4.1 X-ray

A general x-ray uses a modest quantity of radiation to provide an image of the inside organs and structures of the body. An x-ray of the head can occasionally help doctors locate a tumor, but it is insufficient to identify meningioma. By using X-Ray radiograph imaging, osteolysis and hyperostosis results may also be observed [27].

4.2 Computed tomography (CT or CAT)

A CT scan uses head x-rays to acquire photographs of the brain. A computer then combines these data to create a comprehensive, three-dimensional image

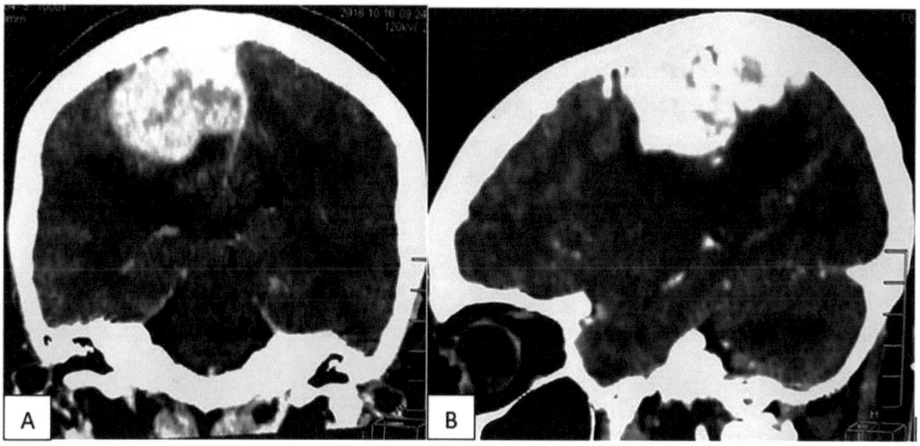

Figure 2.
Post contrast coronal (A) and sagittal (B) CT scan of a 45 year-old lady with histopathologically proven anaplastic meningioma (WHO grade-III) demonstrated an extra-axial heterogeneously contrast enhancing right parasagittal mass, invading the superior sagittal sinus with compression and displacement of falx cerebri towards the left side. The mass had irregular margin with evidence of surrounding vasogenic edema. Beside this, no features of hyperostosis was seen.

that displays any anomalies or tumours, including the size of the tumours. Before a scan, a patient may get an injection of a specific dye called a contrast medium to improve the image's clarity. The most effective method for identifying changes in the skull that a meningioma may produce is a CT scan. When individuals are not appropriate for MRI, particularly when the meningioma is completely ossified or calcified, CT is helpful. The first modality used to assess neurological indications or symptoms is frequently computed tomography (CT), which is also frequently the modality that finds an accidental injury [27]. For the presentation of tumour-induced osseous alterations such remodelling with localized hyperostosis and bone thickening or bone invasion with concomitant osteoblastic response (more rarely osteolysis) in malignant patients, CT continues to be the gold standard alongside MRI [28–30] (**Figure 2**).

4.3 Magnetic resonance imaging (MRI)

The preferred examination for identifying and classifying meningiomas is MRI. Instead than using x-rays, an MRI creates precise pictures of the body using magnetic fields. MRIs often reveal changes in the brain brought on by tumors, such as swelling or places where the tumor has grown, and can produce more comprehensive images than CT scans. The diagnosis may be determined with an extremely high degree of accuracy when both the look and location are usual. However, in other cases, the appearances are uncommon, necessitating careful interpretation in order to determine the proper preoperative diagnosis. Meningiomas' T2-weighted imaging signal intensity corresponds with their histological subtypes. MRI offers excellent contrast definition, soft tissue characterization, and multiplanar reconstructions, making it the gold standard method for meningioma diagnosis and assessment [11] (**Figure 3**). The correlation between DWI and tumor grade is still debatable because no clear-cut statistical relationship between ADC values and tumoral behavior has yet been established. DWI has also been used to depict

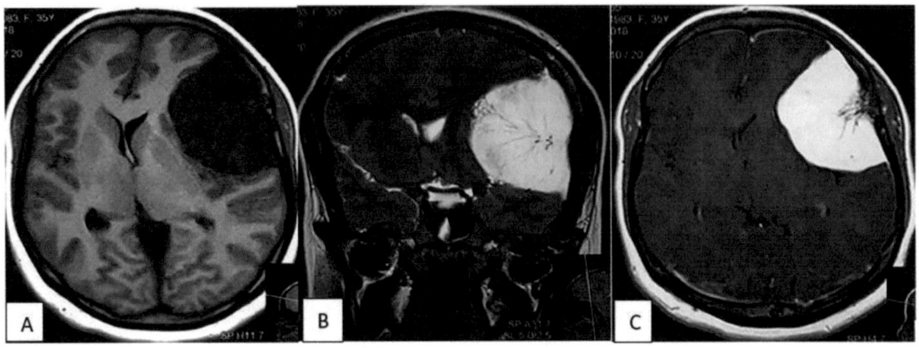

Figure 3.
A lady of 35 year-old with no history of prior radiation, presented with intermittent dull aching localized headache for years. MRI of brain, T1-weighted axial (A) section demonstrated a predominantly hypointense extra-axial dural based mass measuring about 6×5 cm located along the lesser wing of the sphenoid bone. The mass became hyperintense in T2-weighted image with numerous intrinsic flow voids (B). After administration of contrast, there was intense homogenous contrast enhancement (C). Mass effect was evidenced by flattening of the underlying sulci and gyri, compression of the lateral ventricle and midline shifting. However, histopathology demonstrated Chordoid meningioma (WHO grade-II).

higher-grade meningiomas with increased cellularity, which show reduced values on corresponding apparent diffusion coefficient (ADC) maps [31–33]. Unenhanced and contrast-enhanced MR angiography are superior at identifying intra-tumoral dysplastic vasculature. While unenhanced phase-contrast MR venogram (and also black-blood MR imaging) has been shown to be a valid tool in detecting sinus invasion, MR venogram is often employed to evaluate venous sinuses invasion thrombosis or occlusion. For both diagnosis and follow-up, MRI of the spine is the preferred modality; the features are comparable to intracranial meningiomas [28–30].

4.4 Cerebral angiogram

Cerebral angiography reveals the arteries and veins in the brain with specific relationships with the tumor. After a specific dye known as a contrast medium is injected into the major arteries of the brain, CT scans are obtained. An angiography may be necessary to plan surgery because meningioma can obstruct or invade the venous sinuses or vital veins that drain blood from the brain. Additionally, the angiography might show any aberrant arteries that may be feeding the tumor (**Figure 4**). Sometimes, Digital subtraction angiography plays a pivotal role for pre-operative documentation of feeding arteries, involvement of veins, and to assess the extent of cross circulation. Beside this, intraoperative bleeding can be minimized by injecting sclerosing agents into feeding arteries in the same sitting [19].

4.5 Advanced techniques: Possible applications

Conventional MRI often performs well for diagnostic reasons, although it can be exceedingly difficult to differentiate between extra-axial dural-based masses or between various meningioma subtypes. The application of sophisticated imaging techniques can improve tissue characterisation, the identification of key characteristics for surgical planning, and the discovery of prognostic biomarkers.

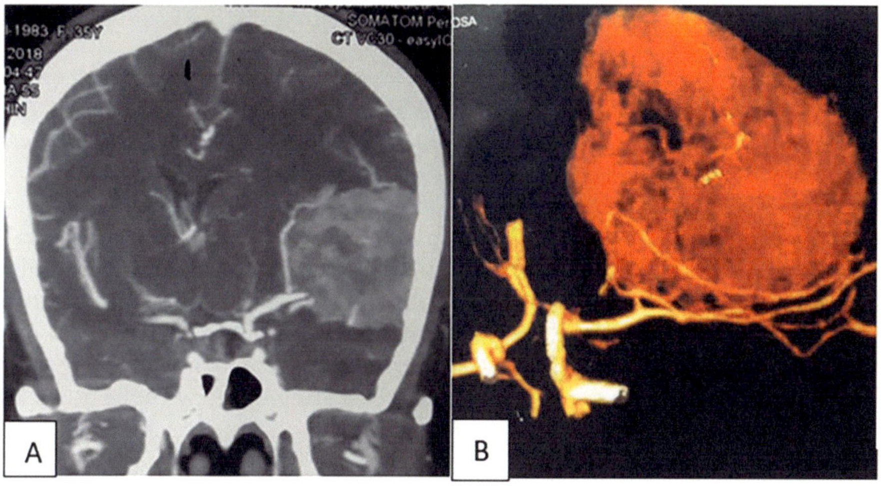

Figure 4.
CT angiogram of cerebral vessels (A) with 3D reconstruction arteriogram (B) demonstrated compression and displacement of M2 and M3 segments of left middle cerebral artery (MCA). This highly vascularized grade-II meningioma was feeded by the branches from M3 and M4 segments of MCA.

4.5.1 Spectroscopy

Spectroscopy is an MRI method used to determine the concentration of metabolites in an area of interest. Conversely, increased alanine has been shown to be unique for meningioma but can be challenging to detect. Meningiomas have high choline and reduced N-acetylaspartate as well as decreased creatinine, a metabolic profile common to other neoplastic processes. Meningiomas have been shown to have an enhanced metabolite peak at 3.8 parts per million, which helps to distinguish them from high-grade gliomas and intracranial metastases. It has been shown that MR spectroscopy cannot distinguish between atypical and normal meningiomas [34–37].

4.5.2 Perfusion imaging

The dynamic susceptibility contrast (DSC) technique and the dynamic contrast enhancement (DCE) approach, both of which call for the injection of intravenous gadolinium, as well as arterial spin labeling, are methods used in MR perfusion to measure blood flow in tissues. When making a differential diagnosis, MR perfusion can be particularly helpful in separating meningiomas from dural-based metastases and from high-grade gliomas that have invaded the dura mater. However, hypervascular metastases, such as those from melanoma, renal carcinoma, or Merkel cell carcinoma, cannot be distinguished by MR perfusion. Meningioma and dural metastases from diverse sources (breast, colon, and prostate) may be distinguished by MR perfusion (increased cerebral blood volume) [38, 39].

A primary glial neoplastic process may be distinguished from intracranial metastases and meningiomas via the analysis of the time-intensity curve. Meningioma vascularity appears to be significantly correlated with cerebral blood flow (CBF) values, and more recently, a significant correlation between CBV and VEGF expression has also been shown, raising the possibility of using perfusion MR to predict resistance to conventional treatment and potential responsiveness to anti-angiogenic therapies [40, 41].

Although peritumoral rCBV often exhibits lower values in meningiomas, probably because of peritumoral vasogenic edema, its values are greater in the case of anaplastic meningiomas (WHO Grade III) compared to the other forms. Similarly, reduced peritumoral CBF can be detected by CT perfusion, which may indicate ischemic tissue that can be salvaged following meningioma excision [42, 43].

By measuring perfusion without the confusing impact of permeability, arterial spine labeling offers the benefit of perhaps enabling the distinction between WHO Grade I and WHO Grades II and III cerebral meningiomas. Vascular permeability was directly measured using the DCE technique and had a role in the grading of meningiomas; atypical meningiomas had greater Ktrans values than benign meningiomas. Additionally, several meningioma subtypes can be distinguished with the use of MR perfusion. In comparison to meningothelial, fibrous, or anaplastic subtypes, angiomatous meningioma has shown increased tumor rCBV [43, 44].

4.5.3 Diffusion tensor imaging

Diffusion tensor imaging (DTI) has been used to distinguish between various meningioma grades due to the ability to measure the amount and directionality of water diffusion. Despite the fact that high-grade meningiomas often have lower ADC values than low-grade ones, there have been some disputed findings, particularly for the other DTI metrics. In terms of predicting preoperative consistency, DTI has demonstrated considerable possibilities. The majority of research have found that hard meningiomas had greater fractional anisotropy (FA) values than soft ones, with a few exceptions. Meningioma consistency has also been found to be predicted by signal intensity on FA and mean diffusivity maps [45–47]. Tractography, derived from DTI data, may give additional information for treatment planning of skull base meningiomas [48].

4.5.4 MR elastography

A promising new method called MR elastography (MRe) may be able to determine the consistency of a tumor and how it interacts with nearby structures. By analyzing the share wave passage through that specific tissue, it offers a measurement of the stiffness of the tissue. A substantial association between the MRe measures and the intraoperative qualitative evaluation of tumor consistency has been shown in recent investigations [36].

4.5.5 Molecular imaging

Due to strong physiological FDG uptake in the cerebral cortex and FDG buildup in inflammatory processes, the most common molecular imaging method in the area of oncology is (18F-FDG)-PET, which employs a glucose analog to identify metabolically active cells. There is no link between FDG uptake and WHO grading, MIB-1 labeling index, or tumor doubling time, despite certain studies showing its capacity to identify benign meningioma from atypical/malignant ones and to separate recurrent/growing meningiomas from static ones [48].

On the other hand, due to the enhanced expression of SSTR II in meningiomas compared to the relatively low expression in bone and brain tissue, a strong meningioma-to-background contrast can be achieved utilizing radiolabeled somatostatin receptors II (SSTR II) ligands. When compared to contrast-enhanced MRI, PET using gallium-68-labeled SSTR-ligands, such as 68Ga-DOTATOC (DOTA-(Tyr3)-octreotid) and 68Ga DOTATATE (DOTA-DPhe1-Tyr3-octreotate), has shown a better sensitivity in identifying meningiomas. When researching optic sheath meningioma, for example, SSTR-PET is helpful for differential diagnosis. Additionally, this method enables the precise delineation of meningioma extent, which is crucial for treatment planning but difficult in cases of complex localization (skull base, orbit, falx cerebri, sagittal, and cavernous sinuses), trans-osseous growth, or in cases of meningiomas that have already received treatment, when MR contrast results are constrained [36, 49–52].

Additionally, SSTR-PET may distinguish between live tumor and scar tissue using a semi-quantitative data analysis since SSTR II expression as determined by immunostaining and semi-quantitative uptake values (SUV) have a strong correlation. Additionally, SSTR-PET may be used if MRI results are unclear since it has been shown to be more accurate at locating residual meningioma. The RANO-PET workgroup has put out an evidence-based recommendation for the use of molecular imaging in meningiomas, even if SSTR II imaging's usefulness still needs to be further validated [53–55].

4.5.6 Future directions

Radiomics is a young branch of study that analyzes medical pictures and extracts several aspects from them. Following lesion segmentation, two types of features—semantic and agnostic—can be retrieved from the region of interest. Semantic characteristics, such as form, position, etc., are frequently employed in radiology to characterize a lesion in detail, but in the discipline of radiomics, they are quantified with computer aid. Because artificial intelligence is better at handling this volume of data than traditional statistics, it may be used with radiology. Artificial intelligence uses algorithms to let computers learn directly from the data and make predictions on unknown datasets [56, 57].

Radiomics and artificial intelligence have showed potential in the study of meningiomas for preoperative assessment, recurrence and outcome prediction, and radiation therapy planning. Planning and monitoring of therapy also greatly benefit from volumetric evaluation of meningiomas. The ability to predict local failure and overall survival in these patients using preoperative radiologic and radiomic characteristics such apparent diffusion coefficient and sphericity has shown to be successful. With promising findings (accuracy 90%), MR radiomics has also been used to predict early progression or recurrence, which define a subgroup of skull base meningiomas. In order to enhance the texture-based distinction of tumor from edema and to distinguish vasogenic from tumor infiltration edema, radiomics has shown effective in the determination of radiation target volume, which constitutes a crucial step in treatment planning [58, 59].

5. Management

Surgery with the aim of full excision is the traditional first-line therapy for all MNs. The recurrence rate for high grade meningiomas is considerable; up to 60% of tumors may return after 15 years following total excision. Due to a lack of available data, there are currently no recognized standard effective therapies [60, 61]. Depending on the tumor grade and the degree of tumor excision as determined by Simpson, current recommendations call for progressive treatment regimens. Treatment and follow-up based on the most recent EANO is recommended widely. For grade I tumors (Simpson grades I–III) that can be completely removed, surveillance is advised. Stereotactic radiosurgery is the adjuvant of choice when complete resection is not possible [62, 63].

The ongoing ROAM/EORTC 1308 experiment is testing whether Simpson grade I resected atypical tumors should be treated with radiation or observation. The recommended follow-up schedule is six months apart for the first five years, then yearly. Given their severe clinical history, Grade III cancers necessitate major surgery and adjuvant radiation. No matter how extensive the surgery, fractionated radiation is recommended (recommendation level B). Anaplastic meningiomas should be followed up with every three to six months. Meningioma metastasis is uncommon, even in WHO grade III malignancies (**Figure 5**) [64, 65].

5.1 Surgical management

The development of endoscopic transsphenoidal methods for skull base meningiomas has led to a recent progression in surgical procedures during the past few decades.

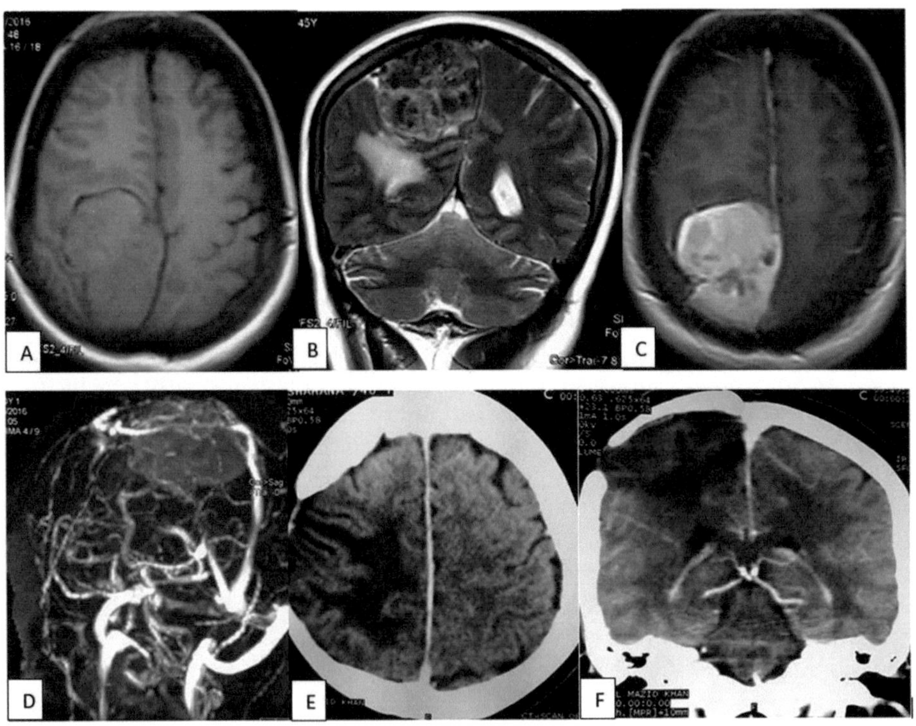

Figure 5.
A 45 year-old lady presented with progressive left sided hemiparesis for 2 years and convulsion for several episodes for the same duration. Pre-operative MRI of brain demonstrated a fairly large (6×5×4.5 cm) lobulated T1 weighted isointense (A), T2 weighted heterogeneously hypointense mass in the right parietal parasagittal location with moderate perilesional edema. The mass showed avid contrast enhancement after administration of the gadolinium (C). Mass effect was evidenced by compression of underlying sulci, lateral ventricle and gross midline shifting (8 mm). Magnetic resonance Venogram demonstrated filling defect at middle part of SSS with development of multiple collaterals (D). Follow up CT scan of brain after 5 years demonstrated no evidence of recurrence with encephalomalachic changes (E, F).

Although it was quite popular, its usage is now in decline because cerebrospinal fluid leaking could result in serious local and neurological consequences [66, 67].

Total removal is not usually feasible due to the tumor's location, infiltration of nearby tissues, and brain parenchyma. Regardless of the histological grade, post-operative Simpson grading based on the surgeon's assessment grades removal from grade 1 (complete) to 5 (simple biopsy) and enables prediction of symptomatic recurrence at 10 years from 10% to 100%. Since it was first reported in 1957, this conclusion has drawn criticism from a number of scientists, particularly given the lack of a systematic postoperative MRI. It has been established that, for grade II meningiomas, patients who undergo Simpson 1 resection had a longer overall and progression-free survival (**Figure 6**) [60, 68].

For grade III meningiomas selectively, the progression-free survival at 5 years is 28% after gross total resection alone, versus 0% after subtotal removal alone. Although the results all tend to favor gross total resection, this goal should not affect the patients' immediate neurological status, and combined strategies could be used to maximize progression-free survival while reducing the neurological risks [69, 70].

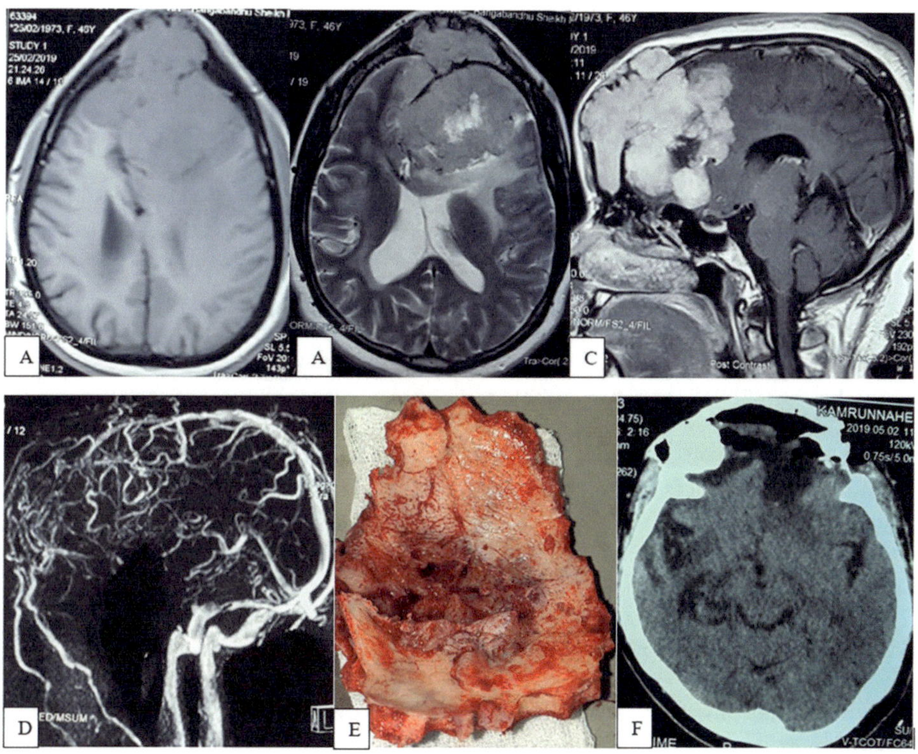

Figure 6.
A 46year-old lady, known case of papillary carcinoma of thyroid, presented with progressive enlargement of palpable hard mass in the frontal region for 2 years and convulsion for several episodes for the same duration. Pre-operative MRI of brain demonstrated a fairly large (7×6×5.5 cm) irregular T1WI iso to hypointense (A) and mixed intensity (B) mass present in both frontal region, having extra and intradural extension and invasion of the brain parenchyma. Mass effect was evident by moderate perilesional edema, compression of ventricles and gross midline shifting. After administration of contrast, there was heterogenous contrast enhancement with central non enhancing necrosed area (C). Magnetic resonance Venogram demonstrated obliteration of the anterior 1/3rd of SSS with development of multiple collaterals (D). Intraoperative photograph showed evidence of bone infiltration as well as osteolysis (E). Follow up CT scan of brain after 6 months demonstrated no evidence of recurrence (F).

Surgical resection is typically the first-line treatment for high-grade meningiomas when the tumor is in an accessible location, and the extent of surgical resection is an important prognostic factor for progression-free and overall survival (OS), with gross tumor resection (GTR) defined as Simpson grade 1–3 and subtotal tumor resection (STR) classified as Simpson grade 4 and 5. However, rates of recurrence are high, especially with STR, and radiotherapy may significantly decrease this risk. For the purposes of this review, we will exclusively focus on the role of RT for high-grade meningiomas. Interstitial brachytherapy can be an effective adjunct to surgical resection and external beam radiotherapy, especially for aggressive, recurrent, and/or large meningiomas, but is associated with high complication rates [71–73].

5.2 Radiation therapy

Radiation therapy has emerged as the first-line treatment for some meningiomas, particularly skull base lesions surrounding the vascular and nerve structures like the optic nerve sheath or the cavernous sinus. Surgery still holds a significant position because it can alleviate the tumor mass effect and establish a histological diagnosis. If imaging results are usual and surgery is not an option, radiation therapy alone may be suggested. These findings, combined with radiation-induced damage, highlight the importance of these therapies for untreatable cancers less than 3 cm. Stereotactic radiotherapy for tiny tumors has few side effects, however there have been occurrences of radionecrosis, and pituitary function must be monitored following skull base irradiation [74–78].

5.3 Targeted therapy

Meningiomas exhibit a modest mutation rate, and there are not many known possible molecular targets. In high-grade MN (80% of cases), NF2 is commonly changed compared to low-grade MN (40%). The majority of the genomic and regulatory changes that have been identified in high grade MN take place in the wake of NF2 protein disruption. Furthermore, the mTOR signaling cascade is one of the primary routes connected to NF2. Natural NF2 functions as a repressor of mTORC1 and mTORC2, and when it is altered, this pathway is uncontrollably activated. This has led to the identification of mTOR and several of its downstream and upstream effectors as potential targets. Research is also being done on other pathways controlled by receptor tyrosine kinases as EGFR, PDGFR, and VEGFR (angiogenesis) [79, 80].

5.4 Adjuvant treatment: Radiotherapy indications

Meningiomas of grades II and III are aggressive tumors that have greater recurrence rates. Adjuvant radiation treatment of the tumor zone could be useful for these cancers even after gross complete resection [68, 81–83]. Based on the grade, size, and location of the tumor, the best form of radiation therapy must be chosen. In the event of a small tumor, stereotactic radiation in a single or series of doses is advised. External beam irradiation is the go-to treatment option for recurring, many, or large lesions, with doses up to 70 Gy for grade II-III meningiomas, whether using 3D conformal radiotherapy or intensity-modulated radiation therapy with or without tomotherapy. Additionally helpful, proton radiation can be utilized in conjunction with photon radiotherapy [84, 85]. Tumor recurrence less likely (2%) with Stereotactic Radiotherapy compared to 12% for surgical treatment [86].

For grade III tumors, it is established that adjuvant radiation improves long-term control and overall survival, even after total gross removal. In contrast, there is conflicting evidence for its role in grade II meningiomas. It has been shown that radiation therapy improves overall and progression-free survival when the tumor has been sub-totally removed, but not after total gross resection. Indeed, reported side-effects of radiotherapy and radiosurgery are usually mild but there is also evidence that radiation increases the risk of malignant transformation [70, 87–89].

After stereotactic radiosurgery for brain malignancies, radiation necrosis is a known consequence that affects 15% of patients. No matter the type of tumor in patients having radiosurgery, large diameter and high doses were reliable independent risk factors that led to more often occurring radiation necroses. Due to the increased risk of developing radiation necrosis, other therapeutic approaches may be taken into account in lesions with a large volume and an anticipated high radiation dosage [90]. Grade III anaplastic meningiomas are malignant (cancerous) and associated with cranial radiation exposure. People with neurofibromatosis type 2 are also at increased risk for developing meningiomas [91]. Radiation exposure during childhood significantly increases the risk of second malignancy as compared to older population. Malignant transformation can occur after radiation treatment in around 2% people due to insufficient killing of cells and some of the surviving cells acquire mutations in genes, such as TP53, that can transform a benign tumour into a malignant one [92, 93].

5.5 Chemotherapy and ongoing clinical trials

In the context of meningioma, chemotherapy is regarded as experimental since there is insufficient data on most drugs or just conflicting findings. As a result, their usage is only advised in anaplastic situations and is preferred within clinical studies. With SMO- and NF2-mutant meningiomas, respectively, targeted therapy studies for SMO and FAK inhibitors are currently being conducted. Only this trial stratifies individuals according to tumor genotype and considers potential driver mutations. Regardless of molecular background, the mTOR inhibitor vistusertib is being examined in phase II research; nonetheless, there may be a benefit to mTOR inhibition in cancers that have PI3K or AKT mutations. Bevacizumab, a number of immune checkpoint inhibitors, and tumor-treating technologies are also being studied [94, 95].

The European Organization for Research and Treatment of Cancer (EORTC) oversaw a phase II research that compared adjuvant postoperative radiation treatment with observation in patients with newly diagnosed grade II or grade III meningiomas between 2008 and 2013. (NCT00626730, Switzerland). Due to significant protocol violations and inclusion issues, this experiment had to be stopped. The second study, the American RTOG 0539 (NCT00895622) trial, involved 244 patients and is still underway. It focuses on observation for low-risk meningiomas and radiation for intermediate and high-risk meningiomas. After three years, preliminary results indicate that patients with totally resected grade II and recurring grade I who received postoperative radiation had a 96% survival rate without progression [68, 96]. A phase II randomized controlled study (ROAM/EORTC-1308) comparing radiation (60 Gy in 30 fractions) with observation after surgical excision of an atypical meningioma was launched in the UK in 2015. Distinct facilities have different treatment decisions in clinical practice. In the United Kingdom, Germany, and France, radiation is administered to patients after subtotal grade II removal by 59%, 74%, and 80% of neurosurgeons, respectively, whereas following grade II gross complete resection by 45-60% of neurosurgeons, immediate adjuvant radiotherapy is recommended [64, 97, 98].

6. Challenges in meningioma management

6.1 Surgical challenges

Due to poor localization of otherwise benign tumors, such as skull base meningiomas, or invasion of healthy brain, which indicates malignancy in the first place, surgery might be challenging. While the first group's neurosurgical procedure improves, anaplastic tumors require adjuvant treatment. It is suggested to employ advanced preoperative and postoperative imaging methods for tumor definition, determining residual tumor mass, and identifying bone or brain invasion [53, 99].

6.2 Radiotherapeutic challenges

Patients with poor clinical outcomes, tumors with complicated morphologies, or cancers in challenging sites are frequently evaluated for primary or adjuvant radiation. Planning for radiation is likewise impacted by all of these variables. It is essential to precisely assess tumor size in order to treat the tumor mass as a whole while sparing normal brain tissue and important systems like the optic nerve. PET imaging employing SSTR ligands (current data indicate 68Ga-DOTATOC) has shown to be helpful in planning the target volume in skull base cancers for stereotactic or intensity-modulated radiotherapy, and may help with both volume definition and dose sparing [100–102].

6.3 Peritumoral edema

Peritumoral edema is a symptom of meningiomas in 40–66% of cases. Particularly for the histological subtype of secretory meningiomas, which are non-NF2 tumors distinguished by the co-occurrence of KLF4 and TRAF7 mutations, life-threatening episodes of peritumoral edema have been observed. Steroids, particularly dexamethasone, are the mainstay of treatment for peritumoral edema, however antiangiogenic therapy may be used in rare circumstances where (long-term) adverse effects or inadequate effectiveness are present. Critical cases, particularly those with secretory meningioma, may necessitate treatment in an intensive care unit with sedation, mechanical breathing, and intracranial pressure monitoring [103–105].

6.4 Meningioma en plaque

En plaque meningiomas are tumors that develop along the dura in a pattern resembling a sheet. They frequently include the orbit, but mostly occur at the sphenoid wing. They often have a noticeable hyperostosis at presentation. With extensive complete resection occurring in 56–83% of cases, their surgical removal is difficult. Therefore, a combination primary strategy with adjuvant radiosurgery may be preferable over extensive resection [106, 107].

6.5 Optic nerve sheath meningioma

1-2% of meningiomas are optic nerve sheath meningiomas (ONSM). When MRI results are ambiguous, 68Ga-DOTATATE-PET molecular imaging should be considered to rule out other possible diagnoses (e.g. lymphoma, optic neuritis, metastasis). OnSM, in particular intracanalicular ONSM, might resemble ocular neuritis. Most of the time, surgery is not an option, particularly when the tumor and the optic nerve share the same blood supply. The suggested treatment of preference is stereotactic fractionated radiation [50, 108, 109].

6.6 Multiple meningiomas

The majority of multiple meningiomas are associated with neurofibromatosis type 2, which is identified by heterozygous NF2 germline inactivation. In NF2, intracranial meningiomas frequently involve numerous tumors, with a median of three tumors. Even though the majority of the evidence predates the difference between sporadic NF2-mutated meningiomas and non-NF2 sporadic cases, meningiomas with neurofibromatosis type 2 are more likely to be atypical or anaplastic than sporadic instances. Young age (30 years) at the time of the initial meningioma presentation should raise the possibility of a germline mutation and may call for molecular testing. Patients with suspected or confirmed neurofibromatosis should be provided genetic counseling due to the disease's high penetrance and potential impact on family planning. Other genetic predispositions to meningioma have been identified in addition to neurofibromatosis type 2. Clear cell meningioma of the spinal cord and intracranially are predisposed by SMARCE1 mutations [25, 110–112].

7. Future research

In bigger trials that stratify between grade-2 and grade-3 meningioma, combination regimens such as ICI with targeted treatments or new therapeutics targeting immunosuppressive myeloid cells will be evaluated. Future investigations that stratify patients based on previous systemic therapies are necessary given the evidence that chemotherapy sensitizes solid tumors to ICI by increasing dendritic-cell activation and decreasing regulatory T-cell and myeloid-derived suppressor-cell responses [113, 114].

The most often used and researched adjuvant treatment for meningiomas is radiotherapy, however there are still a lot of unanswered problems. The majority of experts think that RT has no place in treating WHO grade I cancers, unless they are symptomatic primary or recurring tumors that cannot be surgically removed. Numerous phase II and randomized controlled trials are attempting to shed light on the function of radiation in WHO grade II GTR tumors, despite the fact that this involvement has not yet been completely understood. In a phase II trial (RTOG 0539), it was found that the intermediate risk group's 3-year progression-free survival (PFS) and 3-year overall survival (OS) rates were 98.3% and 96%, respectively, for newly diagnosed WHO grade II GTR (69.2%) and recurrent WHO grade I with any resection extent (30.8%), respectively (OS). Using adjuvant RT at a high dosage of 60 Gy, WHO grade II GTR meningiomas were shown to have an 88.7% 3-year PFS and a 98.2% 3-year OS in another phase II study. Currently, grade II GTR meningiomas receiving adjuvant RT are the subject of the randomized controlled trials ns20191111, NRG-BN003, and the ROAM/EORTC-1308 study, which compares at least 5-year OS and PFS [115–117].

There are clinical trials investigating pathway-directed therapies such as MEK pathway inhibitor, selumetinib (SEL-TH-1601, NCT03095248), CDK-p16-Rb pathway inhibitor, ribociclib (LEE-011, NCT02933736), and mTOR-pathway inhibitor, everolimus (NCT01880749 and NCT01419639), and vistusertib (AZD2014, NCT03071874). The ALTREM clinical trial is investigating the co-administration of phosphoinositide 3-kinase α (PI3Kα) specific inhibitor, alpelisib, and the MEK inhibitor, trametinib (NCT03631953). The phase II CEVOREM trial demonstrated that the coadministration of everolimus and octreotide (SSTR2A agonist) had a 6-month PFS of 55%, and 6- and 12-month OS of 90% and 75%, respectively. The CEVOREM trial showed more than a 50% decrease in the growth rate at 3 months in 78% of tumors and the median tumor growth rate over 3 months decreased from 16.6% before treatment to 0.02% at 3 months and 0.48% at 6 months after treatment. The NCT02831257 trial demonstrated that patients treated with AZD2014 had a 6-month PFS of 88.9 and 5.6% (1/18) of patients experienced a decrease in tumor volume of at least 20% compared to baseline [118].

There are also clinical trials investigating immunotherapy agents such as checkpoint inhibitors PD-1 antagonist, nivolumab (NCT02648997, NCT03173950, and NCT03604978 in combination with ipilimumab), another PD-1 antagonist, pembrolizumab (NCT03279692, NCT03016091, and NCT04659811 in combination with stereotactic radiosurgery), and PD-L1 antagonist, avelumab (NCT03267836 in combination with proton radiotherapy).

The discovery of innovative treatments to combat meningioma is being driven by growing biological understanding of this disease. Additionally, prognostication and trial stratification may benefit from genomic and epigenetic characteristics. Meningioma quantitative radiomic characterizations that are still under development may offer more tumor stratification tools and early tumor behavior prediction at the time of initial diagnosis. Finally, taking into account the multidrug-resistant meningioma's cellular heterogeneity, which cancer stem cells bestow, opens a parallel pathway for therapeutic discoveries.

8. Conclusion

Meningioma development has been linked to particular molecular changes and ionizing radiation. In many cases of high-grade meningioma, current treatment protocols using surgery and/or radiation are sufficient for tumor management. Prospective research is required to confirm potential molecular prognostic indicators and detect negative clinical trends early on. An integrated diagnostic approach can increase the precision of recurrence and outcome forecasting and assist in the development of customized treatment programs for particular patients. Despite the discovery of important mutations and signaling pathways, targeted systemic treatments are still lacking, despite the fact that several clinical studies are now being conducted.

Conflict of interest

The author of the chapter declares that, there was no conflict of interest.

Author details

Nazmin Ahmed
Department of Neurosurgery, Ibrahim Cardiac Hospital and Research Institute (A Centre for Cardiovascular, Neuroscience and Organ Transplant Units), Shahbag, Dhaka, Bangladesh

*Address all correspondence to: nazmin.bsmmu@gmail.com

References

[1] Louis DN, Ohgaki H, Wiestler OD, Cavenee WK, Burger PC, Jouvet A, et al. The 2007 WHO classification of tumours of the central nervous system. Acta Neuropathologica. 2007;**114**:97-109. DOI: 10.1007/s00401-007-0243-4

[2] Huntoon K, Toland AMS, Dahiya S. Meningioma: A review of Clinicopathological and molecular aspects. Frontiers in Oncology. 2020;**10**:579-599. DOI: 10.3389/fonc.2020.579599

[3] Ostrom QT, Cioffi G, Gittleman H, Patil N, Waite K, Kruchko C, et al. CBTRUS statistical report: Primary brain and other central nervous system tumors diagnosed in the United States in 2012-2016. Journal of Neuro-Oncology. 2019;**21**:V1-V100. DOI: 10.1093/neuonc/noz150

[4] Piccardo A, Albert NL, Borgwardt L, Fahey FH, Hargrave D, Galldiks N, et al. Joint EANM/SIOPE/RAPNO practice guidelines/SNMMI procedure standards for imaging of paediatric gliomas using PET with radiolabelled amino acids and [18F]FDG: Version 1.0. European Journal of Nuclear Medicine and Molecular Imaging. 2022. DOI: 10.1007/s00259-022-05817-6

[5] Chukwueke UN, Wen PY. Use of the response assessment in neuro-oncology (RANO) criteria in clinical trials and clinical practice. CNS Oncology. 2019;**8**:CNS28. DOI: 10.2217/cns-2018-0007

[6] Porcu M, Solinas C, Garofalo P, de Azambuja E, Scartozzi M, Willard-Gallo K, et al. Radiological evaluation of response to immunotherapy in brain tumors: Where are we now and where are we going? Critical Reviews in Oncology/Hematology. 2018;**126**:135-144. DOI: 10.1016/j.critrevonc.2018.03.026

[7] Korhonen K, Salminen T, Raitanen J, Auvinen A, Isola J, Haapasalo H. Female predominance in meningiomas can not be explained by differences in progesterone, estrogen, or androgen receptor expression. Journal of Neuro-Oncology. 2006;**80**:1-7. DOI: 10.1007/s11060-006-9146-9

[8] Kshettry V, Ostrom Q, Kruchko C, Al-Mefty O, Barnett G, Barnholtz-Sloan J. Descriptive epidemiology of World Health Organization grades II and III intracranial Meningiomas in the United States. Journal of Neurological Surgery. Part B Skull Base. 2015;**76**. DOI: 10.1055/s-0035-1546468

[9] Meningioma Diagnosis and Treatment. National Cancer Institute. 2021. Available from: https://www.cancer.gov/rare-brain-spine-tumor/tumors/meningioma

[10] Esteban Garcia-Robledo J, Ordóñez-Reyes C, Ruiz-Patiño A, Muñoz Á, Arrieta O, Jiménez E, et al. High grade meningiomas: Current therapy based on tumor biology. 2022. DOI: 10.5772/intechopen.100432

[11] Varlotto JM, Flickinger J, Pavelic MT, Specht CS, Sheehan JM, Timek DT, et al. Distinguishing grade I meningioma from higher grade meningiomas without biopsy. Oncotarget. 2015;**6**:38421-38428. DOI: 10.18632/oncotarget.5376

[12] Brastianos PK, Horowitz PM, Santagata S, Jones RT, Mckenna A, Getz G, et al. Genomic sequencing of meningiomas identifies oncogenic SMO

and AKT1 mutations. Nature Genetics. 2013;**45**:285-289. DOI: 10.1038/ng.2526

[13] Clark VE, Erson-Omay EZ, Serin A, Yin J, Cotney J, Özduman K, et al. Genomic analysis of non-NF2 meningiomas reveals mutations in TRAF7, KLF4, AKT1, and SMO. Science. 2013;**339**:1077-1080

[14] Proctor DT, Ramachandran S, Lama S, Sutherland GR. Towards molecular classification of meningioma: Evolving treatment and diagnostic paradigms. World Neurosurgery. 2018;**119**:366-373. DOI: 10.1016/j.wneu.2018.08.019

[15] Galani V, Lampri E, Varouktsi A, Alexiou G, Mitselou A, Kyritsis AP. Genetic and epigenetic alterations in meningiomas. Clinical Neurology and Neurosurgery. 2017;**158**:119-125. DOI: 10.1016/j.clineuro.2017.05.002

[16] Pereira BJA, Oba-Shinjo SM, de Almeida AN, Marie SKN. Molecular alterations in meningiomas: Literature review. Clinical Neurology and Neurosurgery. 2019;**176**:89-96. DOI: 10.1016/j.clineuro.2018.12.004

[17] Zack TI, Schumacher SE, Carter SL, Cherniack AD, Saksena G, Tabak B, et al. Pan-cancer patterns of somatic copy number alteration. Nature Genetics. 2013;**45**:1134-1140. DOI: 10.1038/ng.2760

[18] Bi WL, Greenwald NF, Abedalthagafi M, Wala J, Gibson WJ, Agarwalla PK, et al. Genomic landscape of high-grade meningiomas. NPJ Genomic Medicine. 2017;**2**:14-17. DOI: 10.1038/s41525-017-0014-7

[19] Ogasawara C, Philbrick BD, Adamson DC. Meningioma: A review of epidemiology, pathology, diagnosis, treatment, and future directions. Biomedicine. 2021;**9**. DOI: 10.3390/biomedicines9030319

[20] Chamoun R, Krisht KM, Couldwell WT. Incidental meningiomas. Neurosurgical Focus. 2011;**31**:112-120. DOI: 10.3171/2011.9.FOCUS11220

[21] Rubin G, Herscovici Z, Laviv Y, Jackson S, Rappaport ZH. Outcome of untreated meningiomas. The Israel Medical Association Journal. 2011;**13**:157-160

[22] Black PM, Morokoff AP, Zauberman J. Surgery for extra-axial tumors of the cerebral convexity and midline. Neurosurgery. 2008;**62**. DOI: 10.1227/01.NEU.0000318093.43855.2A

[23] Oya S, Kim SH, Sade B, Lee JH. The natural history of intracranial meningiomas. Journal of Neurosurgery. 2011;**114**:1250-1256

[24] Dirks MS, Butman JA, Kim HJ, Wu T, Morgan K, Tran AP, et al. Long-term natural history of neurofibromatosis type 2-associated intracranial tumors: Clinical article. Journal of Neurosurgery. 2012;**117**:109-117. DOI: 10.3171/2012.3.JNS111649

[25] Goutagny S, Bah AB, Henin D, Parfait B, Grayeli AB, Sterkers O, et al. Long-term follow-up of 287 meningiomas in neurofibromatosis type 2 patients: Clinical, radiological, and molecular features. Journal of Neuro-Oncology. 2012;**14**:1090-1096. DOI: 10.1093/neuonc/nos129

[26] Kim KH, Kang SJ, Choi JW, Kong DS, Seol HJ, Nam DH, et al. Clinical and radiological outcomes of proactive gamma knife surgery for asymptomatic meningiomas compared with the natural course without intervention. Journal of Neurosurgery. 2019;**130**:1740-1749. DOI: 10.3171/2017.12.JNS171943

[27] Altaş M, Aras M, Bayaroğullari H, Karcioğlu M, Serarslan Y, Yilmaz N.

Giant calvarial meningioma which obliterated superior sagittal sinus: Case report, Ondokuz Mayis Univ. Tip Derg. Journal of Experimental and Clinical Medicine. 2012;**29**:225-228. DOI: 10.5835/jecm.omu.29.03.011

[28] Mariniello G, Malacario F, Dones F, Severino R, Ugga L, Russo C, et al. Sudden post-traumatic sciatica caused by a thoracic spinal meningioma. The Neuroradiology Journal. 2016;**29**:390-392. DOI: 10.1177/1971400916655479

[29] O'Leary S, Adams WM, Parrish RW, Mukonoweshuro W. Atypical imaging appearances of intracranial meningiomas. Clinical Radiology. 2007;**62**:10-17. DOI: 10.1016/j.crad.2006.09.009

[30] Mariniello G, Napoli M, Russo C, Briganti F, Giamundo A, Maiuri F, et al. MRI features of spinal solitary fibrous tumors: A report of two cases and literature review. The Neuroradiology Journal. 2012;**25**:610-616. DOI: 10.1177/197140091202500516

[31] Sanverdi SE, Ozgen B, Oguz KK, Mut M, Dolgun A, Soylemezoglu F, et al. Is diffusion-weighted imaging useful in grading and differentiating histopathological subtypes of meningiomas? European Journal of Radiology. 2012;**81**:2389-2395. DOI: 10.1016/j.ejrad.2011.06.031

[32] Tang Y, Dundamadappa SK, Thangasamy S, Flood T, Moser R, Smith T, et al. Correlation of apparent diffusion coefficient with Ki-67 proliferation index in grading meningioma. American Journal of Roentgenology. 2014;**202**:1303-1308. DOI: 10.2214/AJR.13.11637

[33] Watanabe Y, Yamasaki F, Kajiwara Y, Takayasu T, Nosaka R, Akiyama Y, et al. Preoperative histological grading of meningiomas using apparent diffusion coefficient at 3T MRI. European Journal of Radiology. 2013;**82**:658-663. DOI: 10.1016/j.ejrad.2012.11.037

[34] Zakhari N, Torres C, Castillo M, Nguyen TB. Uncommon cranial meningioma: Key imaging features on conventional and advanced imaging. Clinical Neuroradiology. 2017;**27**:135-144. DOI: 10.1007/s00062-017-0583-y

[35] Gajjar K, Heppenstall LD, Pang W, Ashton KM, Trevisan J, Patel II, et al. Diagnostic segregation of human brain tumours using Fourier-transform infrared and/or Raman spectroscopy coupled with discriminant analysis. Analytical Methods. 2013;**5**:89-102. DOI: 10.1039/c2ay25544h

[36] Shiroishi MS, Cen SY, Tamrazi B, D'Amore F, Lerner A, King KS, et al. Predicting meningioma consistency on preoperative neuroimaging studies. Neurosurgery Clinics of North America. 2016;**27**:145-154. DOI: 10.1016/j.nec.2015.11.007

[37] Tamrazi B, Shiroishi MS, Liu CSJ. Advanced imaging of intracranial Meningiomas. Neurosurgery Clinics of North America. 2016;**27**:137-143. DOI: 10.1016/j.nec.2015.11.004

[38] Kremer S, Grand S, Rémy C, Pasquier B, Benabid AL, Bracard S, et al. Contribution of dynamic contrast MR imaging to the differentiation between dural metastasis and meningioma. Neuroradiology. 2004;**46**:642-648. DOI: 10.1007/s00234-004-1194-2

[39] Newton AT, Pruthi S, Stokes AM, Skinner JT, Quarles CC. Improving perfusion measurement in DSC-MR imaging with multiecho information for arterial input function determination. American Journal of Neuroradiology.

2016;**37**:1237-1243. DOI: 10.3174/ajnr.A4700

[40] Hakyemez B, Erdogan C, Bolca N, Yildirim N, Gokalp G, Parlak M. Evaluation of different cerebral mass lesions by perfusion-weighted MR imaging. Journal of Magnetic Resonance Imaging. 2006;**24**:817-824. DOI: 10.1002/jmri.20707

[41] Kimura H, Takeuchi H, Koshimoto Y, Arishima H, Uematsu H, Kawamura Y, et al. Perfusion imaging of meningioma by using continuous arterial spin-labeling: Comparison with dynamic susceptibility-weighted contrast-enhanced MR images and histopathologic features. American Journal of Neuroradiology. 2006;**27**:85-93. DOI: 10.1016/s0098-1672(08)70493-4

[42] Sergides I, Hussain Z, Naik S, Good C, Miles K, Critchley G. Utilization of dynamic CT perfusion in the study of intracranial meningiomas and their surrounding tissue. Neurological Research. 2009;**31**:84-89. DOI: 10.1179/174313208X331563

[43] Zhang Q, Jia GJ, Bin Zhang G, Wang L, Wu Z, Jia W, et al. A logistic regression model for detecting the presence of malignant progression in atypical Meningiomas. World Neurosurgery. 2019;**126**:e392-e401. DOI: 10.1016/j.wneu.2019.02.062

[44] Qiao XJ, Kim HG, Wang DJJ, Salamon N, Linetsky M, Sepahdari A, et al. Application of arterial spin labeling perfusion MRI to differentiate benign from malignant intracranial meningiomas. European Journal of Radiology. 2017;**97**:31-36. DOI: 10.1016/j.ejrad.2017.10.005

[45] Ortega-Porcayo LA, Ballesteros-Zebadúa P, Marrufo-Meléndez OR, Ramírez-Andrade JJ, Barges-Coll J, Tecante A, et al. Prediction of mechanical properties and subjective consistency of meningiomas using T1-T2 assessment versus fractional anisotropy. World Neurosurgery. 2015;**84**:1691-1698. DOI: 10.1016/j.wneu.2015.07.018

[46] Santelli L, Ramondo G, Della Puppa A, Ermani M, Scienza R, D'Avella D, et al. Diffusion-weighted imaging does not predict histological grading in meningiomas. Acta Neurochirurgica. 2010;**152**:1315-1319. DOI: 10.1007/s00701-010-0657-y

[47] Wang S, Kim S, Zhang Y, Wang L, Lee EB, Syre P, et al. Determination of grade and subtype of meningiomas by using histogram analysis of diffusion-tensor imaging metrics. Radiology. 2012;**262**:584-592. DOI: 10.1148/radiol.11110576

[48] Huang RY, Bi WL, Griffith B, Kaufmann TJ, La Fougère C, Schmidt NO, et al. Imaging and diagnostic advances for intracranial meningiomas. Journal of Neuro-Oncology. 2019;**21**:I44-I61. DOI: 10.1093/neuonc/noy143

[49] Nowosielski M, Galldiks N, Iglseder S, Kickingereder P, Von Deimling A, Bendszus M, et al. Diagnostic challenges in meningioma. Journal of Neuro-Oncology. 2017;**19**:1588-1598. DOI: 10.1093/neuonc/nox101

[50] Klingenstein A, Haug AR, Miller C, Hintschich C. Ga-68-DOTA-TATE PET/CT for discrimination of tumors of the optic pathway. Orbit (London). 2015;**34**:16-22. DOI: 10.3109/01676830.2014.959185

[51] Afshar-Oromieh A, Giesel FL, Linhart HG, Haberkorn U, Haufe S, Combs SE, et al. Detection of cranial meningiomas: Comparison of

68Ga-DOTATOC PET/CT and contrast-enhanced MRI. European Journal of Nuclear Medicine and Molecular Imaging. 2012;**39**:1409-1415. DOI: 10.1007/s00259-012-2155-3

[52] Reimold M, la Fougere C. Molecular imaging in neurological diseases. Der Radiologe. 2016;**56**:580-586

[53] Galldiks N, Albert NL, Sommerauer M, Grosu AL, Ganswindt U, Law I, et al. PET imaging in patients with meningioma—Report of the RANO/PET group. Journal of Neuro-Oncology. 2017;**19**:1576-1587. DOI: 10.1093/neuonc/nox112

[54] Rachinger W, Stoecklein VM, Terpolilli NA, Haug AR, Ertl L, Pöschl J, et al. Increased 68Ga-DOTATATE uptake in PET imaging discriminates meningioma and tumor-free tissue. Journal of Nuclear Medicine. 2015;**56**:347-353. DOI: 10.2967/jnumed.114.149120

[55] Sommerauer M, Burkhardt JK, Frontzek K, Rushing E, Buck A, Krayenbuehl N, et al. 68Gallium-DOTATATE PET in meningioma: A reliable predictor of tumor growth rate? Journal of Neuro-Oncology. 2016;**18**:1021-1027. DOI: 10.1093/neuonc/now001

[56] Koçak B, Durmaz EŞ, Ateş E, Kılıçkesmez Ö. Radiomics with artificial intelligence: A practical guide for beginners. Diagnostic and Interventional Radiology. 2019;**25**:485-495. DOI: 10.5152/dir.2019.19321

[57] Gillies RJ, Kinahan PE, Hricak H. Radiomics: Images are more than pictures, they are data. Radiology. 2016;**278**:563-577. DOI: 10.1148/radiol.2015151169

[58] Zhang Y, Chen JH, Chen TY, Lim SW, Wu TC, Kuo YT, et al. Radiomics approach for prediction of recurrence in skull base meningiomas. Neuroradiology. 2019;**61**:1355-1364. DOI: 10.1007/s00234-019-02259-0

[59] Morin O, Chen WC, Nassiri F, Susko M, Magill ST, Vasudevan HN, et al. Integrated models incorporating radiologic and radiomic features predict meningioma grade, local failure, and overall survival. Neuro-Oncology Advances. 2019;**1**. DOI: 10.1093/noajnl/vdz011

[60] Apra C, Peyre M, Kalamarides M. Current treatment options for meningioma. Expert Review of Neurotherapeutics. 2018;**18**:241-249. DOI: 10.1080/14737175.2018.1429920

[61] Al-Rashed M, Foshay K, Abedalthagafi M. Recent advances in meningioma immunogenetics. Frontiers in Oncology. 2020;**9**:72-83. DOI: 10.3389/fonc.2019.01472

[62] Simpson D. The recurrence of intracranial meningiomas after surgical treatment. Journal of Neurology, Neurosurgery, and Psychiatry. 1957;**20**:22-39. DOI: 10.1136/jnnp.20.1.22

[63] Goldbrunner R, Minniti G, Preusser M, Jenkinson MD, Sallabanda K, Houdart E, et al. EANO guidelines for the diagnosis and treatment of meningiomas. The Lancet Oncology. 2016;**17**:e383-e391. DOI: 10.1016/S1470-2045(16)30321-7

[64] Jenkinson MD, Javadpour M, Haylock BJ, Young B, Gillard H, Vinten J, et al. The ROAM/EORTC-1308 trial: Radiation versus observation following surgical resection of atypical meningioma: Study protocol for a randomised controlled trial. Trials. 2015;**16**. DOI: 10.1186/s13063-015-1040-3. no pagination

[65] Kessler RA, Garzon-Muvdi T, Yang W, Weingart J, Olivi A, Huang J,

et al. Metastatic atypical and anaplastic meningioma: A case series and review of the literature. World Neurosurgery. 2017;**101**:47-56. DOI: 10.1016/j.wneu.2017.01.070

[66] Zada G, Başkaya MK, Shah MV. Introduction: Surgical management of skull base meningiomas. Neurosurgical Focus. 2017;**43**1-14. DOI: 10.3171/2017.10.FocusVid.Intro

[67] Muskens IS, Briceno V, Ouwehand TL, Castlen JP, Gormley WB, Aglio LS, et al. The endoscopic endonasal approach is not superior to the microscopic transcranial approach for anterior skull base meningiomas—A meta-analysis. Acta Neurochirurgica. 2018;**160**:59-75. DOI: 10.1007/s00701-017-3390-y

[68] Durand A, Labrousse F, Jouvet A, Bauchet L, Kalamaridès M, Menei P, et al. WHO grade II and III meningiomas: A study of prognostic factors. Journal of Neuro-Oncology. 2009;**95**:367-375. DOI: 10.1007/s11060-009-9934-0

[69] Sughrue ME, Kane AJ, Shangari G, Rutkowski MJ, McDermott MW, Berger MS, et al. The relevance of Simpson grade I and II resection in modern neurosurgical treatment of World Health Organization grade I meningiomas. Journal of Neurosurgery. 2010;**113**:1029-1035. DOI: 10.3171/2010.3.JNS091971

[70] Dziuk TW, Woo S, Butler EB, Thornby J, Grossman R, Dennis WS, et al. Malignant meningioma: An indication for initial aggressive surgery and adjuvant radiotherapy. Journal of Neuro-Oncology. 1998;**37**:177-188. DOI: 10.1023/A:1005853720926

[71] Ware ML, Larson DA, Sneed PK, Wara WW, McDermott MW, Kondziolka D, et al. Surgical resection and permanent brachytherapy for recurrent atypical and malignant meningioma. Neurosurgery. 2004;**54**:55-64. DOI: 10.1227/01.NEU.0000097199.26412.2A

[72] Gutin PH, Leibel SA, Hosobuchi Y, Crumley RL, Edwards MS, Wilson CB, et al. Brachytherapy of recurrent tumors of the skull base and spine with iodine-125 sources. Neurosurgery. 1987;**20**:938-945. DOI: 10.1097/00006123-198706000-00020

[73] Goldsmith BJ, Wara WM, Wilson CB, Larson DA. Postoperative irradiation for subtotally resected meningiomas. Journal of Neurosurgery. 1994;**80**:195-201

[74] Minniti G, Clarke E, Cavallo L, Osti MF, Esposito V, Cantore G, et al. Fractionated stereotactic conformal radiotherapy for large benign skull base meningiomas. Radiation Oncology. 2011;**6**:6-36. DOI: 10.1186/1748-717X-6-36

[75] Valery CA, Faillot M, Lamproglou I, Golmard JL, Jenny C, Peyre M, et al. Grade II meningiomas and gamma knife radiosurgery: Analysis of success and failure to improve treatment paradigm. Journal of Neurosurgery. 2016;**125**:89-96. DOI: 10.3171/2016.7.gks161521

[76] Cho M, Joo JD, Kim IA, Han JH, Oh CW, Kim CY. The role of adjuvant treatment in patients with high-grade meningioma. Journal of Korean Neurosurgical Association. 2017;**60**:527-533. DOI: 10.3340/jkns.2016.1111.009

[77] Patibandla MR, Lee C, Sheehan J. Stereotactic radiosurgery of central Skull Base Meningiomas—Volumetric evaluation and long-term outcomes. World Neurosurgery. 2017;**108**:176-184. DOI: 10.1016/j.wneu.2017.08.166

[78] Starke RM, Przybylowski CJ, Sugoto M, Fezeu F, Awad AJ, Ding D,

et al. Gamma knife radiosurgery of large skull base meningiomas. Journal of Neurosurgery. 2015;**122**:363-372. DOI: 10.3171/2014.10.JNS14198

[79] Dai J, Ma Y, Chu S, Le N, Cao J, Wang Y. Identification of key genes and pathways in meningioma by bioinformatics analysis. Oncology Letters. 2018;**15**:8245-8252. DOI: 10.3892/ol.2018.8376

[80] Everson RG, Hashimoto Y, Freeman JL, Hodges TR, Huse J, Zhou S, et al. Multiplatform profiling of meningioma provides molecular insight and prioritization of drug targets for rational clinical trial design. Journal of Neuro-Oncology. 2018;**139**:469-478. DOI: 10.1007/s11060-018-2891-8

[81] Walcott BP, Nahed BV, Brastianos PK, Loeffler JS. Radiation treatment for WHO grade II and III meningiomas. Frontiers in Oncology. 2013;**3**:227. DOI: 10.3389/fonc.2013.00227

[82] Palma L, Celli P, Franco C, Cervoni L, Cantore G. Long-term prognosis for atypical and malignant meningiomas: A study of 71 surgical cases. Journal of Neurosurgery. 1997;**86**:793-800. DOI: 10.3171/jns.1997.86.5.0793

[83] Rogers L, Barani I, Chamberlain M, Kaley TJ, McDermott M, Raizer J, et al. Meningiomas: Knowledge base, treatment outcomes, and uncertainties. A RANO review. Journal of Neurosurgery. 2015;**122**:4-23. DOI: 10.3171/2014.7.JNS131644

[84] Boskos C, Feuvret L, Noel G, Habrand JL, Pommier P, Alapetite C, et al. Combined proton and photon conformal radiotherapy for intracranial atypical and malignant meningioma. International Journal of Radiation Oncology, Biology, Physics. 2009;**75**:399-406. DOI: 10.1016/j.ijrobp.2008.10.053

[85] Noël G, Renard A, Valéry C, Mokhtari K, Mazeron JJ. Role of radiotherapy in the treatment of cerebral meningiomas. Cancer Radiothérapie. 2001;**5**:217-236. http://www.ncbi.nlm.nih.gov/pubmed/11446076

[86] Williams BJ, Salvetti DJ, Starke RM, Yen CP, Sheehan JP. Stereotactic radiosurgery for WHO II and III meningiomas: Analysis of long-term clinical and radiographic outcomes. Journal of Radiosurgery SBRT. 2013;**2**:183-191. http://www.ncbi.nlm.nih.gov/pubmed/29296361%0A. http://www.pubmedcentral.nih.gov/articlerender.fcgi?artid=PMC5658810

[87] Yamanaka R, Hayano A, Kanayama T. Radiation-induced Meningiomas: An exhaustive review of the literature. World Neurosurgery. 2017;**97**:635-644.e8. DOI: 10.1016/j.wneu.2016.09.094

[88] Graffeo CS, Leeper HE, Perry A, Uhm JH, Lachance DJ, Brown PD, et al. Revisiting adjuvant radiotherapy after gross total resection of World Health Organization grade II meningioma. World Neurosurgery. 2017;**103**:655-663. DOI: 10.1016/j.wneu.2017.04.095

[89] Park HJ, Kang HC, Kim IH, Park SH, Kim DG, Park CK, et al. The role of adjuvant radiotherapy in atypical meningioma. Journal of Neuro-Oncology. 2013;**115**:241-247. http://ovidsp.ovid.com/ovidweb.cgi?T=JS&PAGE=reference&D=emed11&NEWS=N&AN=2013680382

[90] Kerschbaumer J, Demetz M, Krigers A, Nevinny-Stickel M, Thomé C, Freyschlag CF. Risk factors for radiation necrosis in patients undergoing cranial stereotactic radiosurgery. Cancers

(Basel). 2021;**13**:4736. DOI: 10.3390/cancers13194736

[91] Evans DGR. Neurofibromatosis type 2 (NF2): A clinical and molecular review. Orphanet Journal of Rare Diseases. 2009;**4**:16. DOI: 10.1186/1750-1172-4-16

[92] Dracham CB, Shankar A, Madan R. Radiation induced secondary malignancies: A review article. Radiation Oncology Journal. 2018;**36**:85-94. DOI: 10.3857/roj.2018.00290

[93] Evans DGR, Birch JM, Ramsden RT, Sharif S, Baser ME. Malignant transformation and new primary tumours after therapeutic radiation for benign disease: Substantial risks in certain tumour prone syndromes. Journal of Medical Genetics. 2006;**43**:289-294. DOI: 10.1136/jmg.2005.036319

[94] Kaley T, Barani I, Chamberlain M, McDermott M, Panageas K, Raizer J, et al. Historical benchmarks for medical therapy trials in surgery-and radiation-refractory meningioma: A RANO review. Journal of Neuro-Oncology. 2014;**16**:829-840. DOI: 10.1093/neuonc/not330

[95] Kros JM, Cella F, Bakker SLM, Paz Geuze D, Egeler RM. Papillary meningioma with pleural metastasis: Case report and literature review. Acta Neurologica Scandinavica. 2000;**102**:200-202. DOI: 10.1034/j.1600-0404.2000.102003200.x

[96] Coskun M, Straube W, Hurkmans CW, Melidis C, de Haan PF, Villà S, et al. Quality assurance of radiotherapy in the ongoing EORTC 22042-26042 trial for atypical and malignant meningioma: Results from the dummy runs and prospective individual case reviews. Radiation Oncology. 2013;**8**. DOI: 10.1186/1748-717X-8-23

[97] Marcus HJ, Price SJ, Wilby M, Santarius T, Kirollos RW. Radiotherapy as an adjuvant in the management of intracranial meningiomas: Are we practising evidence-based medicine? British Journal of Neurosurgery. 2008;**22**:520-528. DOI: 10.1080/02688690802308687

[98] Simon M, Boström J, Koch P, Schramm J. Interinstitutional variance of postoperative radiotherapy and follow up for meningiomas in Germany: Impact of changes of the WHO classification. Journal of Neurology, Neurosurgery, and Psychiatry. 2006;**77**:767-773. DOI: 10.1136/jnnp.2005.077974

[99] Raheja A, Couldwell WT. Microsurgical resection of skull base meningioma—Expanding the operative corridor. Journal of Neuro-Oncology. 2016;**130**:263-267. DOI: 10.1007/s11060-016-2197-7

[100] Milker-Zabel S, Zabel-du Bois A, Henze M, Huber P, Schulz-Ertner D, Hoess A, et al. Improved target volume definition for fractionated stereotactic radiotherapy in patients with intracranial meningiomas by correlation of CT, MRI, and [68Ga]-DOTATOC-PET. International Journal of Radiation Oncology, Biology, Physics. 2006;**65**:222-227. DOI: 10.1016/j.ijrobp.2005.12.006

[101] Graf R, Nyuyki F, Steffen IG, Michel R, Fahdt D, Wust P, et al. Contribution of 68Ga-DOTATOC PET/CT to target volume delineation of skull base meningiomas treated with stereotactic radiation therapy. International Journal of Radiation Oncology, Biology, Physics. 2013;**85**:68-73. DOI: 10.1016/j.ijrobp.2012.03.021

[102] Nyuyki F, Plotkin M, Graf R, Michel R, Steffen I, Denecke T, et al. Potential impact of 68Ga-DOTATOC PET/CT on stereotactic radiotherapy

planning of meningiomas. European Journal of Nuclear Medicine and Molecular Imaging. 2010;**37**:310-318. DOI: 10.1007/s00259-009-1270-2

[103] Regelsberger J, Hagel C, Emami P, Ries T, Heese O, Westphal M. Secretory meningiomas: A benign subgroup causing life-threatening complications. Journal of Neuro-Oncology. 2009;**11**:819-824. DOI: 10.1215/15228517-2008-109

[104] Osawa T, Tosaka M, Nagaishi M, Yoshimoto Y. Factors affecting peritumoral brain edema in meningioma: Special histological subtypes with prominently extensive edema. Journal of Neuro-Oncology. 2013;**111**:49-57. DOI: 10.1007/s11060-012-0989-y

[105] Abe T, Black PM, Ojemann RG, Hedley-White ET. Cerebral edema in intracranial meningiomas: Evidence for local and diffuse patterns and factors associated with its occurrence. Surgical Neurology. 1994;**42**:471-475. DOI: 10.1016/0090-3019(94)90075-2

[106] Mirone G, Chibbaro S, Schiabello L, Tola S, George B. En plaque sphenoid wing meningiomas: Recurrence factors and surgical strategy in a series of 71 patients. Neurosurgery. 2009;**65**. DOI: 10.1227/01.NEU.0000345652.19200.D5

[107] Boari N, Gagliardi F, Spina A, Bailo M, Franzin A, Mortini P. Management of spheno-orbital en plaque meningiomas: Clinical outcome in a consecutive series of 40 patients. British Journal of Neurosurgery. 2013;**27**:84-90. DOI: 10.3109/02688697.2012.709557

[108] Shapey J, Sabin HI, Danesh-Meyer HV, Kaye AH. Diagnosis and management of optic nerve sheath meningiomas. Journal of Clinical Neuroscience. 2013;**20**:1045-1056. DOI: 10.1016/j.jocn.2013.03.008

[109] Jackson A, Patankar T, Laitt RD. Intracanalicular optic nerve meningioma: A serious diagnostic pitfall. American Journal of Neuroradiology. 2003;**24**:1167-1170

[110] Kijima C, Miyashita T, Suzuki M, Oka H, Fujii K. Two cases of nevoid basal cell carcinoma syndrome associated with meningioma caused by a PTCH1 or SUFU germline mutation. Familial Cancer. 2012;**11**:565-570. DOI: 10.1007/s10689-012-9548-0

[111] Smith MJ, Wallace AJ, Bennett C, Hasselblatt M, Elert-Dobkowska E, Evans LT, et al. Germline SMARCE1 mutations predispose to both spinal and cranial clear cell meningiomas. The Journal of Pathology. 2014;**234**:436-440. DOI: 10.1002/path.4427

[112] Perry A, Giannini C, Raghavan R, Scheithauer BW, Banerjee R, Margraf L, et al. Aggressive phenotypic and genotypic features in pediatric and NF2-associated meningiomas: A clinicopathologic study of 53 cases. Journal of Neuropathology and Experimental Neurology. 2001;**60**:994-1003. DOI: 10.1093/jnen/60.10.994

[113] Emens LA, Middleton G. The interplay of immunotherapy and chemotherapy: Harnessing potential synergies, cancer. Immunologic Research. 2015;**3**:436-443. DOI: 10.1158/2326-6066.CIR-15-0064

[114] Yeung J, Yaghoobi V, Aung TN, Vesely MD, Zhang T, Gaule P, et al. Spatially resolved and quantitative analysis of the immunological landscape in human Meningiomas. Journal of Neuropathology and Experimental Neurology. 2021;**80**:150-159. DOI: 10.1093/jnen/nlaa152

[115] Weber DC, Ares C, Villa S, Peerdeman SM, Renard L, Baumert BG,

et al. Adjuvant postoperative high-dose radiotherapy for atypical and malignant meningioma: A phase-II parallel non-randomized and observation study (EORTC 22042-26042). Radiotherapy and Oncology. 2018;**128**:260-265. DOI: 10.1016/j.radonc.2018.06.018

[116] Rogers L, Zhang P, Vogelbaum MA, Perry A, Ashby LS, Modi JM, et al. Intermediate-risk meningioma: Initial outcomes from NRG oncology RTOG 0539. Journal of Neurosurgery. 2018;**129**:35-47. DOI: 10.3171/2016.11.JNS161170

[117] Wilson TA, Huang L, Ramanathan D, Lopez-Gonzalez M, Pillai P, De Los Reyes K, et al. Review of atypical and anaplastic Meningiomas: Classification, molecular biology, and management. Frontiers in Oncology. 2020;**10**. DOI: 10.3389/fonc.2020.565582

[118] Graillon T, Sanson M, Campello C, Idbaih A, Peyre M, Peyriere H, et al. Everolimus and octreotide for patients with recurrent meningioma: Results from the phase II CEVOREM trial. Clinical Cancer Research. 2020;**26**:552-557. DOI: 10.1158/1078-0432.CCR-19-2109

Chapter 4

Surgical and Radiosurgical Treatment of the Pituitary Neuroendocrine Tumors

Mustafa Caglar Sahin and Gokhan Kurt

Abstract

Pituitary neuroendocrine tumors (PitNETs) arising from adenohypophyseal cells are generally accepted as benign. It is a very heterogeneous group of tumors according to their origin, biological behavior, and growth patterns. It is the third most common intracranial tumor type after meningiomas and gliomas. Transsphenoidal surgery (TSS) is the primary treatment of choice in all PitNETs except for lactotroph tumors, which are primarily treated with dopamine agonists. In this book section, surgical approaches in the treatment of PitNETs will be explained. In addition, PitNET radiosurgery will be explained in detail by using current literature information.

Keywords: PitNETs, pituitary adenoma, endoscopic surgery, transsphenoidal surgery, radiosurgery

1. Introduction

The new classification clearly distinguishes anterior lobe (adenohypophyseal) from posterior lobe (neurohypophyseal) and hypothalamic tumors. Anterior lobe tumors include (i) well-differentiated adenohypophyseal tumors that are now classified as pituitary neuroendocrine tumors (PitNETs; formerly known as pituitary adenoma), (ii) pituitary blastoma, and (iii) the two types of craniopharyngioma.

Pituitary adenomas usually present with three types of clinical signs. The first type of clinical manifestations includes amenorrhea-galactorrhea syndrome, acromegaly or gigantism, Cushing's disease, and secondary hyperthyroidism because of hypersecretion of prolactin, growth hormone, adrenocorticotropic hormone, and thyroid stimulating hormone (very rare). About 70% of pituitary adenomas are endocrinely active, the presence of hypersecretory endocrine status is the most common presentation.

The second type of clinical manifestations includes pituitary insufficiency and is typically associated with large tumors compressing the nontumoral pituitary gland or stalk. In general, the pituitary gland exhibits outstanding functional resistance, even in chronic compression and distortion. The tolerance of each pituitary axis to chronic compression is different. Gonadotropes are the most susceptible and the first to be affected. After that, thyrotropic, somatotropic, and corticotropic functions are affected respectively. Regardless of the size of the tumor or the degree of compression of the gland or stalk, pituitary adenomas rarely present with posterior pituitary insufficiency; the preoperative presence of this condition almost excludes the diagnosis of pituitary adenoma. The hypopituitarism associated with pituitary adenomas is usually a chronic process, but when pituitary apoplexy is present, it can be acute, unexpected, and immediately life-threatening.

The third type of clinical manifestations includes mass effect symptoms with or without endocrinopathy. Headache is usually the first finding and is attributed to stretching of the diaphragm sella innervated by the trigeminal nerve. The most common objective finding of these tumors is loss of vision, the result of the suprasellar growing tumor pressing on the anterior visual pathways. Although many patterns of visual dysfunctions are seen, asymmetrical bitemporal hemianopsia is the pathognomonic deficit. Visual field disorders decreased visual acuity, afferent pupillary defects, papilledema, optic atrophy, and total blindness can be observed.

Although the suprasellar and lateral areas are difficult to see with the microscope, the transsphenoidal microsurgical approach has yielded results as a surgical treatment for pituitary adenomas. The first transsphenoidal approach for resection of a pituitary lesion was documented by Schloffer in 1906. In 1914, Dr. Harvey Cushing developed the sublabial transseptal technique, which reduces the degree of nasal trauma associated with previous external rhinotomy incisions. The integration of the operative microscope into pituitary surgery by Hardy in the 1960s provided magnification and illumination, enabling more precise tumor resection via the transsphenoidal route, especially for pituitary microadenomas [1].

In 1987, Griffith and Veerapen reviewed the endonasal approach for microscopic pituitary surgery with the placement of a transsphenoidal retractor through the natural nasal airway into the sphenoid rostrum [2]. The first reported use of the endoscope specifically for transsphenoidal surgery was in the sublabial approach by Guiot and colleagues in 1963 [3]. Jankowski et al. performed the first full endoscopic pituitary surgery in 1992 [4]. In 1996, Jho and Carrau described their technique of a pure endoscopic approach in detail, and in 1997, they published their report of endoscopic removal of pituitary adenomas in 44 patients [5, 6]. The continuous development and improvement of endoscopic equipment and surgical instruments have greatly contributed to the advancement of endoscopic surgery as a viable procedure for transsphenoidal approaches to the sella.

2. Pituitary neuroendocrine tumors surgery

2.1 Surgical management and indications

A comprehensive preoperative evaluation is performed after the decision for surgery for resection of the pituitary tumor is made. First, the patient's medical condition should be optimized. Hypertension, heart disease, diabetes, thyroid status, hematological problems, the presence of sleep apnea, and pituitary endocrine function should be carefully evaluated, especially in patients with Cushing's disease or acromegaly. Common comorbid conditions in patients with pituitary tumors require special considerations regarding anesthesia [6, 7]. Prognathism and soft tissue hypertrophy (including macroglossia) in patients with acromegaly and cervico-cranial stoutness in patients with Cushing disease challenge intubation and airway management.

Hypopituitarism is among the important endocrine conditions that require preoperative treatment, especially for hypocortisolism and hypothyroidism. For patients

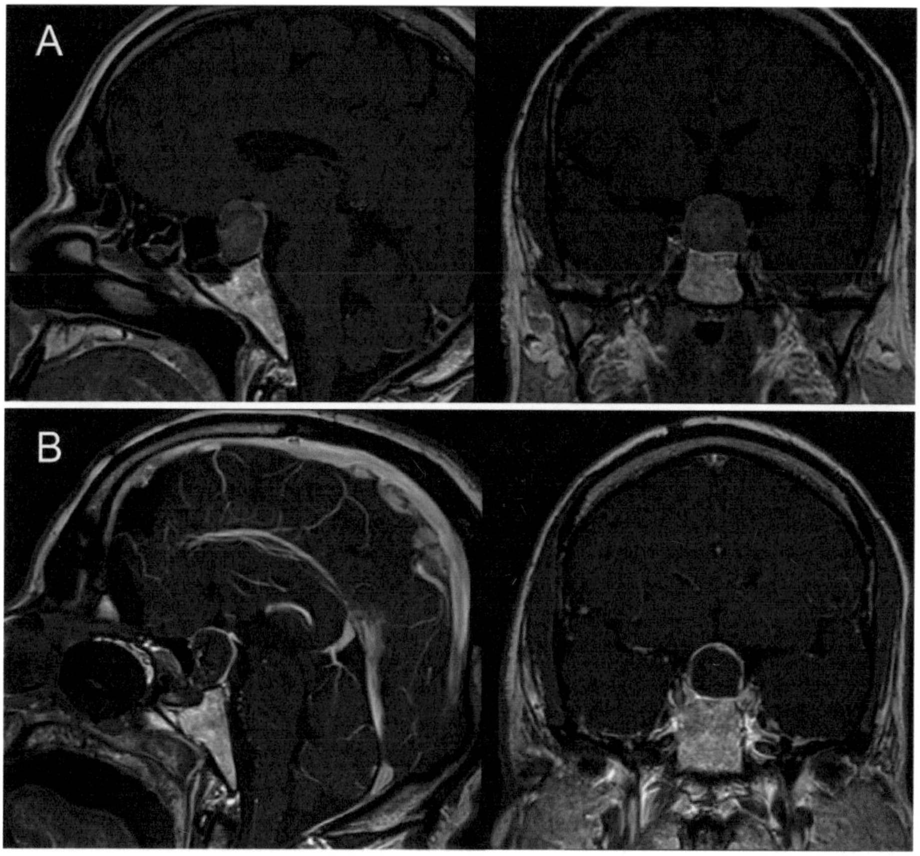

Figure 1.
A: Sagittal and coronal preoperative MRI image in pituitary-focused contrast-enhanced brain MRI of the patient who was operated with the diagnosis of Pitnet B: Sagittal and coronal postoperative MRI image in pituitary-focused contrast-enhanced brain MRI of the patient who was operated with the diagnosis.

with preoperative vision problems or tumors affecting the optic apparatus on MRI, formal neuro-ophthalmologic evaluations are performed with preoperative follow-up eye exams. Brain MRI with pituitary focus, with and without contrast, is the best diagnostic imaging modality of choice for most pituitary adenomas (**Figure 1**). CT imaging with pituitary focus and dynamic contrast protocol may be an alternative for patients who cannot undergo MRI for various reasons. The basic anatomy of the paranasal sinuses and any variation of the patient can be adequately evaluated on MRI for transsphenoidal surgical planning. However, in patients with prior paranasal sinus or transsphenoidal surgery, bone window CT scans with thin-slice axial and coronal views can reveal the bony anatomy of the paranasal sinuses in detail (**Figure 2**).

In the treatment of pituitary adenomas, it is aimed to normalize the excess of hormone secretion, if any, to preserve and even restore normal pituitary function, to eliminate the mass effect, to preserve or restore visual acuity and/or visual field, and to obtain a complete pathological diagnosis. Clinically silent pituitary tumors are primarily treated surgically because the surgical treatment modality is currently the only method that can achieve all the previously mentioned goals. Pituitary apoplexy and visual impairment due to mass effect or cranial nerve palsy can be shown as a general surgical indication for such lesions. Large invasive pituitary tumors and tumors with

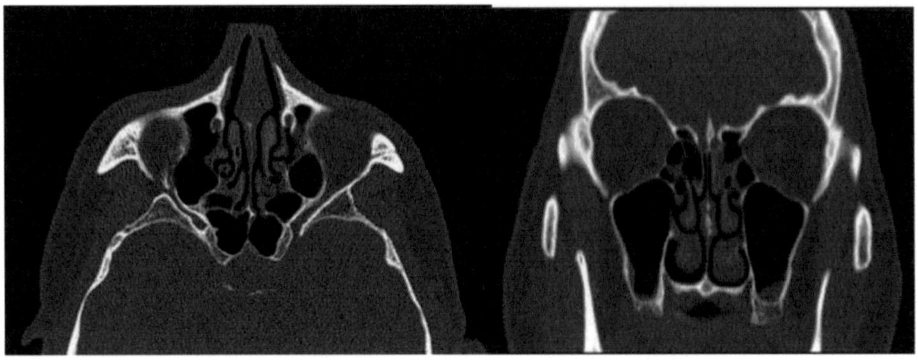

Figure 2.
Detailed view of the paranasal sinuses in thin section axial and coronal sections. Permission has been obtained for the figures used in the book section.

open cavernous sinus invasion are considered difficult to treat independently of the surgical approach, because gross complete removal of the tumor is often not achieved. Patients with hormonally inactive or dysfunctional pituitary adenomas are operated when they have symptomatic findings such as optic chiasm compression, hypopituitarism, pituitary apoplexy, or severe persistent headaches.

Prolactinoma patients are operated on only when they do not respond appropriately to dopaminergic drugs and develop intolerable side effects to drugs. In other hormone-secreting pituitary adenomas, the primary treatment is surgical, not medical.

Clear identification of anatomical landmarks is especially important for a transsphenoidal approach to the sella. The surgeon should be aware of nasal septal deviations, sphenoid septations and their relationship to the carotids, bony defects in the carotid canal, the degree of sphenoid bone pneumatization, and the extent of bone expansion or erosion from an aggressive lesion. The surgeon should try to determine the position of the normal pituitary gland and any deviations in the infundibulum prior to surgery.

2.2 Surgical approaches

2.2.1 Transcranial approaches

There are conditions that limit and sometimes contraindicate the choice of the transsphenoidal approach over the transcranial approach, regarding the anatomy of the surgical route, morphology, or consistency of the lesion. The size of the sella, the size and pneumatization of the sphenoid sinus, and the position and tortuosity of the carotid arteries can significantly increase the difficulty of the transsphenoidal procedure. When such selected indications warrant a transcranial approach, there are several options. These are pterional, subfrontal unilateral, subfrontal bilateral interhemispheric approaches.

2.2.2 Transsphenoidal approaches

Transsphenoidal resection of pituitary masses involves the operating microscope, endoscope, or a combination of both. The microsurgical transsphenoidal technique provides bimanual dexterity during dissection of the tumor from the surrounding neurovascular structures, but the viewing angle may be limited. Endoscopic techniques offer a wider field of view and flexibility to change the viewpoint all the way from the cribriform plate to the cervical junction. Transsphenoidal approaches can be divided into three main stages as nasal, sphenoidal, and sellar.

2.2.2.1 Microsurgical transsphenoidal approaches

Although many different transsphenoidal procedures and variations have been described, there are currently three mains microsurgical transsphenoidal approaches to pituitary tumors. These are the transnasal transseptal transsphenoidal approach, the sublabial transseptal transsphenoidal approach, and the endonasal trans-sphenoidal approach.

The procedure is performed with an operating microscope to visualize, illuminate, and magnify the surgical field. The three mains microscopic transsphenoidal methods differ slightly, mainly in the initial stage up to the exposure of the sphenoid sinus; they then follow the same surgical sphenoidal and sellar steps.

2.2.2.2 Endoscopic endonasal transsphenoidal approach

The main advantages of the endoscopic procedure over microsurgical procedures are the features of the endoscope itself and the absence of a nasal speculum [8, 9]. The nasal speculum forms a fixed tunnel. The endoscope allows a wider view of the surgical field with a close view inside the anatomy. Angle lens endoscopes allow the surgeon to study tumors located in the suprasellar and parasellar regions under direct visual control. The endoscopic endonasal procedure has a lower complication rate than the traditional microsurgical approach [10]. With the endoscopic procedure, microsurgery makes the procedure faster and easier compared to microsurgery, as the submucosal nasal phase of the operation is avoided.

Disadvantages of the endoscopic approach include the unusual anatomy of the nasal cavities and the learning curve to rely on specific endoscopic dexterity. However, after sufficient experience, especially in the case of relapse, the operative time becomes the same or shorter than the time required for transsphenoidal microsurgery. The endoscope offers only two-dimensional vision on the video monitor. The sense of depth can be gained by the surgeon's experience, allowing the endoscope to move in and out. To achieve surgical targets, especially those that angled endoscopes can show special microsurgical endoscopic instruments with secure grip, flat and non-bayonet-shaped, equipped with different and variable-angle tips are required.

In general, endoscopic instruments are long, rotating instruments with a single straight shaft equipped with angled tips. Angled tips on the working ends of many surgical instruments allow for a greater range of motion than standard instruments. The use of straight shaft instruments is preferred in endoscopy compared with the microsurgical technique, which typically uses bayonet instruments to avoid interference with the light source. The endoscope can be inserted into the nostrils with a sheath attached to an irrigation system that allows cleaning the lens without repeatedly removing and reentering the telescope. An endoscope holder can be used during the sellar phase of the procedure to stabilize the view of the surgical field, but its use limits dynamic movement that helps compensate for the loss of depth perception. The use of neuronavigational systems, although not essential, may be helpful in patients with recurrent lesions or abnormal sellar or paranasal sinus anatomy.

Key components of the endoscopic setup include a rigid lens endoscope, a high-resolution camera, a fiberoptic cable and light source, a large high-definition video monitor, and a video recording system. The most used endoscope is 4 mm in diameter and 18 or 30 cm in length. Differences in lens angle exist for certain steps of the operation, including 0-degree binoculars, 30-degree binoculars, and 45-degree binoculars. Wider-angle binoculars, ranging from 70 to 120 degrees, are available, but are rarely required for most endoscopic skull base operations.

2.2.2.2.1 Operational setup in surgery

The video monitor is placed behind the patient's head and, in most cases, in the direct line of sight of the surgeon standing on the right side of the patient. The anesthesiologist is on the left side of the patient. The head of the bed is turned approximately 120 degrees away from the anesthesiologist, and the patient is placed in a semi-recumbent position with the thorax elevated to 15 degrees to optimize venous flow. The head is positioned with a slight degree of rotation toward the surgeon, approximately 10 degrees, with the midline of the patient's head parallel to the side walls of the operating room and the patient's nose bridge parallel to the floor. The degree of flexion/extension of the patient's head depends on the location of the lesion. Lesions located primarily in the clivus, or sphenoid sinus, often require slight flexion of the head to allow working space for the endoscope. More anteriorly located lesions, such as the planum sphenoidale, require the head to be neutral or slightly hyperextended.

2.2.2.2.2 Patient preparation

Nasal decongestion facilitates pituitary procedures in most patients, except for patients with a history of hypertension and coronary artery disease. Before and immediately after induction of anesthesia, patients are given a 0.05% spray solution of oxymetazoline (Afrin) intranasally. During positioning, bayonet forceps are used to insert cotton pads soaked in oxymetazoline, followed by pads soaked in 1:200,000 epinephrine and 1% lidocaine between the middle turbinates and septum. The pads are allowed to remain in contact with the nasal mucosa for 5–10 minutes. The nostrils are then wiped with an aqueous solution of antibiotics such as chlorhexidine. A broad-spectrum antibiotic is given perioperatively with a nasal packing attached. If the results of the preoperative adrenal axis test suggest adrenal insufficiency, intravenous hydrocortisone is given before induction of anesthesia. Steroids are avoided in patients with Cushing's disease to allow postoperative evaluation of successful resection. Leg fascia lata area or lower quadrant abdominal area is prepared in all patients to allow potential fat grafting in case of encountering cerebrospinal fluid (CSF).

2.2.2.2.3 Nasal stage

The aim of the nasal phase is to reach the sphenoid sinus through the sphenoid ostium and posterior nasal septectomy, which can be achieved with different strategies for manipulation of the mucosa and nasal septum. The endoscopic endonasal transsphenoidal technique begins with the insertion of a 0-degree endoscope into one nostril to identify the nasal cavity floor for orientation, the inferior turbinate laterally, the nasal septum medially, and the choana posteroinferiorly. The inferior and middle turbinates, which are the main barriers to the sphenoid ostium, should be carefully lateralized with blunt pressure to avoid excessive mucosal damage. Some surgeons choose to remove part of the middle or upper turbinate, but this is not usually necessary for resection of most pituitary tumors. After creating an appropriately wide working corridor, the sphenoid ostium is defined 1.5 cm above the choana.

The sphenoid ostium is sometimes hidden by mucous membranes or a thin layer of bone, in which case it may be helpful to first try to identify the ostium on the opposite side. Use of neuronavigational can also be helpful in confirming the pathway to the sphenoid sinus, then a small dissector instrument can be used to gently probe for the ostium and enter the sinus. If a pedicled nasoseptal flap is being prepared, it should be done at this stage. Once the ostium has been identified, its mucosal edges are coagulated using light monopolar cautery, which can be extended toward the medial and inferior surfaces of the sphenoid cusp. Avoiding inferolateral cauterization and dissection helps prevent arterial bleeding from septal branches of the sphenopalatine artery. Local anesthesia (epinephrine 1:100,000 to 1% lidocaine) is then injected medially into the posterior nasal septum using a spinal needle with a 20-degree bend.

Placement of the mucosal incision is dependent on expected closure needs and whether a nasoseptal flap is required to close the skull base. An incision can be made at the junction of the bony and cartilage septum and moved inferiorly and posteriorly in a standard transsphenoidal approach for an intrasellar lesion. Extended transsphenoidal approaches for complex sellar, parasellar, and suprasellar lesions often result in high-flow CSF leaks. In this situation, a vascularized nasoseptal flap closure is important to take advantage of natural wound healing mechanisms. While preparing the nasoseptal flap, parallel incisions can be made along the maxillary crest, inferiorly and superiorly caudal to the olfactory epithelium, with an anteriorly connected vertical incision [11]. The size of the flap can be adjusted according to the size of the expected defect. The flap remaining at the base of the sphenopalatine artery is compressed into the nasopharynx or, in some extended approaches, into the maxillary sinus for protection during the operation.

A posterior bite instrument can be used to extend the posterior septectomy further forward as needed to improve communication between both sides of the nasal cavity, improve visualization and instrument mobility, and minimize the possibility of instrument collision. The lateral and superior soft tissue and bony prominence of the sphenoid rostrum and sinus may be resected to provide sufficient space to position the endoscope superolateral at the 10 o'clock position. The bony rostrum is raised to the level of the floor of the sphenoid sinus to create a working area for the endoscope and two instruments.

2.2.2.2.4 Sphenoid stage

The sphenoid surface of the pneumatized sinus can be entered after dilation of the ostium or resection of the vertical plate. In a presellar or conchal sphenoid sinus, the bone is removed with a chisel or drill. Care must be taken to avoid injury to the sphenopalatine artery as it arises near the inferolateral vomer. This is particularly important when a pedicled nasoseptal flap is envisioned for reconstruction at the end of the procedure, called the salvage flap. The mucosa within the sphenoid sinus is often removed to reduce the risk of postoperative mucocele. Septations within the sphenoid sinus are also removed. The surgical view at this point should encompass the sellar floor at the center, the rostral clivus inferiorly, the planum sphenoidale superiorly, the bulge of the internal carotid siphon immediately juxtaposed to the sella, the wings of the optic nerves coursing superolaterally with respect to the sella, and the opticocarotid recess in between the optic nerve canal and the carotid protuberance.

2.2.2.2.5 Sellar stage

To safely perform bimanual microdissection for the sellar phase of the operation, two surgeons switch to the "four-handed" technique. Alternatively, the endoscope can be secured with the endoscope holder so that a single surgeon can operate with both hands. When the base of the sella is enlarged and thinned by an intrasellar lesion, it can usually be fractured using a pituitary rongeur or blunt microdissector. In some cases, a thicker sellar floor prevents this maneuver and requires the use of an osteotome, drill, or ultrasonic bony curette. A sellar bone defect is then performed, typically extending from one cavernous sinus to the other. In addition to defining the cavernous sinuses laterally, the anterior intercavernous sinus is often defined in the rostral aspect of exposure. A micro-Doppler probe and neuro-navigation can be routinely used to check the location of the internal carotid arteries and to confirm the location of the planned dural opening. The carotid artery may be ectatic within the sella, especially in acromegalic patients. Macroadenomas often compress the venous plexus between the two leaves of the dura, allowing a relatively bloodless opening. In contrast, intact venous channels between the dura and intercavernous sinuses may surround smaller tumors and should be thoroughly investigated prior to tumor resection.

Dural clearance differs according to surgeon preference; A rectangular opening allows dural pathology to be obtained for pathological examination when dural invasion is suspected. If the gland needs to be separated from an underlying lesion, the first vertical incision preserves blood flow. Care should be taken to remove as many tumors as possible for pathology and/or tissue banking. After sufficient specimen has been collected, curettes and aspiration can be used to remove the remainder of the tumor. The arachnoid may descend into the field of view at this point and should be carefully manipulated and protected with a cotton swab to avoid direct aspiration. Venous cavernous sinus bleeding may be encountered following tumor removal and temporary gelatin foam filling and/or injection may be given. A 30- or 45-degree endoscope may be inserted to look laterally and superiorly into the cavernous sinuses to assess the remaining tumor. In cases of macroadenoma with large suprasellar extension, the tumor will often subside spontaneously with mild curettage given sufficient time. Intrasellar and cavernous sinus hemostasis can be achieved, typically by temporary packing with a gelatin sponge followed by coating the tumor cavity with oxidized cellulose (Surgicel).

2.2.2.2.6 Closure

After tumor resection is complete and hemostasis is achieved, the closure phase begins with the goal of reconstructing the skull base defect and repairing any possible CSF leak. Many methods are available to perform reconstruction, including conventional repairs with autologous or artificial grafts, vascularized pedicled nasoseptal flap formation and rotation, and multilayer closure techniques using dural and bone substitutes.

CSF leaks may result from tumor removal from a thinned or inadequate diaphragm, from traction applied during dissection, or from deliberate opening of the diaphragm to access suprasellar lesions. High-flow CSF leakage is expected, especially in tumors that extend into the suprasellar compartment or the third ventricle. In the absence of significant CSF leakage, the Valsalva maneuver can be performed to detect minimal CSF leakage. A drip of dark liquid against the background of venous bleeding indicates a hidden leak.

For smaller defects, the sellar base can be reconstructed with allograft bone, cartilage, or ideally a biosynthetic substitute placed in the sellar extradural space. Alternative reconstruction techniques include the gasket-seal method and the use of synthetic grafts reinforced with fascia lata or fibrin sealant [12, 13]. For large CSF leaks, in addition to the maneuvers mentioned above, a vascularized flap provides the most effective closure.

2.2.2.3 Extended endoscopic endonasal transsphenoidal approach

Medial cavernous sinus tumor surgery can be performed with an extended transsphenoidal transsellar approach. This approach involves puncturing the bone over the carotid siphon and removing the medial opticocarotid recess. However, this only provides limited access to the medial cavernous sinus wall. The ethmoids need to be opened using the transethmoidal corridor to gain better access to the cavernous sinus. Additional lateral access can be achieved using the transmaxillary corridor. This approach can be used for cavernous sinus tumors or lateral sphenoid pathology.

The extended endoscopic endonasal approach does not require brain and optic nerve manipulation compared with transcranial approaches. It provides a direct view of the suprasellar region. Because of this advantage, the risk of worsening postoperative vision is much less than with transcranial approaches. However, the extended endoscopic endonasal approach is technically much more difficult and can be performed by experienced surgeons.

2.3 Complications

Despite the minimally invasive nature of transsphenoidal approaches to sella turcica, complications can occur. Complications encountered in the nasal cavity during the approach include anosmia, nasal septal perforation, crusting, saddle nose deformity, orbital fracture, cribriform plate injury with CSF leakage, and epistaxis. Complications occurring within the sphenoid sinus include sinusitis, mucocele formation, and optic nerve or carotid artery injury resulting from sphenoid body fracture. Potential complications associated with tumor resection and the sellar phase include CSF leakage, hypopituitarism, diabetes mellitus, meningitis, postoperative hematoma, carotid artery or other vascular injury, optic nerve injury, ophthalmoplegia, subarachnoid hemorrhage, vasospasm, and tension pneumocephalus. The most common non-endocrine complications for both microscopic and endoscopic transsphenoidal surgery are CSF leakage, meningitis, and sinusitis [14, 15].

2.4 Postoperative care and follow-up

Patients should be observed very closely following endoscopic transsphenoidal pituitary surgery. Most patients are discharged home on the second or third day after surgery. In most patients, serum sodium levels and urine output are monitored every 6–8 hours for the first 48 hours. Patients with any new evidence of hypocortisolemia should receive adequate replacement therapy. Patients with functional pituitary adenomas typically undergo basic non-stimulation hormonal testing (e.g., serum prolactin, cortisol, or growth hormone) on the first and second postoperative days. If nasal packing is used, it is usually removed on the first postoperative day. The patient is usually discharged from the hospital on the second or third postoperative day and is expected to see an endocrinologist for hormonal follow-up. The patient will be evaluated in the outpatient clinic 3 months later with sellar contrast MRI postoperatively.

3. Pituitary neuroendocrine tumors radiosurgery

Especially in macroadenomas and tumors invading the cavernous sinus, total resection is not always possible. Total resection rate in pituitary adenomas remains below 70% [15]. Tumor control rates with microsurgery between 50 and 80% vary [16]. Another factor limiting the effectiveness of surgical treatment in pituitary adenomas is recurrence in 11.5% of radiologically resected pituitary adenomas [17].

Pituitary adenomas are very suitable lesions for radiosurgery if suprasellar and parasellar neural tissues can be preserved because they are in a well-circumscribed environment. For this reason, radiosurgery has been applied as an adjuvant treatment method for many years to provide hormonal normalization and control of tumor growth. It has been proven that a single dose of stereotactic radiosurgery can effectively provide tumor control and hormonal normalization as adjuvant therapy [18]. It can even be applied as a primary treatment method in cases where surgical and medical treatment cannot be applied.

The aim of radiosurgery of pituitary adenomas is to normalize abnormal levels of hormone, reduce the size of the tumor, or at least control its growth, without damaging neural tissues, especially the optic apparatus, and without causing pituitary insufficiency.

The marginal dose should be at least 12 Gray (gy) to achieve tumor control. Otherwise, even if growth control is achieved, hormonal recovery may not be possible. It has been reported that small lesions at some distance from optic nerves marginal doses about up to 30–35 Gy. Although it is recommended to avoid doses of more than 8–10 Gy to protect the optic nerve, there are series in which the median maximum dose of the optic apparatus is increased up to 12 Gy [19, 20].

Hormone-suppressing drugs should be quitted 1–2 months ago because of the possibility of affecting tumor cell cycle and metabolism and reducing sensitivity to radiation. There is no consensus on the time of initiation after radiosurgery [21].

The effectiveness of conventional radiotherapy in pituitary adenomas is well known. Although different results have been reported between series, it generally provides approximately 90% tumor control and 40–70% hormonal control [22]. However, in addition to this efficacy, it has disadvantages such as toxicity in temporomesial and hypothalamic structures, high pituitary insufficiency rate, optic neuropathy, long treatment time, and long time required for the effect to occur [16].

3.1 Tumor growth and hormonal control

Pituitary adenomas are already very slow growing tumors. For this reason, long-term follow-ups should be made after radiosurgery to decide that the growth is under control. This rate has been reported as 83–100% in series with a follow-up period of 4 years or more. This rate includes not only patients with reduced tumor volume, but also patients with growth arrest. For growth control of hormone-active tumors compared with nonfunctional adenomas, higher doses are needed.

Volumetric shrinkage may vary depending on the pathology of the tumor. Growth hormone-secreting adenomas tend to shrink more than prolactinomas and nonfunctional adenomas [23].

In the series published by Park et al. in 2011, in which they applied radiosurgery to 125 cases of nonfunctional adenoma, the 1-year control rates were 99%, while this rate decreased to 94% in 5 follow-ups and to 76% at the end of 10-year follow-up [24].

The onset of hormonal recovery after radiosurgery takes an average of 2 years (3 months–8 years). Hormone remission rate varies according to which hormone the adenoma secretes, how much maximum and marginal dose is applied, and whether antisecretory drugs are used during radiosurgery. If infundibulum damage develops during surgery and/or radiosurgery due to the compression of the tumor, it should be kept in mind that a decrease in prolactin level can be observed regardless of the adenoma [25].

The hormone remission rate after radiosurgery is the lowest in prolactinomas (25–30%). The most important factor here is thought to be the long-term dopaminergic treatment of the patients. Therefore, it is recommended to quitting antisecretory therapy at least 1–2 months before radiosurgery.

In tumors that secrete growth hormone, the hormonal response is obtained after an average of 2 years. The aim of radiosurgery is to reduce the GH level below 1 ng/ml. In big series with long follow-up, it has been reported that the hormonal cure rate between 20 and 96% varies. Also, it is thought that using somatostatin analogue reduces the response radiosurgery by changing the cell cycle. For this reason, it is recommended to stop or reduce the treatment at least 1 month before the radiosurgery.

Although hormone remission starts a little earlier in Cushing's disease (14–18 months), they reported remission rates varying between 17 and 83% in big series.

3.2 Non-functional adenomas and stereotactic radiosurgery

Since non-functional adenomas are usually asymptomatic until signs of compression appear, they are found to be larger than functional adenomas at the time of diagnosis, and surgical resection is the first choice. However, the development of residual or recurrent tumors after surgery is substantial. For these cases, radiosurgery has become a comfortable and very effective treatment option, protecting patients from the risks of revision surgery. In non-functional microadenomas or macroadenomas that do not create optic pressure, follow-up is the strategy that should be considered first, and treatment should be planned in case of tumor growth.

There are many studies in the literature showing the efficacy of radiosurgery in non-functional adenomas. When the data of 512 patients with non-functional adenomas from nine Gamma Knife centers were analyzed, 94% had a history of previous surgical treatment, 6% had a history of prior radiotherapy. In the series, where the mean dose was 16 Gy and the mean follow-up was 36 months, the tumor control rate was 98, 95, 91, and 85% at the 3rd, 5th, 8th, and 10th years, respectively. The rate of pituitary insufficiency after radiosurgery was 21%, new or progressive cranial nerve deficit was 9%, and new or progressive optic nerve dysfunction was 6.6%. When the factors associated with cranial nerve deficit were examined, it was revealed that young age, increased volume, and the presence of previous radiation therapy increased the risk [26].

In the review of Kim et al., tumor marginal dose ranges between 13 and 24 Gy and 83–100% tumor control are reported in Gamma Knife series. The authors, who did not detect a significant relationship between tumor control and dose, reported a decrease in these rates as the follow-up period increased. Tumor shrinkage ranged from 42–89% [27].

In a large series evaluating Gamma Knife radiosurgery results in non-functional adenomas, visual side effects were found to be 0.8%, and cranial nerve deficit rate was 1.6%. This series shows that tumor control rates decrease as the tumor volume grows, the follow-up period increases, and the treatment dose decreases. In addition, there was no difference in outcome between operated and unoperated cases [24].

In the long-term follow-up (80.5 months mean) series of Gopalan et al. 48 cases, the tumor control rate was 83% and the new hormone deficit was 39%. Hormone deficits were found to be 8% for corticotropin deficiency, and as 4.2% for thyroid hormone deficiency with 20.8% gonadotropin deficiency, respectively. A decrease in tumor control rate and an increase in complications were found to be associated with the size of the irradiated tumor volume [28].

It has been shown that Gamma Knife radiosurgery at doses ranging from 10 to 25 Gy provides tumor control at a rate of 94–95% in 5–7 years of follow-up, and these rates decrease to 76% at the end of 10-year follow-ups [20, 29].

Effective tumoral control can be achieved with 12–15 Gy in non-functional adenomas. Therefore, in non-functional adenomas, radiosurgery can be applied even in some cases where the tumor meets the optic apparatus. Another option for large tumors is hypo-fractionated radiosurgery, and it is possible to better protect the optic structures by dividing the total dose 3–4 times.

As can be seen, radiosurgery provides more than 90% tumor control in non-functional adenomas. Since hormonal remission is not targeted, the fact that lower doses are frequently administered ensures that the rates of pituitary insufficiency and visual complications are lower than in the functional adenomas. In cases where it is thought that complete removal cannot be achieved due to cavernous sinus invasion or other reasons, surgical strategies that will reduce the tumor below 3 cm and remove it from the optic structures can make patients suitable for radiosurgery and provide an effective and safe treatment.

3.3 Functional adenomas and radiosurgery

Despite advances in surgical techniques and medical agents, endocrine remission, or recurrences are observed in a significant proportion of pituitary adenomas. In such difficult cases, the option of radiosurgery is often on the agenda. The literature clearly reveals hormonal remission rates with radiosurgery, endocrine cure is between 20 and 30% in prolactinomas, 50% in growth hormone adenomas, and 40–65% in ACTH-secreting adenomas.

The ideal dose for functional adenomas has not been determined, yet. However, the chance of achieving hormonal normalization at doses below 16 Gy is low. The chance of success increases with doses up to 30 Gy. Doses between 20 and 25 Gy are frequently preferred [16]. The possibility of pituitary insufficiency increases, especially at doses above 24 Gy [30].

The major disadvantage in radiation therapy of pituitary adenomas is the length of time required for biochemical remission. Sheehan et al.'s study of 418 cases found the mean time required for remission to be 48.9 months. They reported that this time was inversely proportional to the dose received by the tumor and directly proportional to the tumor volume [21].

3.3.1 Cushing's disease

The first and most effective treatment for Cushing's disease is surgery. However, there is a significant group of patients who cannot be cured by surgery, and radiosurgery has become an effective option for these patients. Recurrence develops in 30% of patients after successful surgery in Cushing's disease [31]. In these patients, radiosurgery is one of the treatment options.

Jaganathan et al. evaluated the results of 49 Cushing's patients who applied Gamma Knife and followed up for an average of 45 months and reported that the tumor shrank 80%. The average dose in this series is 23 Gy. In this study, in which the criterion of successful endocrinological response was determined as the normal level of free cortisol in 24-hour urine, successful endocrinological results were obtained in 54% of the patients in 13 months average. In 27 months, average, 20% of the patients relapsed and new hormonal deficits occurred in 22% of the patients. In this study, no relationship was found between tumor volume and endocrine response to radiosurgery. Hormonal normalization after radiosurgery varies between 7.5 and 58 months [13, 20]. In series where the marginal dose ranged from 15 to 30 Gy, it was reported that an average of 20 Gy accelerated the clinical and endocrine cure response. Cushing's disease's radiosurgery response develops more rapidly than other functional tumors. Although hormonal normalization has been reported between 10 and 87%, the success rate in most series is between 40 and 65%. Tumor control is reported in 80–100%, and shrinkage is reported in 10–70% of cases [16]. As with other adenomas, the response to radiosurgery is higher in ACTH-secreting microadenomas [32].

3.3.2 Prolactinomas

Surgery and radiosurgery options should be considered in a group of patients who are resistant or intolerant to medical treatment.

In the study of Jezkova et al. examining the role of radiosurgery in prolactinomas with 35 cases with an average follow-up of 75 months, normoprolactinemia was achieved in 37%, and dopamine agonist use was discontinued in 43% of cases. The time required for hormone normalization has been reported as 96 months. The tumor control rate was found to be 97% [33].

In the series of 38 cases with 22 years of follow-up, published by Sheehan et al. in 2015, it was reported that 55% of the patients used dopamine agonists before radiosurgery. In this series with an average follow-up of 43 months, endocrine remission was reported as 50% without using dopamine agonists. Pituitary insufficiency secondary to radiosurgery was found to be 30%. In this study, it is reported that medical treatment before radiosurgery worsens hormone normalization results [34].

Although a higher dose (mean marginal dose of 25Gy) is applied in the radiosurgical treatment of prolactinomas compared with other functional adenomas, the endocrine remission rate is lower. In addition, 80% of the patients have a decrease in prolactin level [16].

3.3.3 Growth-hormone-secreting adenomas

In the study by Franzin et al., in which they examined the Gamma Knife radiosurgery results in 103 patients with acromegaly, 58.3% of the 63 patients who were followed up for an average of 71 months achieved remission in 58.3%, while 14.6% of the patients achieved remission with somatostatin analogues. The rate of hormonal deficit was found 7.8% [6]. It has been determined that the most important factor affecting the success of radiosurgery is low GH and/or IGF-I levels during treatment. IGF-1 lower than 2.25 times normal is a positive prognostic factor [16].

In the series of Jagannathan et al.'s 95 cases, which were followed up 57 months average and underwent radiosurgery after unsuccessful surgery, a successful result was accepted as IGF-I normalization, and a successful result was obtained in 53%

of the patients after an average of 30 months after radiosurgery. In this study, where the mean treatment dose was 22Gy, reduction in tumor volume was found in 92% of patients, and new endocrinological deficits occurred in 34% of patients. This study also shows that the duration of hormonal remission is faster in radiosurgery than radiotherapy. Researchers recommended that hormone-suppressing therapy should be discontinued 2 months before radiosurgery and not used for 6 weeks afterwards [35].

3.4 Radiosurgery in cavernous sinus invasive adenomas

Cavernous sinus invasion is observed in 7–42% of the cases in pituitary adenomas. Post-surgical residual tumor in pituitary adenomas is most frequently observed in tumors that have spread to the cavernous sinus. Neurovascular complex and venous hemorrhage in this region reduce the chance of surgeons to intervene in this area, and morbidity may be 27–50% because of intervention in this area. For this reason, radiosurgery is frequently the option for residual tumors in this region.

In 89 patients with recurrent or residual pituitary adenomas located in the cavernous sinus, who underwent radiosurgery by Hayashi et al., 97% tumor control was achieved at a mean 36-month follow-ups. Tumor shrinkage was detected in 64% of them. 18.2 Gy average was applied in non-functional adenomas, and 25.2 Gy average was applied in functional adenomas, and transient cranial nerve dysfunction was observed in 2% of cases. In this series, hormonal normalization was found in 39% of cases. Radiosurgery-related morbidity is less than 1% in lesions invading the cavernous sinus [36].

3.5 Complications

The main problems that may arise in radiosurgery of pituitary adenomas are pituitary insufficiency, optic neuropathy, and other cranial nerve paralysis.

The most important risk factors in the development of optic neuropathy are the contact of the tumor with the optic nerve, the size of the tumor, and the inability to clearly evaluate the relationship between the tumor and the optic apparatus in operated cases. After radiosurgery, a decrease in visual acuity and/or narrowing of the visual field may occur due to the proximity of the residual mass to the optic nerve. This rate is 1–6% and decreases further with advanced MRI. It is known that the cranial nerves in the cavernous sinus are more radioresistant than the optic nerve. In big series, damage to other cranial nerves (CN III, IV, V, VI, VII) is 2–3%.

Diabetes insipidus development due to neurohypophysis or infundibulum damage is approximately 1–2% in big series [19, 28]. Very rarely, narrowing of the carotid artery has been observed after radiosurgery, but it is even rarer to cause symptoms [26].

Stereotactic radiosurgery is an effective and safe alternative or supportive treatment to conventional treatments in the treatment of pituitary adenomas. Due to the risks of radiation, it should be applied in the right indications, considering the appropriate dose-volume relationship, and protecting critical structures. While the short duration of the treatment is advantageous, the most important risks that may develop after the procedure are pituitary insufficiency and vision problems due to optic nerve damage. Neurosurgeons, endocrinologists, and ophthalmologists should take a multidisciplinary approach together both in the evaluation of the efficacy of the treatment and in the management of its complications.

After radiosurgery, patient follow-up should continue for a long time, both to evaluate the effectiveness of the treatment and to develop complications after a long time.

Conflict of interest

The authors declare no conflict of interest.

Acronyms and abbreviations

PitNET	Pituitary Neuroendocrine Tumors
CSF	Cerebrospinal fluid
Surgicel	oxidized cellulose
Gy	Gray

Author details

Mustafa Caglar Sahin* and Gokhan Kurt
Gazi University Faculty of Medicine Department of Neurosurgery, Ankara, Turkey

*Address all correspondence to: dr.mcaglarsahin@gmail.com

References

[1] Jane JA, Han J, Prevedello DM, Jagannathan J, Dumont AS, Laws ER. Perspectives on endoscopic transsphenoidal surgery. FOC. 2005;**19**(6):1-10

[2] Griffith HB, Veerapen R. A direct transnasal approach to the sphenoid sinus: Technical note. Journal of Neurosurgery. 1987;**66**(1):140-142

[3] Guiot J, Rougerie J, Fourestier M, Fournier A, Comoy C, Vulmiere J, et al. Intracranial endoscopic explorations. Presse Médicale. 1893;**1963**(71):1225-1228

[4] Jankowski R, Auque J, Simon C, Marchai JC, Hepner H, Wayoff M. Endoscopic pituitary tumor surgery. The Laryngoscope. 1992;**102**(2):198-202

[5] Jho HD, Carrau RL. Endoscopy assisted transsphenoidal surgery for pituitary adenoma: Technical note. Acta Neurochirurgica. 1996;**138**(12):1416-1425

[6] Nemergut EC, Dumont AS, Barry UT, Laws ER. Perioperative management of patients undergoing transsphenoidal pituitary surgery. Anesthesia & Analgesia. 2005;**101**(4):1170-1181

[7] Lim M, Williams D, Maartens N. Anaesthesia for pituitary surgery. Journal of Clinical Neuroscience. 2006;**13**(4):413-418

[8] Cappabianca P, Cavallo LM, de Divitiis E. Endoscopic endonasal transsphenoidal surgery. Neurosurgery. 2004;**55**(4):933-941

[9] Cappabianca P, Cavallo LM, Colao A, de Divitiis E. Surgical complications associated with the endoscopic endonasal transsphenoidal approach for pituitary adenomas. Journal of Neurosurgery. 2002;**97**(2):293-298

[10] Hadad G, Bassagasteguy L, Carrau RL, Mataza JC, Kassam A, Snyderman CH, et al. A novel reconstructive technique after endoscopic expanded endonasal approaches: Vascular pedicle nasoseptal flap. The Laryngoscope. 2006;**116**(10):1882-1886

[11] Leng LZ, Brown S, Anand VK, Schwartz TH. "GASKET-SEAL" watertight closure in minimal-access endoscopic cranial base surgery. Operative. Neurosurgery. 2008;**62**(5):ONSE342-ONSE343

[12] Kassam A, Carrau RL, Snyderman CH, Gardner P, Mintz A. Evolution of reconstructive techniques following endoscopic expanded endonasal approaches. FOC. 2005;**19**(1):1-7

[13] Ciric I, Ragin A, Baumgartner C, Pierce D. Complications of transsphenoidal surgery: Results of a national survey, review of the literature, and personal experience. Neurosurgery. 1997;**40**(2):225-237

[14] Zada G, Kelly DF, Cohan P, Wang C, Swerdloff R. Endonasal transsphenoidal approach to treat pituitary adenomas and other sellar lesions: An assessment of efficacy, safety, and patient impressions of the surgery. Journal of Neurosurgery. 2003;**98**(2):350-358

[15] Laws ER, Sheehan JP, Sheehan JM, Jagnathan J, Jane JA Jr, Oskouian R. Stereotactic radiosurgery for pituitary adenomas: A review of the literature. Journal of Neuro-Oncology. 2004;**69**(1-3):257-272

[16] Kim JW, Kim DG. Stereotactic radiosurgery for functioning pituitary adenomas. World Neurosurgery. 2014;**82**(1-2):58-59

[17] Shin M, Kurita H, Sasaki T, Tago M, Morita A, Ueki K, et al. Stereotactic radiosurgery for pituitary adenoma invading the cavernous sinus. Journal of Neurosurgery. 2000;**93**(supplement_3):2-5

[18] Grant RA, Whicker M, Lleva R, Knisely JPS, Inzucchi SE, Chiang VL. Efficacy and safety of higher dose stereotactic radiosurgery for functional pituitary adenomas: A preliminary report. World Neurosurgery. 2014;**82**(1-2):195-201

[19] Hasegawa T, Kobayashi T, Kida Y. Tolerance of the optic apparatus in single-fraction irradiation using stereotactic radiosurgery: Evaluation in 100 patients with Craniopharyngioma. Neurosurgery. 2010;**66**(4):688-695

[20] Pollock BE, Cochran J, Natt N, Brown PD, Erickson D, Link MJ, et al. Gamma knife radiosurgery for patients with nonfunctioning pituitary adenomas: Results from a 15-year experience. International Journal of Radiation Oncology *Biology* Physics. 2008;**70**(5):1325-1329

[21] Sheehan JP, Pouratian N, Steiner L, Laws ER, Vance ML. Gamma knife surgery for pituitary adenomas: Factors related to radiological and endocrine outcomes: Clinical article. JNS. 2011;**114**(2):303-309

[22] Minniti G, Brada M. Radiotherapy and radiosurgery for Cushing's disease. Arquivos Brasileiros de Endocrinologia e Metabologia. 2007;**51**(8):1373-1380

[23] Pamir MN, Kiliç T, Belirgen M, Abacioğlu U, Karabekiroğlu N. Pituitary adenomas treated with gamma knife radiosurgery: Volumetric analysis of 100 cases with minimum 3 year follow-up. Neurosurgery. 2007;**61**(2):270-280

[24] Park KJ, Kano H, Parry PV, Niranjan A, Flickinger JC, Lunsford LD, et al. Long-term outcomes after gamma knife stereotactic radiosurgery for nonfunctional pituitary adenomas. Neurosurgery. 2011;**69**(6):1188-1199

[25] Höybye C, Grenbäck E, Rähn T, Degerblad M, Thorén M, Hulting AL. Adrenocorticotropic hormone-producing pituitary tumors: 12- to 22-year follow-up after treatment with stereotactic radiosurgery. Neurosurgery. 2001;**49**(2):284-292

[26] Sheehan JP, Starke RM, Mathieu D, Young B, Sneed PK, Chiang VL, et al. Gamma knife radiosurgery for the management of nonfunctioning pituitary adenomas: A multicenter study: Clinical article. JNS. 2013;**119**(2):446-456

[27] Pouratian N, Kim W, Clelland C, Yang I. Comprehensive review of stereotactic radiosurgery for medically and surgically refractory pituitary adenomas. Surgical Neurology International. 2012;**3**(3):79

[28] Gopalan R, Schlesinger D, Vance ML, Laws E, Sheehan J. Long-term outcomes after gamma knife radiosurgery for patients with a nonfunctioning pituitary adenoma. Neurosurgery. 2011;**69**(2):284-293

[29] Pollock BE, Brown PD, Nippoldt TB, Young WF. Pituitary tumor type affects the chance of biochemical remission after radiosurgery of hormone-secreting pituitary adenomas. Neurosurgery. 2008;**62**(6):1271-1278

[30] Loeffler JS, Shih HA. Radiation therapy in the Management of

Pituitary Adenomas. The Journal of Clinical Endocrinology & Metabolism. 2011;**96**(7):1992-2003

[31] Patil CG, Prevedello DM, Lad SP, Vance ML, Thorner MO, Katznelson L, et al. Late recurrences of Cushing's disease after initial successful transsphenoidal surgery. The Journal of Clinical Endocrinology & Metabolism. 2008;**93**(2):358-362

[32] Kobayashi T. Long-term results of stereotactic gamma knife radiosurgery for pituitary adenomas. In: Yamamoto M, editor. Progress in Neurological Surgery. Basel: KARGER; 2008. pp. 77-95. Available from: https://www.karger.com/Article/FullText/163384 [cited: July 14, 2022]

[33] Ježková J, Hána V, Kršek M, Weiss V, Vladyka V, Liščák R, et al. Use of the Leksell gamma knife in the treatment of prolactinoma patients. Clinical Endocrinology. 2009;**70**(5):732-741

[34] Cohen-Inbar O, Xu Z, Schlesinger D, Vance ML, Sheehan JP. Gamma knife radiosurgery for medically and surgically refractory prolactinomas: Long-term results. Pituitary. 2015;**18**(6):820-830

[35] Jagannathan J, Sheehan JP, Pouratian N, Laws ER, Steiner L, Vance ML. Gamma knife radiosurgery for acromegaly: Outcomes after failed transsphenoidal surgery. Neurosurgery. 2008;**62**(6):1262-1270

[36] Hayashi M, Chernov M, Tamura N, Nagai M, Yomo S, Ochiai T, et al. Gamma knife robotic microradiosurgery of pituitary adenomas invading the cavernous sinus: Treatment concept and results in 89 cases. Journal of Neuro-Oncology. 2010;**98**(2):185-194

Chapter 5

Craniopharyngioma

Gökhan Kurt and Ayfer Aslan

Abstract

Craniopharyngioma (CP) is a rare, benign, slow-growing, but clinically aggressive tumor located mainly in the sellar and suprasellar regions. While it occurs equally in children and adults, there are two peaks in the age distribution: first in 5–14 years of age and second in 45–74 years of age. The clinical presentation varies according to the age of patients, while the predominant symptoms are visual disturbances, headache, and endocrine dysfunctions. CPs are topographically classified in several subgroups based on the relationship of the tumor to the sella, diaphragma sellae, optic chiasm, stalk, and third ventricle; whereas the pathological classification includes two types: adamantinomatous (aCP) and papillary (pCP). Distinctive features of aCP are cysts with content of "motor-oil" fluid, calcification, wet keratin, peripheral palisading of basal cells, stellate reticulum, and mutations in CTNNB1/β-catenin gene; and those of Pcp are regular stratified squamous epithelium, devoid of cilia, papillary projections, no calcification, rare cyst with a clear fluid, and mutations in BRAF V600E. The surgical approaches include transcranial (subfrontal, pterional, transcallosal, and transcortical-transventricular) and transsfenoidal approaches, having different selection criteria, advantages, and disadvantages. Despite complete resection and radiotherapy, CPs are inclined to recur causing high morbidity and mortality.

Keywords: adamantinomatous, craniopharyngioma, papillary, sellar tumor, suprasellar tumor, surgery

1. Introduction

New information about tumor types and subtypes based on molecular studies were introduced first by 2016 update, and then lately by 2021 update of the World Health Organisation (WHO) Classification of Tumors of the Central Nervous System (CNS) [1]. One of the updated tumors is Craniopharyngoma (CP), particularly in the aspects of molecular pathology. We aim to review CPs with the new updates by 2016 and 2021 WHO classification systems highlighting important implications for clinical practice including diagnosis and management. We also intend to include a brief consideration of epidemiology and demographics, clinical manifestations, morphologic and molecular features, behavior, and prognosis of craniopharyngioma along with the current treatment modalities – surgery, radiosurgery, radiation therapy – with a thorough review of the literature.

IntechOpen

2. Terminology and staging

Craniopharyngioma (CP) is a benign primary brain tumor originating from epithelial remnants of craniopharyngeal duct (Rathke's pouch, a diverticulum arising from the embryonic buccal cavity and rising to form the anterior pituitary gland) [2].

CP is a WHO grade I neoplasm often with a low proliferation index (MIB-1 < 10%) [1]. Although it is classified as a benign tumor, it has a tendency to recur due to its invasive nature, and inability to complete excision, particularly when MIB-1 is higher than 7% [3].

Despite its current WHO grade I classification with no malignant subtype, more and more case reports of a malignant form of CP occurring de novo or transforming from a benign variant have been published in recent years [4–10]. The exact pathogenesis and biological behavior of malignant change in CP are not yet clear; however, some reports have suggested that radiation may be a contributing factor to carcinogenesis [4, 6, 7, 9] though such a link has not been proven yet by any studies with high level of evidence [8, 11, 12]. Although malignant CP is still a rare clinical entity with less than 40 reported cases in the current literature, it may induce a new update in the WHO classification system in the future.

3. Epidemiology

CP is overall rare accounting for 1.2–4.6% of all brain tumors; [2, 13] yet, its incidence is higher in children, accounting for 5–13% of all pediatric brain tumors [14–16]. The overall incidence of CP was reported as 0.13 per 100,000 person-years in the USA with no difference between genders or races [17]. CPs occur almost equally in children and adults, and there is a bimodal age distribution with the first peak in children at the age of 5–14 years, and the second peak in older adults aged 45–74 years [14, 17, 18]. Between two types of CPs (adamantinomatous and papillary), the adamantinomatous CP (aCP) occurs predominantly in children, while papillary (pCP) is seen almost exclusively in adults [19, 20]. About 90% of CPs are aCP, and 10% are pCPs [14, 19].

4. Anatomy

4.1 Location

CPs may originate from anywhere along the pituitary stalk, extending from the tuber cinereum to the pituitary gland, where the remnants of an incompletely involuted hypophyseal-pharyngeal duct may locate [21, 22]. Most frequently, CPs originate in the suprasellar location; while some cases can be exclusively intrasellar or extend in any direction to encompass crucial structures, such as pituitary stalk, optic chiasm, optic tracts, third ventricle, hypothalamus, and thalamus [14, 15].

4.2 Topographical classification

CP has been anatomically classified based on the relationship of the tumor to the sella, diaphragma sellae, optic chiasm, stalk (infundibulum), and third ventricle mainly to assist in planning optimal surgical approach [21, 23]. The first classification was introduced by Gazi Yaşargil based on his microsurgical experience with CPs [23]. According to his scheme, type A is confined within the sella (intrasellar infra diaphragmatic); type B is both intra- and suprasellar, infra- and supradiaphragmatic; type C is supradiaphragmatic, parachiasmatic, and extraventricular; type D is intra- and extraventricular; type E is paraventricular with respect to the third ventricle; type F is purely intraventricular [24].

Upon the development of endoscope and advances in transsphenoidal endoscopic surgeries, Kassam et al [25] have suggested a different classification system based on the relationship of the lesion to the infundibulum, which is the key anatomical consideration determining the amount of additional exposure needed in expanded endonasal approach (EEA). Accordingly, type I is preinfundibular, type II is transinfundibular, type III is post- or retroinfundibular, and type IV is isolated third ventricular. However, CPs are rarely restricted to only one location but spread widely engulfing the entire suprasellar and prepontine cisterns. In the latter case, the authors of this classification suggest surgeons consider the predominant site in which the greater part of the solid component is located to be the primary target when determining the specific EEA module [25]. Later, Jamshidi et al. [26] added an additional subtype to this scale, called type 0, which describes fully subdiaphragmatic tumors located within the sella.

Recently, Fan et al [27] also suggest a new classification system, called QST, based on tumor origin. They classified CPs into three types as follows: infrasellar/subdiaphragmatic CPs (Q-CPs), subarachnoidal CPs (S-CPs), and pars tuberalis CPs (T-CPs). Q-CPs arise from the subdiaphragmatic infrasellar space with an enlarged pituitary fossa, and the gland is scarcely recognizable; S-CPs arise from the middle or inferior segment of the stalk and tend to extend among cisterns, and the entire stalk can be recognized on MRI; and T-CPs arise in the top of the pars tuberalis, mainly extend upward, and occupy the space of the third ventricle [27]. This new scheme has been proposed to guide the surgeons in choosing the best surgical approach between endoscopic endonasal and transcranial surgery and to predict the outcomes.

Despite the several topographical classifications of CPs, there has not been a consensus on a standard reference classification system [28].

5. Diagnosis

5.1 Clinical presentation

The origin and size of CPs and the patient's age significantly affect the symptoms and signs. Clinical presentations are generally related to the mass effect, high intracranial pressure, and hypothalamic and endocrinologic dysfunctions. Overall, the most frequent symptoms are headache and visual problems due to pressurized optic structures and obstructive hydrocephalus. Patients with CP frequently exhibit the manifestations of hypothalamic-pituitary axis dysfunction, including growth hormone deficiency, adrenocortical insufficiency, central hypothyroidism, hypogonadism, precocious puberty, hyperprolactinemia, central diabetes insipidus, and hypothalamic obesity [14, 19, 20, 29, 30]. Fatigue, nausea/vomiting, somnolence, and memory impairment are the other signs of the clinical presentation related to CPs [2].

5.2 Microscopic histopathology

CP is known to be arising from rest of pharyngeal epithelium remaining from embryogenesis. Histopathologically, two types of CPs are recognized: adamantinomatous and papillary. The distinction between the two types is made by the encapsulating epithelial lining [15].

Adamantinomatous CP (aCP) has internal layers of stratified squamous epithelium anastomosing with the basal layer of columnar cells and forming stellate reticulum. The surface of aCP is usually irregular and infiltrative, with long epithelial extensions penetrating the adjacent neuroglial tissue. Dysmorphic calcification, lamellar keratin formation ("wet keratin"), and fibrosis can be often noted [14, 15, 31]. It generally has multi-cysts with contents of cholesterol crystals giving the fluid a dark, "motor-oil" appearance [19].

Papillary CP (pCP) has a more regularly stratified mature squamous epithelium, with papillary projections of epithelial cords into the surrounding tissues, but without significant infiltration [15, 31]. They are more commonly solid, with rare cyst formation and no calcification, and if cystic, the contents are clear without significant cholesterol crystals [19, 20].

5.3 Molecular pathology

Owing to advances in technology, the genetic mutations of CPs have been identified. Wnt/β-catenin signaling pathway in particular is important in the development of pituitary [32]. aCP and pCP also differ genetically, as BRAF V600E mutations are detected in pCP and CTNNB1 mutations in aCP [1, 2, 19, 33–35]. CTNNB1 gene encodes β-catenin, mutations of which have been found in 70–90% of aCPs and seem to play important role in the tumorigenesis of aCP [34, 36, 37]. BRAF V600E is reported to be the most common mutation in pCPs (65–100%) [34, 35]. These findings have important implications for the diagnosis and treatment of these neoplasms.

5.4 Macroscopic features

The typical macroscopic appearance of aCP is a small solid portion and large single or multiple cysts containing dark, viscous, "motor-oil" colored fluid rich in cholesterol crystals. aCP has calcification and irregular surfaces adhered to the surrounding normal structures [14]. On the other hand, pCP is usually solid, has a smooth surface and a cauliflower-like appearance, is rarely cystic, and if so filled with clear fluid [14].

5.5 Imaging features

Radiological appearances of aCPs and pCPs also differ due to their distinct histopathological features. aCPs present with 90% calcifications, 90% enhancement, and 90% cysts containing cholesterol-rich fluid; whereas, pCPs appear mostly solid, rarely cystic, with more homogeneous enhancement and without calcifications [2, 13, 38].

5.5.1 Computed tomography (CT)

A large conglomerate suprasellar mass with an area of calcification is a common computed tomography (CT) finding in CPs [13]. CT is superior to magnetic resonance imaging (MRI) in detecting the presence of calcification, and therefore, seems more specific in establishing the diagnosis of CP (**Figure 1**) [39]. It may present as a suprasellar ring lesion with a peripheral rim of increased enhancement after contrast administration. CPs are generally mixed solid and cystic tumors, the former having well defined hyperdense appearance, while the latter presenting an area of low density on CT [13]. The sella turcica is usually intact or only minimally enlarged, suprasellar cistern is distorted, and hydrocephalus is common [13].

5.5.2 Magnetic resonance imaging (MRI)

MRI is the preferred method in the evaluation of tumor extent and recurrence. MRI is valuable in preoperative and radiation therapy planning due to its multiplanar capabilities [39]. Signal intensity on MRI varies with cyst contents [14]. CPs mostly demonstrate high signal intensity on both T2- and T1-weighted images (**Figures 2** and **3**) [38, 39]. High intensity on T1-weighted images corresponded to high cholesterol content or presence of methemoglobin in cystic lesions. Tumors lacking significant cholesterol or blood show moderate intensity (hypo- or iso intensity) on T1-weighted images [39]. While the CP cysts are variably hyperintense on FLAIR scan, the solid portion of the lesion does not suppress (**Figure 2**) [14]. CPs generally appear as mixed solid and cystic, lobulated lesions extending superiorly with the third ventricle compression, and reticular enhancement of the solid portion (**Figures 2** and **3**) [40].

5.6 Differential diagnosis

Most common lesions involving intrasellar and suprasellar regions include pituitary adenoma, CP, and Rathke cleft cyst. Pituitary adenoma has often a snowman shape, solid characteristics with less cystic changes, and more homogenous contrast enhancement; while CPs frequently present with superiorly lobulated shape, cystic changes, calcification, and heterogeneity of enhancement with enhancing solid

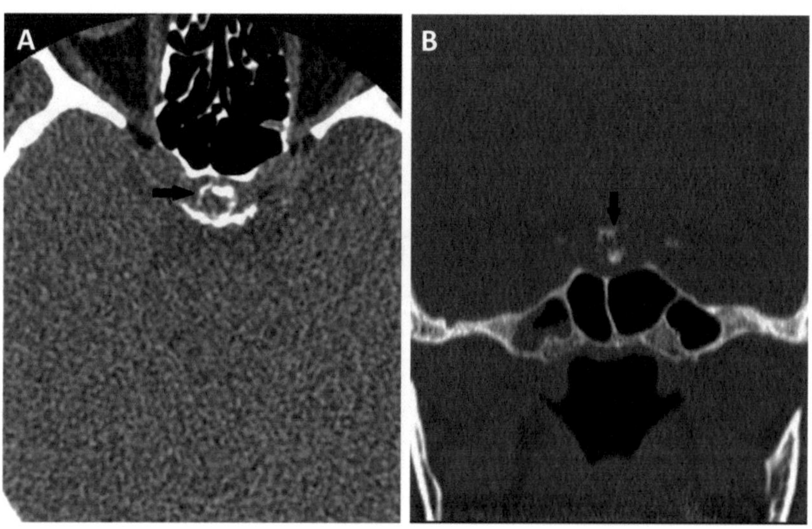

Figure 1.
Axial (A) and coronal (B) non-enhanced CT shows suprasellar dispersed calcifications (black arrow) in a patient with adamantinomatous craniopharyngioma.

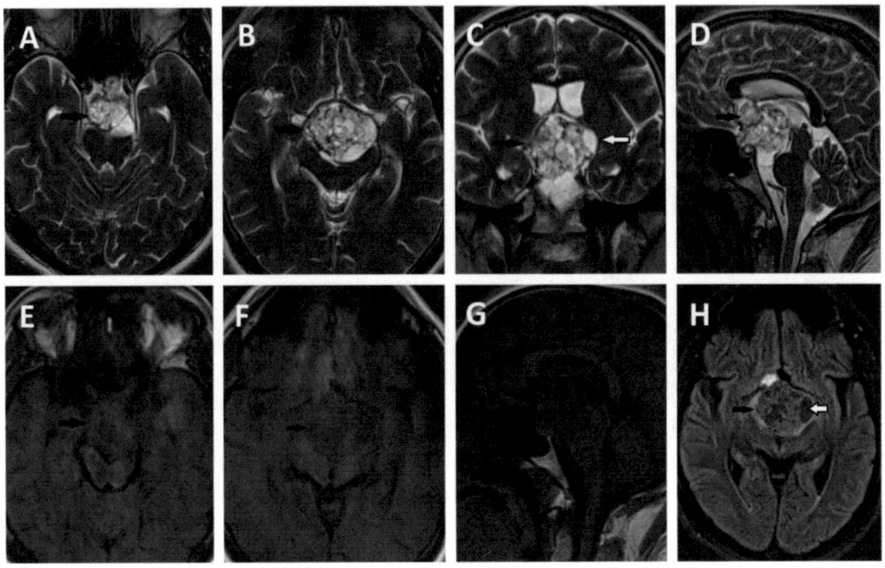

Figure 2.
The MRI of a 33-year-old man shows a lobulated sellar and suprasellar mass that is hyperintense on axial (A, B), coronal (C) and sagittal (D) T2-weighted scans; and nearly isotense or slightly hyperintense on axial (E, F) and sagittal (G) T1-weighted, and FLAIR scans (black arrow) with some small cystic areas (white arrow), radiologically suggesting craniopharyngioma.

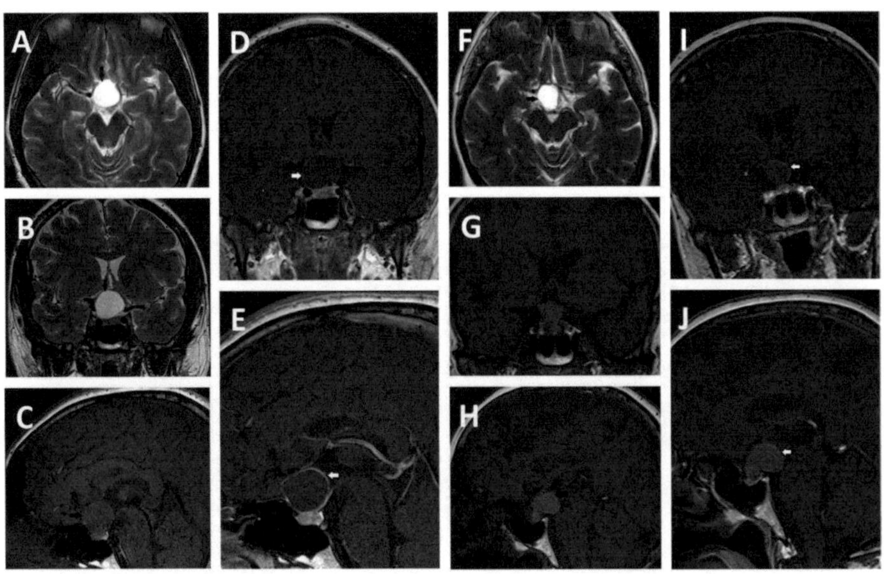

Figure 3.
The sellar and suprallar masses appear hyperintense on axial (A, F) and coronal (B) T2-weighted images; isointense and slightly hiperintense on sagittal (C, H) and coronal (G) T1-weighted images (black arrow). Coronal (D, I) and sagittal (E, J) contrast enhanced T1-weightes scans show thin rim enhancement around the mass with a small tumor nodule at the base of the mass (white arrow).

portion and unenhanced areas on contrast-enhanced T1WI [38, 40]. On the other hand, Rathke cleft cysts are in ovoid shape, with cystic lesions with no or thin cyst wall enhancement without calcification [14, 40].

6. Management

Because of the high variability in the manifestations of CPs, the management strategy should be tailored to the patient. The important parameters for treatment planning are the volumes of the solid and cystic parts of the tumor, its proximity and adhesion to the hypothalamus and optical structures, and the neurological and endocrinological state of the patient [41]. Moreover, the management of CP should be carried out by multidisciplinary teams including neurosurgeons, endocrinologists, ophthalmologists, and oncologists.

6.1 Observation alone

Although the mere observation of the tumor without treatment is currently not recommended, it gives the opportunity to observe natural course of the disease. Nevertheless, the natural growth of the CP seems unpredictable. In the literature, there have been a few case reports of CPs presented with long-term survival (up to 60 years), in spite of receiving no treatment and having some degree of morbidity [42, 43]. In these cases, tumors were mostly calcified, had low proliferative activity, and with partly cessation growth.

6.2 Surgical treatment

Microsurgical resection should be preferred when the solid part of the tumor is large and if the resection is feasible with a low risk of morbidity and mortality. The position of optic chiasm in relation to the sella is an important criterion for the selection of an approach. The chiasm may be above the tuberculum (prefixed), above the diaphragm or the middle of the sellae (normal), or above the dorsum sellae (post-fixed) [44].

Postoperative care is vital in CP management. Endocrine dysfunctions often ensue from the surgery. Therefore, following the removal of a CP, patients must be carefully monitored, including for their urination as total removal of a CP frequently leads to diabetes insipidus. To overcome the risk of hypocortisolism, preoperative doses of dexamethasone should be continued for a period of time and tapered off without causing insufficiency. Thyroid function, sexual function, and growth should be carefully observed, as a replacement therapy may be needed [22].

The ideal surgical approach is still controversial. However, some criteria can guide surgeons to choose the best approach to surgery.

6.2.1 Transcranial Approaches

6.2.1.1 Subfrontal approach

CPs that are considered prechiasmatic can be more easily resected via subfrontal approach. A right-sided unilateral frontal craniotomy usually suffices and a unilateral approach along the falx provides approximately equal visualization of both sides of the optic chiasm [45]. Osmotic diuretics and lumbar drainage of cerebrospinal fluid can be used to minimize the retraction of the frontal lobe. If there is a need for approaching the tumor through lamina terminalis behind the optic chiasm, the necessity of removing a small strip of the undersurface of the frontal lobe from the frontal pole to the chiasm along the falx might arise, which is the main limitation of subfrontal approach [45]. Moreover, inevitable dissection of the olfactory nerves brings about the risk of olfaction impairment [46].

6.2.1.2 Pterional approach

The pterional approach has been traditionally used most frequently because it allows early identification of the stalk, anterior circulation, and protection of the chiasm while giving access to virtually all parts of even very large tumors [24, 46]. The exposure through pterional craniotomy can be widened by adding the resection of the orbital rim and zygoma, which gives access to the skull base and minimize brain retraction [46]. Dissection can be performed through several corridors in the parachiasmal spaces: prechiasmatic, opticocarotid (between carotid artery and optic nerve), and carotidotentorial triangles (superior to the carotid artery bifurcation) or through the opening of the lamina terminalis [24, 46]. The main limitation of the pterional approach is the tumor extending into the upper part of the third ventricle and retrosellar region [46]. When tumors extend superiorly in the third ventricle, the pterional approach can be combined with the transcallosal approach because the pure pterional approach may be insufficient for proper dissection of the superior and posterior portions of the tumor within the third ventricle [23, 24]. CPs are usually subarachnoid tumors; therefore, they may be easily dissected from the surrounding structures covered with their own arachnoid layers. Nevertheless, great care should be paid to differentiating the tumor from hypothalamus and pituitary stalk. To avoid dreadful hypothalamic and infundibular injuries, tumor removal should be done stepwise, starting with the most easily accessible tumor portions, through internal decompression and dissection of the capsular-arachnoid plane [24, 46].

6.2.1.3 Transcallosal approach

Transcallosal approach is used for tumors primarily involving the third ventricle. Following a unilateral paramedian frontal craniotomy, the brain is retracted away from the falx and the corpus callosum will be exposed. A small callosal incision is made and intraventricular parts of the tumor can be removed through foramen of Monro [24]. With the pure transcallosal approach, optic chiasm and pituitary stalk cannot be identified early, and the anterosuperior portions of the tumor under chiasm and lamina terminalis may not be visible, in case of which a combined pterional-transcallosal approach is recommended [24, 46].

6.2.1.4 Transcortical-transventricular approach

Transcortical-transventricular approach via a frontal craniotomy was first introduced by Busch in 1944 mainly for tumors of the third ventricle [47]. It was used for CPs with giant cysts extended to the dorsal surface of the frontal lobe; nevertheless, it is unfavorable for the risk of producing porencephalic cyst or postoperative epilepsy [24].

6.2.2 Transsphenoidal Approach

If predominant portion of the tumor is intrasellar, the approach should be transsphenoidal (TS). TS approaches were traditionally reserved only for intrasellar infradiaphragmatic tumors; [24] yet, with technological developments, new transsphenoidal approaches, such as expanded endonasal approach (EEA), the exclusive or additional use of the endoscope, have been introduced also for the resection of suprasellar craniopharyngiomas [25, 48]. Nevertheless, TS approach can be combined with the pterional approach in cases of CPs with supradiaphragmatic extensions to achieve a total resection (**Figure 4**) [24]. Reconstruction of the sellar floor is one of the most crucial steps of TS as it was associated with a high incidence of cerebrospinal fluid (CSF) leak [49]. To prevent this complication, autologous grafts, such as fascia, muscle, or adipose tissue can be fixed with fibrin glue and patched to the base of the sella. On the other hand, shorter hospital stays, and a higher rate of preservation of pituitary function are its main advantages [50, 51].

6.2.2.1 Expanded endonasal approach (EEA)

Exposure of suprasellar tumor components is improved with the development of EEA [46]. Currently, EEA is considered the first-line therapy when the distance between the optic chiasm and the surface of the pituitary gland is large, the lateral extension does not go beyond the internal carotid artery, and there is no extension beyond the posterior clinoid process; whereas, poorly developed sphenoid sinus, the pituitary stalk traveling anterior to the tumor, and CPs predominantly in the third ventricle are limitations of EEA [48].

In EEA, the bone of the sellar floor, tuberculum sellae, and planum sphenoidale are removed; while the optic canals mark the lateral limits, and the posterior ethmoidal arteries mark the anterior limit of the bony resection. The medial opticocarotid recess is a very important landmark marking the medial aspect of carotid and

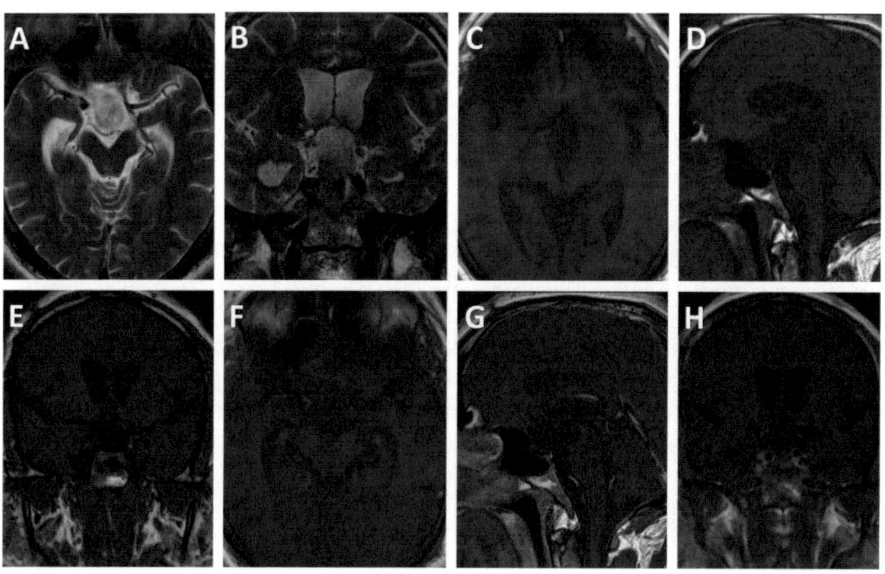

Figure 4.
The postoperative MRI of the patient on the ***Figure 2*** *following the surgery by combined transsphenoidal and pterional approach reveals total resection without residue or recurrence after 5 years. Papillary craniopharyngioma was diagnosed at histopathology. (A) axial T2-, (B) coronal T2-, (C) axial T1-, (D) sagittal T1-, (E) coronal T1, (F) axial contrast enhanced T1-, (G) sagittal contrast enhanced T1-, (H) coronal contrast enhanced T1-weighted images.*

optic canals [52]. In CPs confined to the sella, removal of the anterior sella wall only would suffice, while preinfundibular tumors require larger bone resection over tuberculum sella and planum sphenoidale, rather than the anterior sellar wall. Whereas, in transinfundibular CPs, additional bone removal from the anterior sella; and in retroinfundibular CPs, extensive bone removal from the sellar floor, posterior clinoid processes, and dorsum sella may be needed [52].

6.3 Radiation therapy

Due to the proximity and adhesiveness of CP to critical structures, including the optic chiasm, pituitary stalk, and hypothalamus, a complete removal is not always feasible, which increases the risk of recurrence. Postoperative radiation therapy (RT) is beneficial in patients with subtotal resection and recurrence, increasing the 10-year progression-free survival rates from 30 to 50% (of incomplete excision alone) to 75–90% (of incomplete excision followed by conventional RT) [20, 53]. Moreover, the tumor control rates were reported over 90% with newer higher precision techniques such as fractionated stereotactic conformal radiotherapy [53–56]. Radiation-related toxicities include impairment of endocrinological functions and vision, necrosis, radiation-induced tumors, and cognitive decline.

6.3.1 Conventional radiation therapy

The standard conventional radiotherapy technique is fractionated 3-dimensional (3D) conformal external beam radiotherapy (3DCRT) using computerized 3D treatment planning coupled with imaging for conforming to the shape of the tumor and delivering photons through a linear accelerator under precise immobilisation [53]. A more complex computerized treatment planning, called intensity-modulated radiotherapy (IMRT), using the modulation of the intensity of radiation can be preferred for more individualized beam shaping, particularly for the avoidance of some critical normal structures [53].

6.3.2 Stereotactic radiosurgery

Stereotactic radiosurgery (SRS) is an efficient option of radiotherapy for recurrent CPs following the surgical removal, ensuring tumor shrinkage and clinical improvement, without significant complications [57, 58]. Radiation can be delivered using gamma rays from multiple cobalt sources arranged in a hemisphere focused through a static collimator system onto the tumor (defined as Gamma Knife Radiosurgery) [53]. In this treatment modality, the use of a fixed frame entails completing the treatment in one day with a single fraction. Hypofractionated SRS may be useful for protecting the visual nerve and neuroendocrine function [58].

6.3.3 Fractionated stereotactic radiotherapy

Fractionated stereotactic conformal radiotherapy was developed to provide more localized irradiation administered in fractions over weeks with a steeper dose gradient between the tumor and surrounding normal structures compared to conventional radiotherapy [54]. This method has been found as effective and safe adjuvant therapy in the treatment of cystic CPs [55, 56].

6.3.4 Intracavitary irradiation

Stereotactic intracavitary brachytherapy with injection of colloidal phosphorus-32 (P-32) is a minimally invasive treatment modality for patients with cystic CP, resulting in improvement of symptoms and cyst regression [59, 60]. Some reports suggested that stereotactic intracavitary irradiation should be considered as the initial surgery for cystic CPs since it seems a safe and effective treatment [59, 60].

6.4 Chemotherapy

Chemotherapy is an option of adjuvant therapy in cases of multiple recurrences of CP despite surgical and radiotherapeutic treatments. Systemic chemotherapy includes vincristine, procarbazine, cisplatin, etoposide, anthracyclines (Adriamycin/doxorubicin), and nitrourea-derivates (BCNU, CCNU/lomustine) can be administered at six weeks intervals and found to be effective in preventing recurrence [61–63].

In cases of subtotal resection, injection of some chemotherapeutical agents such as bleomycin, and interferon alpha into the remaining tumor has been also introduced as a postoperative adjuvant therapy [64–68]. The intratumoral chemotherapy was found to reduce the volume of cystic CPs, and was considered a new therapeutic alternative, proposed to be more advantageous than total excision for cystic-type CPs; [64–69] still, it is not without serious risks of side effects due to its probable toxicity on deep brain structures [70].

7. Outcomes and prognosis

CPs may behave aggressively despite their benign histological nature. Tumor recurrence is very common because of their location and tendency to invasion into surrounding structures, such as the hypothalamus, pituitary gland, and optic apparatus, which makes total resection difficult [18]. Even after complete resection and radiotherapy, CPs have a propensity to recur. Most recurrences appear during the first five years following the first surgery, and during the first three years following repeated surgery [29]. Recurrence rates were reported between 5% and 59% in some series [24, 71].

The recurrence rate and outcomes are mainly dependent on the extent of surgical resection. Katz [72] reported the surgical outcomes of a case series of 34 surgically treated for the first time and 24 reoperated patients with CP. In their series, they noted 74% of cure rate without recurrence after radical primary excision and 16% of cure after reoperation. In the follow-up of 31 living patients of this series, the quality of survival was reported as 39% excellent, 29% good, 29% fair, and 3% poor [72]. In another study among patients with limited surgery (biopsy or removal of less than 25% of the tumor) followed by conventional radiotherapy, the outcomes were good in 50%, poor in 43%, and death in 7% [73]. Yaşargil [24] reported 90% complete resection, with 16% mortality and 7% recurrence rates in their case series of 144 CPs, suggesting that primary total removal of CPs yields the best long-term outcome for the patients.

Perioperative mortality rates were reported between 0% and 25% with higher rates in repeated surgeries [24, 29, 72]. Overall, one- and three-year survival rates are 91% and 86%, respectively [18].

Some studies suggested some potential predictor factors for poor prognosis including histopathological subtype of adamantinous pattern, higher proliferative index (MIB-1/Ki67 > 7%), nuclear atypia, hyperchromatic nuclei of basaloid cells, vascular invasion, coagulative necrosis, and p53 expression pattern [3, 71, 74]. Younger age, smaller tumor size, subtotal resection, and radiation therapy were associated with prolonged survival [17, 18].

The quality of life during follow-up after surgery is closely associated with the extent of removal during surgery. Total and near total resections have more risks of complications, such as hypothalamic syndrome (intellectual impairment, increased appetite, and weight gain) and hypopituitarism (hypogonadism, growth hormone deficiency, hypothyroidism, and hypocortisolemia) [51, 75, 76]. Furthermore, the incidence of CSF leak is much higher after EEA, reaching up to 58% [49].

8. Conclusions

CPs are histopathologically benign, but clinically aggressive suprasellar masses arising from Rathke's pouch. Despite its rarity overall, it is the most common non-glial brain tumor in childhood. It may present with visual and endocrine disturbances, growth retardation, secondary sexual dysfunction, weight gain, polyuria, headache, nausea, and vomiting. aCPs are lobulated, calcified, cystic with cholesterol-rich fluid, and infiltrative lesions; while pCPs are mostly solid, without significant infiltration to the surrounding tissue. Although the management of CPs is controversial, the current consensus is that surgical resection is the first-line therapy for primary and recurrent tumors, while radiation therapy and chemotherapy should be considered adjuvant treatments for subtotal or limited resected and recurrent tumors. Based on individual characteristics and selection criteria; pterional, transsfenoidal, transcallosal, or transcortical-transventricular approaches may be preferred for surgery. Radiation therapy includes the options of conventional radiotherapy, stereotactic radiosurgery, or intracavitary irradiation. Finally, if needed, chemotherapy can be administered intravenously or intralesionally. Owing to the advances in diagnostic and treatment modalities, the outcomes and survival rates have increased despite their inclination to recur.

Acknowledgements

No financial support or benefits have been received by any of the authors from any commercial source which is related directly or indirectly to the scientific work presented.

Conflict of interest

The authors declare no conflict of interest between any person/persons or institution/institutions and the authors in this study. The materials used in the study are extracted from the archives of the authors and have not been published before. The authors declare no conflict of interest for the materials used in the study.

DOI: http://dx.doi.org/10.5772/intechopen.106635

Author details

Gökhan Kurt[1] and Ayfer Aslan[2*]

1 Gazi University Faculty of Medicine, Ankara, Turkey

2 Hitit University Faculty of Medicine, Erol Olçok Training and Research Hospital, Çorum, Turkey

*Address all correspondence to: ayferaslan86@gmail.com

References

[1] Louis DN, Perry A, Wesseling P, Brat DJ, Cree IA, Figarella-Branger D, et al. The 2021 WHO classification of tumors of the central nervous system: A summary. Neuro-Oncology. 2021;**23**:1231-1251

[2] Müller HL, Merchant TE, Warmuth-Metz M, Martinez-Barbera J-P, Puget S. Craniopharyngioma. Nature Reviews. Disease Primers. 2019;**5**:75

[3] Nishi T, Kuratsu J, Takeshima H, Saito Y, Kochi M, Ushio Y. Prognostic significance of the MIB-1 labeling index for patient with craniopharyngioma. International Journal of Molecular Medicine. 1999;**3**:157-161

[4] Wang F, He Y, Li C, Wang Y, Zhong L. Malignant craniopharyngioma: A report of seven cases and review of the literature. World Neurosurgery. 2020;**135**:e194-e201

[5] Mezmezian MB, Fernandez Ugazio G, Paparella ML. Histopathological features of malignant craniopharyngioma: Case report and literature review. Clinical Neuropathology. 2020;**39**:25-31

[6] Gao S, Shi X, Wang Y, Qian H, Liu C. Malignant transformation of craniopharyngioma: Case report and review of the literature. Journal of Neuro-Oncology. 2011;**103**:719-725

[7] Kristopaitis T, Thomas C, Petruzzelli GJ, Lee JM. Malignant craniopharyngioma. Archives of Pathology & Laboratory Medicine. 2000;**124**:1356-1360

[8] Sofela AA, Hettige S, Curran O, Bassi S. Malignant transformation in craniopharyngiomas. Neurosurgery. 2014;**75**:306-314

[9] Ishida M, Hotta M, Tsukamura A, Taga T, Kato H, Ohta S, et al. Malignant transformation in craniopharyngioma after radiation therapy: A case report and review of the literature. Clinical Neuropathology. 2010;**29**:2-8

[10] Lauriola L, Doglietto F, Novello M, Signorelli F, Montano N, Pallini R, et al. De novo malignant craniopharyngioma: Case report and literature review. Journal of Neuro-Oncology. 2011;**103**: 381-386

[11] Signorelli F, D'Alessandris QG, Maira G, Pallini R, Lauretti L. Letter: Malignant craniopharyngioma and radiotherapy: The missing link. Neurosurgery. 2015;**76**:E358-E359

[12] Elarjani T, Alhuthayl MR, Alhindi H, Kanaan IN. The effect of radiation therapy and chemotherapy on malignant craniopharyngioma: A review. Surgical Neurology International. 2021;**12**:539

[13] Danziger A, Price HI. Protean appearance of craniopharyngioma on computed tomography. South African Medical Journal. 1979;**55**:338-339

[14] Salzman KL, Osborn AG. Sellar neoplasms and tumor-like lesions. In: Osborn AG, Hedlund G, Salzman KL, editors. Osborn's Brain: Imaging, Pathology, and Anatomy. 2nd ed. Philadelphia: Elsevier; 2018. pp. 771-818

[15] May JA, Krieger MD, Bowen I, Geffner ME. Craniopharyngioma in childhood. Advanced in Pediatrics. 2006;**53**:183-209

[16] Rickert CH, Paulus W. Epidemiology of central nervous system tumors in

childhood and adolescence based on the new WHO classification. Child's Nervous System. 2001;**17**:503-511

[17] Bunin GR, Surawicz TS, Witman PA, Preston-Martin S, Davis F, Bruner JM. The descriptive epidemiology of craniopharyngioma. Journal of Neurosurgery. 1998;**89**:547-551

[18] Zacharia BE, Bruce SS, Goldstein H, Malone HR, Neugut AI, Bruce JN. Incidence, treatment and survival of patients with craniopharyngioma in the surveillance, epidemiology and end results program. Neurology and Oncology. 2012;**14**:1070-1078

[19] Larkin SJ, Ansorge O. Pathology and pathogenesis of craniopharyngiomas. Pituitary. 2013;**16**:9-17

[20] Crotty TB, Scheithauer BW, Young WFJ, Davis DH, Shaw EG, Miller GM, et al. Papillary craniopharyngioma: A clinicopathological study of 48 cases. Journal of Neurosurgery. 1995;**83**:206-214

[21] Wang K-C, Hong SH, Kim S-K, Cho B-K. Origin of craniopharyngiomas: Implication on the growth pattern. Child's Nervous System. Official Journal of the International Society for Pediatric Neurosurgery. 2005;**21**:628-634

[22] Hoffman HJ. Surgical management of craniopharyngioma. Pediatric Neurosurgery. 1994;**21**(Suppl. 1):44-49

[23] Magill ST, Jane JA, Prevedello DM. Craniopharyngioma classification. Journal of Neurosurgery. 2021;**135**: 1293-1295

[24] Yaşargil MG, Curcic M, Kis M, Siegenthaler G, Teddy PJ, Roth P. Total removal of craniopharyngiomas. Approaches and long-term results in 144 patients. Journal of Neurosurgery. 1990;**73**:3-11

[25] Kassam AB, Gardner PA, Snyderman CH, Carrau RL, Mintz AH, Prevedello DM. Expanded endonasal approach, a fully endoscopic transnasal approach for the resection of midline suprasellar craniopharyngiomas: A new classification based on the infundibulum. Journal of Neurosurgery. 2008;**108**:715-728

[26] Jamshidi AO, Beer-Furlan A, Prevedello DM, Sahyouni R, Elzoghby MA, Safain MG, et al. A modern series of subdiaphragmatic craniopharyngiomas. Journal of Neurosurgery. 2018;**131**:526-531

[27] Fan J, Liu Y, Pan J, Peng Y, Peng J, Bao Y, et al. Endoscopic endonasal versus transcranial surgery for primary resection of craniopharyngiomas based on a new QST classification system: A comparative series of 315 patients. Journal of Neurosurgery. 2021;**2021**:1-12

[28] Lubuulwa J, Lei T. Pathological and topographical classification of craniopharyngiomas: A literature review. Journal of Neurological and Surgical Report. 2016;**77**:e121-e127

[29] Bao Y, Pan J, Qi S-T, Lu Y-T, Peng J-X. Origin of craniopharyngiomas: Implications for growth pattern, clinical characteristics, and outcomes of tumor recurrence. Journal of Neurosurgery. 2016;**125**:24-32

[30] Zhou Z, Zhang S, Hu F. Endocrine disorder in patients with craniopharyngioma. Frontiers in Neurology. 2 Dec 2021;**12**:737743

[31] Okada T, Fujitsu K, Ichikawa T, Mukaihara S, Miyahara K, Kaku S, et al. Coexistence of adamantinomatous and squamous-papillary type

craniopharyngioma: Case report and discussion of etiology and pathology. Neuropathology. 2012;**32**:171-173

[32] Zhu X, Gleiberman AS, Rosenfeld MG. Molecular physiology of pituitary development: Signaling and transcriptional networks. Physiological Reviews. 2007;**87**:933-963

[33] Apps JR, Martinez-Barbera JP. Molecular pathology of adamantinomatous craniopharyngioma: Review and opportunities for practice. Neurosurgical Focus. 2016;**41**:E4

[34] Brastianos PK, Taylor-Weiner A, Manley PE, Jones RT, Dias-Santagata D, Thorner AR, et al. Exome sequencing identifies BRAF mutations in papillary craniopharyngiomas. Nature Genetics. 2014;**46**:161-165

[35] Kassab C, Zamler D, Kamiya-Matsuoka C, Gatalica Z, Xiu J, Spetzler D, et al. Genetic and immune profiling for potential therapeutic targets in adult human craniopharyngioma. Clinical Oncological Research. 2019;**2**:2-8

[36] Buslei R, Nolde M, Hofmann B, Meissner S, Eyupoglu IY, Siebzehnrübl F, et al. Common mutations of beta-catenin in adamantinomatous craniopharyngiomas but not in other tumours originating from the sellar region. Acta Neuropathologica. 2005;**109**:589-597

[37] Sekine S, Shibata T, Kokubu A, Morishita Y, Noguchi M, Nakanishi Y, et al. Craniopharyngiomas of adamantinomatous type harbor beta-catenin gene mutations. The American Journal of Pathology. 2002;**161**:1997-2001

[38] Zhang Y, Chen C, Tian Z, Xu J. Discrimination between pituitary adenoma and craniopharyngioma using MRI-based image features and texture features. Japanese Journal of Radiology. Dec 2020;**38**(12):1125-1134

[39] Pusey E, Kortman KE, Flannigan BD, Tsuruda J, Bradley WG. MR of craniopharyngiomas: Tumor delineation and characterization. AJR. American Journal of Roentgenology. 1987;**149**:383-388

[40] Choi SH, Kwon BJ, Na DG, Kim J-H, Han MH, Chang K-H. Pituitary adenoma, craniopharyngioma, and Rathke cleft cyst involving both intrasellar and suprasellar regions: Differentiation using MRI. Clinical Radiology. 2007;**62**:453-462

[41] Trippel M, Nikkhah G. Stereotactic neurosurgical treatment options for craniopharyngioma. Frontier in Endocrinology (Lausanne). 2012;**3**:63

[42] Inenaga C, Kakita A, Iwasaki Y, Yamatani K, Takahashi H. Autopsy findings of a craniopharyngioma with a natural course over 60 years. Surgical Neurology. 2004;**61**:536-540

[43] Vlajic I, Wappenschmidt J, Nocke-Finck L. Observation of the course of craniopharyngioma. Neurochirurgia (Stuttg). 1976;**19**:260-264

[44] Rhoton D. The Sellar Region. Neurosurgery. 2002;**51**:S335-S374

[45] Patterson RHJ, Danylevich A. Surgical removal of craniopharyngiomas by the transcranial approach through the lamina terminalis and sphenoid sinus. Neurosurgery. 1980;**7**:111-117

[46] Buchfelder M, Schlaffer S-M, Lin F, Kleindienst A. Surgery for craniopharyngioma. Pituitary. 2013;**16**:18-25

[47] Busch E. A new approach for the removal of tumors of the third ventricle.

Acta Psychiatrica Scandinavica. 2007;**19**:57-60

[48] Matsuo T, Kamada K, Izumo T, Nagata I. Indication and limitations of endoscopic extended transsphenoidal surgery for craniopharyngioma. Neurologia Medico-Chirurgica (Tokyo). 2014;**54**(Suppl. 3):974-982

[49] Gardner PA, Kassam AB, Snyderman CH, Carrau RL, Mintz AH, Grahovac S, et al. Outcomes following endoscopic, expanded endonasal resection of suprasellar craniopharyngiomas: A case series. Journal of Neurosurgery. Jul 2008;**109**(1):6-16

[50] Lin Y, Hansen D, Sayama CM, Pan I-W, Lam S. Transfrontal and transsphenoidal approaches to pediatric craniopharyngioma: A national perspective. Pediatric Neurosurgery. 2017;**52**:155-160

[51] Chakrabarti I, Amar AP, Couldwell W, Weiss MH. Long-term neurological, visual, and endocrine outcomes following transnasal resection of craniopharyngioma. Journal of Neurosurgery. Apr 2005;**102**(4):650-657

[52] Sankhla SK, Jayashankar N, Khan GM. Extended endoscopic endonasal transsphenoidal approach for retrochiasmatic craniopharyngioma: Surgical technique and results. Journal of Pediatric Neurosciences. 2015;**10**:308-316

[53] Aggarwal A, Fersht N, Brada M. Radiotherapy for craniopharyngioma. Pituitary. 2013;**16**:26-33

[54] Minniti G, Saran F, Traish D, Soomal R, Sardell S, Gonsalves A, et al. Fractionated stereotactic conformal radiotherapy following conservative surgery in the control of craniopharyngiomas. Radiotherapy and Oncology : Journal of the European Society for Therapeutic Radiology and Oncology. 2007;**82**:90-95

[55] Combs SE, Thilmann C, Huber PE, Hoess A, Debus J, Schulz-Ertner D. Achievement of long-term local control in patients with craniopharyngiomas using high precision stereotactic radiotherapy. Cancer. 2007;**109**:2308-2314

[56] Schulz-Ertner D, Frank C, Herfarth KK, Rhein B, Wannenmacher M, Debus J. Fractionated stereotactic radiotherapy for craniopharyngiomas. International Journal of Radiation Oncology, Biology, Physics. 2002;**54**:1114-1120

[57] Burgess L, Chakraborty S, Malone S. Effective salvage of recurrent craniopharyngioma with fractionated stereotactic radiotherapy. Radiological Case Report. 2020;**15**:1750-1755

[58] Iwata H, Tatewaki K, Inoue M, Yokota N, Baba Y, Nomura R, et al. Single and hypofractionated stereotactic radiotherapy with CyberKnife for craniopharyngioma. Journal of Neuro-Oncology. 2012;**106**:571-577

[59] Yu X, Christ SM, Liu R, Wang Y, Hu C, Feng B, et al. Evaluation of Long-Term Outcomes and Toxicity After Stereotactic Phosphorus-32-Based Intracavitary Brachytherapy in Patients With Cystic Craniopharyngioma. International Journal of Radiation Oncology, Biology, Physics. 2021;**111**:773-784

[60] Pollack IF, Lunsford LD, Slamovits TL, Gumerman LW, Levine G, Robinson AG. Stereotaxic intracavitary irradiation for cystic craniopharyngiomas. Journal of Neurosurgery. 1988;**68**:227-233

[61] Lippens RJ, Rotteveel JJ, Otten BJ, Merx H. Chemotherapy with Adriamycin (doxorubicin) and CCNU (lomustine)

in four children with recurrent craniopharyngioma. European Journal of Paediatric Neurology : EJPN : Official Journal of the European Paediatric Neurology Society. 1998;**2**:263-268

[62] Plowman PN, Besser GM, Shipley J, Summersgill B, Geddes J, Afshar F. Dramatic response of malignant craniopharyngioma to cis-platin-based chemotherapy. Should craniopharyngioma be considered as a suprasellar "germ cell" tumour? British Journal of Neurosurgery. 2004;**18**:500-505

[63] Bremer AM, Nguyen TQ, Balsys R. Therapeutic benefits of combination chemotherapy with vincristine, BCNU, and procarbazine on recurrent cystic craniopharyngioma. A case report. Journal of Neuro-Oncology. 1984;**2**:47-51

[64] Dastoli PA, Nicácio JM, Silva NS, Capellano AM, Toledo SRC, Ierardi D, et al. Cystic craniopharyngioma: Intratumoral chemotherapy with alpha interferon. Arquivos de Neuro-Psiquiatria. 2011;**69**:50-55

[65] Takahashi H, Nakazawa S, Shimura T. Evaluation of postoperative intratumoral injection of bleomycin for craniopharyngioma in children. Journal of Neurosurgery. 1985;**62**:120-127

[66] Cavalheiro S, Dastoli PA, Silva NS, Toledo S, Lederman H, da Silva MC. Use of interferon alpha in intratumoral chemotherapy for cystic craniopharyngioma. Child's Nervous System : ChNS : Official Journal of the International Society for Pediatric Neurosurgery. 2005;**21**:719-724

[67] Savas A, Arasil E, Batay F, Selcuki M, Kanpolat Y. Intracavitary chemotherapy of polycystic craniopharyngioma with bleomycin. Acta Neurochirurgica. 1999;**141**:547-548

[68] Cavalheiro S. Use of bleomycin in intratumoral chemotherapy for cystic craniopharyngioma. Case report. Journal of Neurosurgery. 1996;**84**:124-126

[69] Cavalheiro S, di Rocco C, Valenzuela S, Dastoli PA, Tamburrini G, Massimi L, et al. Craniopharyngiomas: Intratumoral chemotherapy with interferon-alpha: A multicenter preliminary study with 60 cases. Neurosurgical Focus. 2010;**28**:E12

[70] Savas A, Erdem A, Tun K, Kanpolat Y. Fatal toxic effect of bleomycin on brain tissue after intracystic chemotherapy for a craniopharyngioma: Case report. Neurosurgery. 2000;**46**:213-217

[71] Szeifert GT, Sipos L, Horváth M, Sarker MH, Major O, Salomváry B, et al. Pathological characteristics of surgically removed craniopharyngiomas: Analysis of 131 cases. Acta Neurochirurgica. 1993;**124**:139-143

[72] Katz EL. Late results of radical excision of craniopharyngiomas in children. Journal of Neurosurgery. 1975;**42**:86-93

[73] Sanford RA. Craniopharyngioma: Results of survey of the American Society of Pediatric Neurosurgery. Pediatric Neurosurgery. 1994;**21**(Suppl. 1): 39-43

[74] Boongird A, Laothamatas J, Larbcharoensub N, Phudhichareonrat S. Malignant craniopharyngioma; case report and review of the literature. Neuropathology. 2009;**29**:591-596

[75] Pierre-Kahn A, Recassens C, Pinto G, Thalassinos C, Chokron S, Soubervielle JC, et al. Social and

psycho-intellectual outcome following radical removal of craniopharyngiomas in childhood. A prospective series. Child's Nervous System. Aug 2005;**21**(8-9):817-824

[76] Symon L, Pell MF, Habib AHA. Radical excision of craniopharyngioma by the temporal route: A review of 50 patients. British Journal of Neurosurgery. 1991;**5**(6):539-549

Chapter 6

Overview of Brain Metastasis and Treatment Modalities

Edwina Ayaaba Ayabilah, Andrew Yaw Nyantakyi and Joseph Daniels

Abstract

Brain metastasis (BM) is the commonest form of intracranial malignancy, historically considered a single disease entity with a gloomy outcome, often resulting in a palliative approach to clinical management. Primary cancers that most frequently spread to the brain are lung, breast, and renal carcinomas as well as malignant melanomas. Global incidence of brain metastasis is on the rise but may still be underestimated. About 67% of patients with BM present with either generalized or focal symptoms and sometimes both. A thorough clinical workup and application of verified prognostic scores lead to optimal stratification and strongly influences therapeutic decisions and patients' outcomes. Management is multidisciplinary and involves symptomatic treatment, use of best supportive care, radiotherapy, surgery as well as targeted therapy.

Keywords: brain metastasis, cancer, brain tumors, neurological symptoms, whole brain radiotherapy, stereotactic radiosurgery

1. Introduction

Brain metastasis (BM) is the commonest group of intracranial tumors and is considered a direct neurological complication of cancer. It is 10 times more frequent than primary brain neoplasms [1], occurring at a median time of 8.5–12 months from primary diagnosis. About 20–40% of adult cancer patients develop brain metastases, with 40% of these presenting with a limited number of lesions (i.e., 1–4 lesions whereas 60% present with multiple lesions. Brain metastasis is the direct cause of death in 30–50% of cases [2]. Improved cancer survival is one of the key reasons for the rise in prevalence of brain metastasis (Reference). Brain metastasis generally has poor prognosis, causes significant morbidity and is fatal if left untreated. Median survival time ranges from 4.9 to 16.4 months [3]. Localization of brain metastases is influenced by the arterial blood flow distribution with about 80% localized in the cerebral hemispheres, 15% in the cerebellum and 5% in the brainstem [4]. Research has shown a strong correlation between the localization of brain metastases and clinical outcomes, as such infratentorial metastases though not frequent have the worst prognosis [5].

IntechOpen

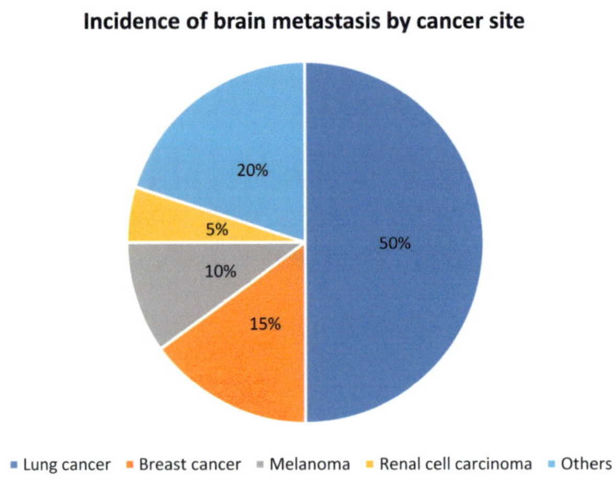

Figure 1.
Distribution of incidence of brain metastasis by cancer site [8].

2. Epidemiology

Population-based studies show global incidence ranging from 8.3 to 14.3 per 100,000 population per year. This is likely underestimated owing to significant inaccuracies associated with these population and pathologic studies [6]. Any type of cancer can metastasize to the brain, however the three commonest primary tumors associated with brain metastases are lung (20–56%), breast (5–20%) and malignant melanomas (7–16%) [2, 6, 7]. Data from the Surveillance, Epidemiology, and End Results (SEER) Program indicate that patients with either small cell lung cancer (SCLC) or non-small cell lung cancer (NSCLC) have the highest rates of brain metastases at diagnosis, whilst patients with malignant melanomas have the highest risk of presenting with metastatic brain disease. By contrast cancers of the prostate, head and neck, skin (non-melanoma skin cancer), and esophagus rarely metastasize to the brain (**Figure 1**) [6].

3. Risk factors

Tumor site and molecular subtype of primary tumors are important factors that influence the risk of distant brain metastases among cancer patients. Some tumors have very high propensity to metastasize to the brain whereas other tumors rarely spread to the brain. For instance, ALK-rearranged NSCLC specifically metastasizes to the brain. Patients with human epidermal growth factor receptor 2 (ERBB2 or HER2) amplification or triple-negative breast cancers (TNBC) have a higher risk of developing brain metastases than those with other molecular subtypes of breast cancer [9]. Other risk factors include advanced age, sex, ethnicity, and geographic location.

4. Pathobiology

The blood-brain barrier (BBB) protects the brain from the effect of chemicals in the blood circulatory system. The BBB maintains normal brain function by tight regulation of transfer of molecules and ions between blood and the brain. The BBB is made up of endothelial cells. Its basement membrane is adjoined by tight cell-to-cell junction proteins with specific transport mechanisms and pinocytic vesicles. The endothelium is further surrounded by cellular elements including pericytes and astroglia foot processes (end foot processes), forming an additional continuous stratum that reinforces the barrier [10]. This barrier permits only small uncharged compounds to diffuse from blood into the brain without a specific transporter.

Metastasis of cancer cells is a multifaceted process that has been simplified in several critical steps. It involves epithelial to mesenchymal transition (EMT) of cancer cells at their primary site, extracellular matrix modulation, intravasation, circulation, extravasation, homing, formation of the premetastatic niche for organotypic colonization and mesenchymal-epithelial transition (MET) at the secondary site. This stepwise process takes into account the interaction between the tumor and the tumor micro-environment, host immunity and secondary site micro-environment.

Multiple hypotheses have been proposed to explain metastatic patterns observed among different primary cancers. Two longstanding theories on the metastatic spread of cancer are the "seed and soil" hypothesis and mechanical theory [11, 12].

The "seed and soil hypothesis" seems to best explain the pathophysiology of brain metastases with the following steps.

1. A normal cell undergoes multiple genetic mutations or epigenetic changes to transform into a malignant cell.

2. The transformed cell proliferates uncontrollably and undergoes angiogenesis.

3. There is invasion of normal tissue stroma and intravasation of tumor cells into blood vessels or lymph channels.

4. Tumor cells in blood vessels overcome the shear stress of blood circulation and evade immune cells.

5. Surviving tumor cells get to the capillary bed and then gain access to arterial circulation.

6. Extravasation and seeding of the brain, usually at the gray-matter/white-matter junction.

7. If the "soil" (brain) microenvironment is favorable, the tumor cells may leave brain capillaries form a metastatic brain lesion.

BM requires synergy between cancer cells and the parenchymal tissue of the central nervous system (CNS). Different primary tumors are characterized by distinct patterns of brain metastasis. Clonal cells of primary tumors undergo a series of genetic changes as they accumulate more and more mutations in their DNA with subsequent divisions and damage of repair mechanisms. This contributes to genomic instability which is associated with the activation of genes that promote abnormal cellular growth and the silencing of genes that regulate the cell cycle. Ultimately, this culminates in the immortalization of cancer cells. This is classically seen in the inactivation of the Retinoblastoma (Rb) protein and destruction of the p53 protein which plays a key role in the pathogenesis of Human Papilloma Virus 16 (HPV 16)-associated head and neck cancers as well as HPV-positive cervical cancers [13]. Mutations downstream from the parent stem cell with subsequent mutations result in a heterogeneous tumor with some cells having the propensity to metastasize. As tumors continue to proliferate and increase in size, increased demand for nutrition and oxygenation to maintain growth triggers angiogenesis. Switch for angiogenesis requires a tip of the balance between pro and anti-angiogenic factors towards the former. This occurs as hypoxia sets in at tumor regions far from blood supply. Under hypoxic conditions, Hypoxia Inducible Factor (HIF) is activated. HIF-1a is stabilized because of the lack of oxygen and dimerizes with HIF-1beta to bind to the hypoxia response element (HRE; 50 -G/ACGTG30). HIF-1 activates the transcription of target genes by interacting with co-activator CBP/p300. These genes regulate and promote glucose transporters and glycolysis, angiogenesis, proliferation, invasion and metastasis [14]. HIF controls the activity of VEGF over-expression promoting angiogenesis; however, blood vessels are poorly formed and defective. Newly formed blood vessels are tortuous and dilated with endothelial cells forming a monolayer and resting on a basement membrane of variable thickness and pericytes forming loose associations of endothelial cells [14, 15]. This results in leakiness of the vessel formed and gives rise to chronic hypoxia in the tumor. This leakiness in the newly formed vasculature also serves as an easy portal for cancer cells to circulate in the bloodstream. HIF-dependent upregulation of transcription repressors of E-cadherin, such as zinc finger protein SNAI1 (SNAIL), twist related protein 1 (TWIST1), transcription factor 3 (TCF3), zinc finger E-box-binding homeobox 1 and 2 (ZEB1 and ZEB2) results in loss of receptors [14, 16]. E-cadherin among others is a major component of adherent junctions that maintain the integrity of the epithelium. This loss is a functional requirement for EMT [14].

EMT is a natural phenomenon that is employed during embryogenesis. Cancer cells employ this principle to aid distant spread. It is a biochemically stimulated process during which epithelial cells acquire a mesenchymal phenotype through EMT transcription factors (these repress epithelial genes and promote mesenchymal genes) [15]. It encompasses changes in multiple phenotypic characteristics including but not limited to apicobasal polarity, cell-cell adhesion, cytoskeleton remodeling and cell-matrix adhesion as well as the gain of mesenchymal markers such as vimentin and alpha smooth muscle actin (αSMA) [16]. All these changes promote the detachment of cancer cells from the parent tumor into the extracellular matrix. Using proteolytic enzymes such as metalloproteinase degrades the extracellular matrix and travels through the extracellular matrix to reach blood and lymphatic vessels [17].

Neo-vascularization by tumor is ineffective as described earlier hence cancer cells easily enter the lumen of blood vessels. In areas where blood vessels do not have the defect of leakiness, intravasation is achieved by use the of enzymes such as heparinase which degrades the basement membrane of vessels and allows cancer cells to enter circulation. Circulation is not a friendly environment for the cell because of host immune system that attacks and lyses these cancer cells. Cancer cells have developed strategies for evasion of host immune defense mechanisms through immune mimicry [15]. This is achieved by upregulating specific receptors such as integrins and protein death ligand 1 (PD-L1) that bind to platelets and host leukocytes to form a complex structure which facilitates immune evasion and also protects cancer cells from mechanical damage [17].

Metastatic tumor cells travel along blood vessels and can get trapped in smaller vessels (end arteries of the brain). Here they adhere to the endothelial lining and have to break through the BBB described earlier. There are various hypotheses that have been generated over the years to explain how this occurs. Three of these hypotheses are; First, tumor adhere to proteins expressed by endothelial cells allowing them to cross the BBB into the perivascular space; Second, tumor cells adhere to systemic immune cells via receptor-ligand interactions and cross through the BBB with the "hijacked" cells; Third, tumor cells modify the endothelial cell wall by stimulating expression of matrix metalloproteases (MMPs), allowing extravasation into the perivascular space [10]. Hereafter there is local extracellular matrix (ECM) remodeling to suit the tumor cells and this is achieved through paracrine interactions between the brain stromal, endothelial wall and invading tumor cells [18]. Proteolytic degradation of the ECM by enzymes such as heparinase concentrated mainly around the region of the advancing cancer cell membrane promotes the breakdown of the endothelial wall into the brain parenchyma. Astedt et al noted urokinase-type plasminogen activator (uPA) is produced and released from cancer cells. Also, tumor associated serine protease plasmin, its activator uPA, the receptor uPA-R (CD87), and plasminogen activator inhibitor type 1 and 2 (PAI-1/2) are linked to cancer invasion and metastasis [19]. At the BBB Urokinase converts the zymogen plasminogen to plasmin, a trypsin-like enzyme with broad substrate specificities. uPA binds to the surface of the cell membrane and causes localized cell surface proteolytic activity, which is required for the destruction of the ECM. PA1-1 modulates the activity of uPa. Plasmin on the other hand activates the other proteolytic enzymes (such as metalloproteases) and degrades components of the ECM as well [18]. In the brain perivascular or parenchymal space, tumor cells adhere for survival through the E-cadherin-catenin complex. This process is a reversal of the epithelial to mesenchymal transition that was seen at the initial stages of metastasis [10]. Through interaction between the tumor cells, ECM and stroma, multiple cytokines, growth factors and enzymes are secreted by microglia and macrophages to promote inflammation, growth and survival of the tumor cells. For instance, vascular endothelial factor (VEGF) promotes angiogenesis, epidermal growth factor (EGF) promotes tumor proliferation and matrix metalloproteases promotes further invasion of tumor cells in the brain. Vessels are poorly formed in this process as described earlier and this results in leakage of water, proteins, and inflammatory mediators at the site of metastasis resulting in edema (perilesional edema as seen on imaging studies).

Specifically in malignant melanoma, expression of programmed death ligand 1 (PD-L1) by microglia promotes invasion of tumor cells and inhibits cytotoxic T cell activity [20]. Furthermore, there is production of proinflammatory chemokine CXCL10 and release of Interleukin 23 (IL-23) as a result of interaction between tumor cells and astrocytes. CXCL10 chemokine attracts T lymphocyte cells as well as tumor cells via CXC3R. Thus, malignant melanoma is the seed and astrocytes make the brain a suitable soil for metastasis. Both malignant melanoma and neural cells originate from neural crest cells hence express neurotrophin receptors (such as P75NRT and TrkC) [21]. This is regulated by neural growth factor (NGF) and neurotrophin 3 secreted by astrocytes and resulting in promoting invasion [20].

Brain tissue uniquely appears to downregulate the expression of the tumor suppressor "phosphatase and tensin homolog" (PTEN) culminating in the growth of tumor in the brain microenvironment in lung cancer. MicroRNA (specifically miR-19) released from astrocytes plays a role in downregulating PTEN expression in invading tumor cells [22]. Over-expression of a disintegrin and metalloprotease 9 (ADAM9) protein promotes migration and expression of integrin 1 on lung cancer cells. This results in adhesion to endothelial cells. It may also increase the activity of tissue plasminogen activator (tPA) culminating in angiogenesis, tumor invasion and proliferation [23]. The chemokine CXCL12 binds the G-protein-coupled receptor

CXCR4 and stimulates the pathways leading to chemotaxis, enhanced intracellular calcium, tumor growth, invasion, homing, angiogenesis and metastasis [24].

In breast cancer, activation of the AKT/MAPK signaling pathway stimulates upregulation of interleukin 6 and 8 (IL-6 and IL-8), B-cell lymphoma 2L1 (BCL2L1), TWIST1, and glutathione S-transferase A5 (GSTA5) anti-apoptotic genes that are responsible for breast cancer metastases to the brain [25]. Phospholipid-binding proteins such as annexin A1 (ANXA1 or lipocortin) ignite CXCR4- mediated migration of breast cancer cells in response to stromal cell derived factor 1α (SDF-1α) which incorporates with CXCR4 [26]. This promotes penetration of breast cancer cells into human brain microvascular endothelial cells [27].

Wyler et al. studied the chemokine and chemoreceptors in 246 autopsy specimens that could explain the frequency and patterns of brain metastasis in renal cell carcinoma (RCC) at autopsy [28]. In all, 15% of the sample had brain metastasis. CXCR4 expression levels were 85.7% and 91.7% in primary RCC and brain metastases respectively. CCR2 and CCL7 expression were 52.1% and 75% respectively metastatic brain cells as compared with primary tumors (15.5% and 16.7%, respectively; $P<0.0001$ each). CD68+ tumor-associated macrophages (TAMs) were similar in primary RCC and brain metastases. However, TAMs were more frequently CCR2-positive in brain metastases than in primary RCC ($P < 0.001$) [28]. This further confirms the changes seen in chemokine and chemoreceptor expression seen in metastatic brain tumor cells.

There is uneven distribution of metastatic lesions in the brain. This distribution is partly explained by the tissue volume in these areas. The lesions are distributed along the grey-white matter junctions and tumor emboli lodges in capillary beds with smaller diameter (thus the watershed distribution). However, it should be noted that the within the cerebral hemisphere, distribution in the frontal and parietal region is higher than the temporal and occipital region as related to the mass of these regions. In the cerebrum, some literature have suggested that the Batson venous plexus via a retrograde pathway through the basilar plexus of veins plays a role in the preferential metastasis of abdominal and pelvic primary lesions [29]. The incidence of vertebral bone metastasis also via this pathway is well documented in literature for prostate, renal, breast, lung and colon cancers [30].

Stephen Paget first proposed that metastatic development was a consequence of particular tumor cells ('seeds') finding a suitable environment ('soil') in order to develop and grow. James Ewing on the other hand proposed that circulatory patterns between the primary tumor and specific secondary organs are sufficient to explain the majority of organ-specific metastatic spread thus the mechanical hypothesis. Interplay between tumor molecular, epigenetic, genetic factors and that of secondary site all contribute to the metastasis of specific tumors to the brain. Presented here is a brief overview of this in-depth picture.

5. Clinical presentation

The clinical manifestation of distant metastatic brain lesions is associated with a wide array of signs and symptoms that are influenced by the region of the brain involved as well as the extent of peritumoral edema. There is a need for high index of suspicion among cancer patients because some of these symptoms can be as vague as mild headaches or mood changes and may be easily taken for granted. Some lesions may be asymptomatic and discovered as incidental findings on brain imaging studies done for other unrelated reasons. Progression of intraparenchymal metastasis may lead to leptomeningeal spread [31]. Leptomeningeal spread occurs in both adults and children especially those with acute leukemia and lymphomas. Intracranial metastasis can present as hemorrhagic or cystic lesions on imaging. The former is likely to occur in cancer types such as renal cell carcinoma, choriocarcinoma, thyroid carcinoma as well as malignant melanoma whereas the latter is predominantly associated with gastro-intestinal malignancies. Common signs and symptoms presented by patients include the following.

5.1 Headache

Headache is a common presenting complaint among 32% - 54% of cancer patients who are diagnosed with brain metastasis [31, 32]. As many as 71% of brain neoplasms are associated with tension headache. Under normal physiologic conditions, the brain is largely insensate demonstrated in neurosurgical procedures in which stimulation of the brain parenchyma in awake patients caused no pain. Projections from the trigeminal [33] and upper cervical dorsal root ganglia innervate the pial, dural, and extracranial blood vessels. Therefore, metastatic brain lesions with their associated peritumoral edema cause pressure and stretching of the pia and dura matter resulting in stimulation of the unmyelinated C fibers (afferent neurons). These fibers transmit the nociceptive information mediated by glutamate through the trigeminal ganglia to synapses on second-order neurons within the trigeminal nucleus. Headache associated with increased ICP typically worsens in the morning and is aggravated with coughing, carotid massage, or Valsalva maneuver. Multiple brain lesions and localization in the posterior cranial fossa are associated with more frequent headaches.

5.2 Increased intracranial pressure (ICP)

The skull bone provides a fixed space that accommodates a person's brain tissue and associated meninges, CSF and vasculature. The presence of a lesion that is increasing size increases the ICP in this fixed space. As a result, there are symptoms that occur due to increased ICP such as altered level of consciousness (confusion), headache, nausea, vomiting and visual disturbance in the form of blurred vision or diplopia. Vomiting is more common with children than adults.

5.3 Seizure

Seizures are potential life-threatening complications of brain metastases; and are a presenting symptom in up to 40% of patients [34]. The risk of developing a seizure is influenced by the tumor type, the location and its proximity to the cortical gray-matter. Prophylactic anticonvulsants are not recommended for routine use by the ASCO guidelines in patients with brain metastases who have not undergone surgical resection and who are otherwise seizure free. It's routine use in the post craniotomy setting for seizure-free patients with brain metastases is not recommended either (Level 3 evidence).

5.4 Cerebrovascular accident (CVA)

Hemorrhagic strokes can occur from metastatic brain lesions with intralesional bleeding, vascular invasion, or embolization of tumor cells. Cancers such as malignant melanoma, choriocarcinoma, thyroid and renal carcinoma are associated with this kind of presentation.

5.5 Altered level of consciousness

The reticular activating system (RAS) is a component of the reticular formation, found in the brainstem. The reticular formation receives afferent neurons from the spinal cord, sensory pathways, thalamus, and cortex and has efferent connections throughout the nervous system. The RAS is composed of four groupings of nuclei namely locus coeruleus, raphe nuclei, posterior tuberomammillary hypothalamus and pedunculopontine tegmentum. The locus coeruleus is located within the upper dorsolateral pons [35] whiles raphe nuclei are located midline throughout the brainstem within the pons, midbrain, and medulla [36]. The tuberomammillary nucleus is located within the posterior aspect of the hypothalamus [37]. The lateral and dorsal pedunculopontine tegmentum lies within the midbrain and pons [38]. Each is unique in the neuropeptides they release, however these centers are largely activated by the lateral hypothalamus (LH), via the release of the neuropeptide orexin in response to the light hitting the eyes, which then stimulates arousal and the transition from sleep to waking [39]. Disruption and inactivation of the intricate network of the RAS decreases the release of neurotransmitters (serotonin, histamine, norepinephrine and nitric oxide) needed for arousal and wakefulness. This results in altered level of consciousness manifested by inattentiveness, drowsiness, decreased cognition, memory impairment, confusion and even hallucinations.

5.6 Focal neurological symptoms

Focal neurological symptoms may manifest on the side of the body opposite to the location of the lesion in the brain. Metastatic brain lesions are usually located in cerebral cortex (80%), cerebellum (15%) and brainstem (5%) [40, 41]. Focal symptoms may manifest as unilateral limb weakness known as Todd's paralysis. Some neurological symptoms are directly dependent on the exact localization of metastatic lesions in the lobes of the brain.

5.6.1 Frontal lobe lesions

Tumor metastasis in the frontal lobe can affect motor function, speech, attention, planning, change in personality and ability to solve problems. Focal weakness is common.

5.6.2 Parietal lobe

Parietal lobe lesions can affect one or several of the core functions of the parietal lobe namely, vision, perception, sensation and spatial-visual coordination. This results in symptoms such as apraxia, right-left confusion, inability to read, write or complete simple calculations.

5.6.3 Temporal lobe

Important cerebral structures in the temporal lobe include the hippocampus, auditory cortex as well as Wernicke's area. Lesions in the temporal lobe may affect the function of these structures leading to receptive aphasia, impaired speech recognition and inability to store new memories.

5.6.4 Occipital lobe

The occipital lobes house's the visual cortex. Metastatic lesions affecting this lobe can result in hemianopsia or cortical blindness.

6. Clinical workup

The initial workup of patients with metastatic brain lesions must include a complete history and physical examination. Immediate relatives and close friends are also a good source of information concerning changes in mental state which the patient may not appreciate as important. During this exercise, the clinician probes into the onset and clinical course of symptoms as well as any history of a previous diagnosis of cancer, previous surgeries and their indication and biopsy taken. A high index of suspicion is present if patient has a known history of cancer and presents with a change in mentation. Physical examination is performed to document firstly the patient's current neurologic deficit and this serves as a baseline for assessment to treatment responds later.

Imaging studies help to confirm a lesion in the brain. Magnetic resonance imaging (MRI) with a gadolinium (Gd)-containing contrast agent is the imaging modality of choice for brain metastasis. Gd-based contrast leaks into parenchyma in areas with BBB breakdown, and the paramagnetic properties of Gd generate hyperintense signal on T1 weighted images. These images are better at demonstrating the anatomy and areas of contrast enhancement just like a contrast enhanced CT scan (which in place of MRI is helpful in a low resource setting) however a better tumor delineation is seen on MRI. T2 weighted and FLAIR images are more sensitive for detecting edema and tumor infiltration.

Computed tomography (CT) scan can be used in situations in which MRI is contraindicated, such as implanted pacemaker, metal fragment or metallic implants. In low-resource countries, a Ct scan done in a planning position saves cost as this can be used to confirm diagnosis radiologically and for radiation treatment. A biopsy of the primary lesion and further immunohistochemistry is essential in the management of brain metastasis as this helps determine the choice of treatment and may predict the responds to treatment.

Examination of blood and serum should include full blood count, renal and liver function tests, and, if any risk factors are present such as HIV antibody status.

7. Prognostic classification

Prognostic classification of brain metastatic disease patients has important implications for patient education and choice of treatment approach. A recursive partitioning analysis of 1200 patients enrolled in one of three consecutive Radiation Therapy Oncology Group (RTOG) trials established three classes (I -III) of patients with different survival estimates based on four key prognostic factors: age, Karnofsky performance status (KPS), evidence of control of the primary tumor and the status of extracranial metastases.

Additional prognostic classification systems have provided an initial framework for estimating a patient's overall survival. These systems include firstly, the Score

Index for Radiosurgery (SIR), which was developed for the classification of patients undergoing Stereotactic radiosurgery (SRS) and hence placed importance on the number and the volume of brain metastases [42]. Secondly, the Basic Score for Brain Metastases in which Karnofsky Performance Score, control of the primary tumor and presence of extracranial disease are used to estimate survival [43].

8. Management

The management of metastatic brain disease requires a multimodality approach involving radiation oncologists, neurosurgeons, neurologists and clinical psychologists amongst others. Treatment options for brain metastases include whole brain radiation therapy (WBRT), stereotactic radiosurgery (SRS), conventional surgery, and systemic therapies (chemotherapy, immunotherapy).

8.1 General management

The general management of patients with metastatic brain lesions includes control of increased intracranial pressure (ICP) and seizures. ICP is due the lesion growing in a fixed space with associated perilesional edema. This manifests as headaches, blurred vision or diplopia, nausea, vomiting and seizures as seen in primary brain lesions. If left unresolved increased ICP can eventually result in coning. Steroids are employed to control the neurologic signs and symptoms associated with cerebral edema caused by metastatic brain lesions.

Kofman first used prednisone for the management of perilesional edema due to brain metastasis in 1957 [44]. Years afterwards, dexamethasone revolutionized care of brain lesions by alleviating cerebral edema. Dexamethasone like other glucocorticoids interacts with the glucocorticoid receptor (GR) which is encoded by a gene located on chromosome 5 [45]. Ligand binding of GR can result in a direct induction or repression of target gene expression and this in turn gives rise to a multitude of steroid exerted effects. The result is a reduction of perilesional edema and a decrease in the permeability of the blood brain barrier [46]. Though there are other medications in this group, dexamethasone is the most commonly used. It has a biological half-life of more than 30 hours with minimal mineralocorticoid effect as compared to hydrocortisone, prednisone, cortisone and methylprednisolone [45]. Steroids are metabolized in the liver in a cytochrome P450-dependent manner therefore a p450 inducer affects the bioavailability of the medication as seen in combined use with anti-seizure medication such as phenytoin carbamazepine and phenobarbital [47]. Non-enzyme-inducing anticonvulsants, such as levetiracetam, lacosamide, lamotrigine, and pregabalin, are preferred in the management of seizures associated with brain metastasis.

Veicht et al in a randomized trial compared 8 mg dexamethasone versus 16 mg dexamethasone or 4 mg versus 16 mg in patients with brain metastases [48]. A similar improvement of the Karnofsky performance status was observed in all groups. However, side effects were significantly more frequent in patients treated with 16 mg dexamethasone per day. Steroids can be stopped without tapering down for a short period of time however prolonged administration lasting for weeks or months requires tapering over a longer period of time to avoid hypocortisolism due to suppression of adrenal function [49]. Effects of long-term use of steroids include osteoporosis, steroid-induced diabetes, myopathy, thromboembolic event, psychiatric disorders and immunosuppression. Furthermore, Patients on glucocorticoids may experience symptoms of gastric irritation which may not translate into an increased risk of peptic ulcer disease (PUD) with only 0.4% of this group developing it [50]. However, the combination of glucocorticoids with nonsteroidal anti-inflammatory medication increases the risk for PUD [51]. Proton pump inhibitors are started to counter this effect.

8.2 Radiotherapy

Different types of cancers have different sensitivities to radiation. Small cell lung cancer and germ cell tumors are very sensitive to radiation whereas lung and breast cancers are only moderately sensitive to radiation. Malignant melanoma and renal cell carcinoma are less sensitive to radiation.

8.2.1 WBRT

WBRT involves irradiating the entire brain and is considered to be a standard of care in select patients with diffuse brain metastasis (≥5 brain metastases). It is also considered for patients in whom surgery or stereotactic radiosurgery (SRS) is not recommended, for example, those with leptomeningeal disease, innumerable metastases, low RTOG DS-GPA scores or medical contraindications. It has the advantage of simplicity of delivery and the ability to treat both local and distant intracranial disease. There is no consensus on the optimal dose and fractionation schedule for WBRT, despite multiple studies to determine the optimal delivery.

An updated Cochrane review from 2018 support the use of a biologically effective WBRT doses, with respect to consequences for survival and improvement in neurological function. WBRT dose of 30 Gy in 10 fractions, as opposed to a lower total of 30 Gy in 10 fractions or 37.5 Gy in 15 fractions continue to remain the standard for a vast majority of patients receiving WBRT. Nieder et al. reported the radiographic overall response rate with this fractionation scheme to be 59%. For patients with poor performance status, and/or uncontrolled extracranial disease, a shorter fractionation scheme (e.g., 20 Gy in 5 fractions) or best supportive care can be considered.

A phase III randomized, noninferiority study, the QUARTZ (Quality of Life after Treatment of Brain Metastases) trial, compared the Quality Adjusted Life Years (QALY) between optimal supportive care (OSC) alone and OSC + WBRT (20 Gy in 5 daily fractions) for NSCLC patients with brain metastases unsuitable for resection or stereotactic radiotherapy. OSC consisted of dexamethasone titrated based on patient's symptoms as well as patient access to palliative care clinicians and nurses. Results revealed a difference in mean QALY of 4.7 days (46.4 QALY days for OSC + WBRT vs. 41.7 QALY days for OSC), which was within the prespecified noninferiority margin of 7 days. Overall survival was not significantly different between randomization arms (OSC + WBRT: 9.2 weeks vs. OSC alone: 8.5 weeks). Subgroup analysis suggested a survival benefit in favor of OSC + WBRT for patients younger than 60, KPS ≥ 70, and controlled extracranial primary disease.

The role of surgery and WBRT in patients with a single metastatic lesion in the brain has been demonstrated to improve both OS and local control (LC) in several trials. In a study by Patchell et al, the efficacy of biopsy sampling plus WBRT was compared with that of WBRT and complete resection in 48 patients with a single metastatic lesion in the brain. Both OS (median 40 weeks versus 15 weeks; $P < 0.01$) and local control (median 38 weeks versus 8 weeks; $P<0.005$) were improved with surgical resection [52]. In another study by Noordijk et al. similar outcomes were reported in a trial involving 63 patients randomized to either surgical resection plus WBRT or to WBRT alone (median OS 10 months versus 6 months; P = 0.04), with those with controlled extracranial disease having the best outcomes [53].

Acute adverse effects of WBRT include skin erythema, alopecia, fatigue, serous otitis and an altered sense of smell and taste. Late-onset adverse effects, such as memory loss, confusion and leukoencephalopathy. The late effects are of most concern to patients, caregivers and health care providers. Effects of WBRT on neurocognitive function (NCF) are best assessed using objective psychometric tests such as Hopkins Verbal Learning Tests (HVLT), Controlled Oral Word Association, Grooved Pegboard test, and Trail Making Tests Parts A and B.

Strategies to mitigate neurocognitive decline from WBRT include the use of Memantine (a non-competitive NMDA receptor antagonist that retains activated NMDA receptors in an open-channel state, thus preserving long-term potentiation) and hippocampal avoidance (HA-WBRT).

In the RTOG 0614 trial, Memantine was started once daily with WBRT and increased to 10 mg twice daily over a few weeks, for a total of 24 weeks. The primary end point was preservation of cognitive function particularly memory function, which was assessed using the revised HVLT (HVLT-R) to measure changes in delayed recall at 24 weeks. Patients in the memantine arm had less decline in performance on HVLT-R delayed recall at 24 weeks: median decline was 0 in the memantine arm versus –0.9 in the placebo arm at 24 weeks, although this difference was not statistically significant (P = 0.059) [54].

8.2.2 Stereotactic radiosurgery

Stereotactic radiosurgery (SRS) is a minimally invasive treatment option in the management of brain metastases with efficacy demonstrated in several randomized trials and multi-institutional studies. It is associated with similarly high efficacy for both radiosensitive and radioresistant tumors. SRS is a preferred option mainly because of the limited area irradiated. It is however limited by its small therapeutic ratio in lesions ≥ 4cm and/or tumor localization in the brainstem. This limitation has recently been solved with the use of fractionated SRS given in 3–7 fractions which typically results in a good therapeutic ratio with high local control rates (75–85%) and lower toxicity rates for large lesions.

SRS can be used alone or as a combined modality with WBRT or surgery. SRS has demonstrated superior local tumor control and functional autonomy for patients with brain metastases when combined with WBRT compared with WBRT alone. Patients with single metastatic brain lesions also experience longer survival with the use of SRS combined with WBRT. The reported survival for patients with RPA prognostic class I is 18–24 months, RPA class II from 9 to 11 months and RPA class III only 3 months.

Postoperative SRS is an alternative to WBRT for patients who undergo resection of brain metastases, with a reduced risk of neurocognitive decline; however, preoperative SRS might be favored given the lower risks of radiation necrosis and leptomeningeal disease. SRS is highly recommended in the American Society of Radiation Oncology (ASTRO) and International Stereotactic Radiosurgery Society (ISRS) consensus guidelines owing to the absence of compromise in survival outcomes with no increase in neurocognitive toxicities, unlike with WBRT. SRS is now the primary treatment for patients with either limited or multiple brain metastases, with potential synergistic effects when combined with certain immunotherapeutic agents or targeted therapies.

8.3 Principles of surgical management

Cancer patients with single metastatic lesions have been shown to benefit more from treatment with surgical resection plus radiotherapy compared to radiotherapy alone. This benefit includes incidence of fewer recurrences, better quality of life and longer overall survival time [52]. Surgery offers rapid and effective symptom control for patients with large tumors or those associated with significant peritumoral edema or mass effect. For patients with active extracranial disease or older age > 60years, surgery has not been shown to provide benefit. Even though age has been identified as a risk factor for high surgery related mortality, it has not been demonstrated to be a strict basis for withholding surgical treatment [53, 55]. Surgical complications encountered include infection, post-op CVA and intracranial bleeding.

Prior to the early nineties, surgery only had a controversial role in the management of brain metastasis. The benefit of surgery as a modality for treatment of brain metastasis was established by two randomized prospective trials published by Patchell et al and Vecht et al. in 1990 and 1994 respectively [48, 51]. Clinical studies show that about 30–50% of all patients with brain metastasis present with multiple lesions [16, 56]. Multiple lesions are known to have poorer prognosis as compared to singular or solitary metastatic brain lesions. Surgery is indicated for patients with single lesions ≤3 cm whereas SRS is preferred for larger lesions [51]. Tumors must be located outside the speech and motor cortices with controlled extracranial disease to be deemed resectable. Surgery is contraindicated for multiple brain lesions and patients who have serious comorbidities as there is no class I evidence in support of surgery among patients with multiple metastatic brain lesions [57].

Microsurgical resection of metastatic brain lesions is effective in relieving brainstem compression and reducing peritumoral edema as well as decreasing ICP caused by "mass effect" of the gross tumor in the brain parenchyma. This translates into improved functional state and overall survival of patients [3, 58, 59]. Microsurgical resection followed by whole brain radiation therapy (WBRT) has been shown to result in prolonged median overall survival compared with WBRT alone in patients with brain metastasis [48, 51]. Furthermore, microsurgical resection results in improvement of neurological function. It enhances quality of life of patients with brain metastasis and may lead to improvement of performance status as evaluated with the Karnofsky score as well as improvement in Recursion Partition Analysis (RPA) score [60]. This benefit is more in elderly patients with symptomatic metastatic brain tumors. Eradication of the gross macroscopic lesion also contributes to the normalization of brain microenvironment further reducing patient's symptoms. Microsurgical brain tumor resection also serves the purpose of tissue sampling for histological, molecular and mutational analysis.

Surgical resection of metastatic brain lesions is associated with a morbidity rate of 2–10%. In the past, this rate was as high as 24.8% [48, 51, 55, 57, 61–65]. The observed reduction in morbidity associated with brain surgery is due to improved surgical techniques, prophylactic anticoagulation, appropriate seizure prophylaxis as well as availability of contemporary imaging modalities [66, 67]. The commonest complications are postoperative hemorrhage (2.7%), pulmonary embolism (2.2%), CSF leakage (0.8%) and cardiovascular accident (0.6%) [61]. Permanent neurological complications range from 6% to 11% [59, 61, 65]. These events are associated more with tumors in eloquent areas of the brain. Contrary to what was previously thought, advanced age > 65 years has not been found to be associated with significantly higher morbidity rate for patients who undergo brain microsurgery [55]. Surgical mortality rates used to be as high as 8–11% but have been shown in recent studies to have improved to about 2–4% [48, 62, 63].

9. Conclusions

BM is a heterogeneous group of diseases with increasing prevalence. The three most common cancers associated with brain metastasis are lung cancer, breast cancer and malignant melanoma. Use of prognostic functional scales such as KPS, RPA and GPA are necessary for the comprehensive evaluation of patients with brain metastasis. Control of extracranial malignant disease is an important survival factor in the management of these patients. The therapeutic decision for each patient must be individualized and a multi-disciplinary approach applied.

Acknowledgements

We wish to express our sincere gratitude to all our friends and loved ones who provided the motivation and encouragement to see this work through to the end.

Conflict of interest

The authors declare no conflict of interest.

Author details

Edwina Ayaaba Ayabilah*, Andrew Yaw Nyantakyi and Joseph Daniels
National Centre for Radiotherapy, Oncology and Nuclear Medicine, Korle Bu Teaching Hospital, Accra, Ghana

*Address all correspondence to: edwina.ayaaba@gmail.com

References

[1] Tsao MN et al. Whole brain radiotherapy for the treatment of newly diagnosed multiple brain metastases. Cochrane Database of Systematic Reviews. 2018;**1**(1):CD003869

[2] Cagney DN et al. Incidence and prognosis of patients with brain metastases at diagnosis of systemic malignancy: A population-based study. Neuro-Oncology. 2017;**19**(11): 1511-1521

[3] Bindal AK et al. Surgery versus radiosurgery in the treatment of brain metastasis. Journal of Neurosurgery. 1996;**84**(5):748-754

[4] Wen PY, Loeffler JS. Management of brain metastases. Oncology. 1999;**13**(7):941-954

[5] Dou Z et al. The infratentorial localization of brain metastases may correlate with specific clinical characteristics and portend worse outcomes based on Voxel-Wise Mapping. Cancers (Basel). 2021;**2021**:13

[6] Martin AM et al. Brain metastases in newly diagnosed breast cancer: A population-based study. JAMA Oncology. 2017;**3**(8):1069-1077

[7] Tabouret E et al. Recent trends in epidemiology of brain metastases: An overview. Anticancer Research. 2012;**32**(11):4655-4662

[8] Lin B et al. Distribution of brain metastases: Low-risk metastasis areas may be avoided when treating with whole-brain radiotherapy. Cancer Imaging. 2020;**20**(1):1-7

[9] Macaluso M, Paggi MG, Giordano A. Genetic and epigenetic alterations as hallmarks of the intricate road to cancer. Oncogene. 2003;**22**(42):6472-6478

[10] Nathoo N et al. Pathobiology of brain metastases. Journal of Clinical Pathology. 2005;**58**(3):237-242

[11] Puduvalli VK. Brain metastases: Biology and the role of the brain microenvironment. Current Oncology Reports. 2001;**3**(6):467-475

[12] Kumar V, Abbas A, Aster J. Robbin's Basic Pathology. 10th ed. Philadelphia: Elsevier; 2017

[13] Lu X, Kang Y. Hypoxia and hypoxia-inducible factors: Master regulators of metastasishypoxia and HIFs in cancer metastasis. Clinical Cancer Research. 2010;**16**(24):5928-5935

[14] Hanahan D, Weinberg RA. Hallmarks of cancer: The next generation. Cell. 2011;**144**(5):646-674

[15] Jolly MK, Celià-Terrassa T. Dynamics of phenotypic heterogeneity associated with EMT and stemness during cancer progression. Journal of Clinical Medicine. 2019;**8**(10):1542

[16] Gavrilovic IT, Posner JB. Brain metastases: Epidemiology and pathophysiology. Journal of Neuro-Oncology. 2005;**75**(1):5-14

[17] Svokos KA, Salhia B, Toms SA. Molecular biology of brain metastasis. International Journal of Molecular Sciences. 2014;**15**:9519-9530

[18] Åstedt B, Holmberg L. Immunological identity of urokinase and ovarian carcinoma plasminogen activator released in tissue culture. Nature. 1976;**261**(5561):595-597

[19] Delattre JY et al. Distribution of brain metastases. Archives of Neurology. 1988;**45**(7):741-744

[20] Salvati L, Mandala M, Massi D. Melanoma brain metastases: Review of histopathological features and immune-molecular aspects. Melanoma Manag. 2020;**7**(2):MMT44

[21] Klein A et al. Astrocytes facilitate melanoma brain metastasis via secretion of IL-23. The Journal of Pathology. 2015;**236**(1):116-127

[22] Zhang L et al. Microenvironment-induced PTEN loss by exosomal microRNA primes brain metastasis outgrowth. Nature. 2015;**527**(7576):100-104

[23] Ebben JD, You M. Brain metastasis in lung cancer: Building a molecular and systems-level understanding to improve outcomes. The International Journal of Biochemistry & Cell Biology. 2016;**78**:288-296

[24] Chatterjee S, Behnam Azad B, Nimmagadda S. The intricate role of CXCR4 in cancer. Advances in Cancer Research. 2014;**124**:31-82

[25] Kim SW et al. Role of the endothelin axis in astrocyte-and endothelial cell-mediated chemoprotection of cancer cells. Neuro-Oncology. 2014;**16**(12):1585-1598

[26] Kim S-J et al. Astrocytes upregulate survival genes in tumor cells and induce protection from chemotherapy. Neoplasia. 2011;**13**(3):286-298

[27] Tayyeb B, Parvin M. Pathogenesis of breast cancer metastasis to brain: A comprehensive approach to the signaling network. Molecular Neurobiology. 2016;**53**(1):446-454

[28] Wyler L et al. Brain metastasis in renal cancer patients: Metastatic pattern, tumour-associated macrophages and chemokine/chemoreceptor expression. British Journal of Cancer. 2014;**110**(3):686-694

[29] Grossman SA, Krabak MJ. Leptomeningeal carcinomatosis. Cancer Treatment Reviews. 1999;**25**(2):103-119

[30] Brook R, Tung K, Oeppen R. Batson's plexus and retrograde venous spread of malignancy—A pictorial review. Cancer Imaging. 2014;**14**(1):1-1

[31] Argyriou A et al. Headache characteristics and brain metastases prediction in cancer patients. European Journal of Cancer Care. 2006;**15**(1):90-95

[32] Chalk J et al. Phenytoin impairs the bioavailability of dexamethasone in neurological and neurosurgical patients. Journal of Neurology, Neurosurgery & Psychiatry. 1984;**47**(10):1087-1090

[33] Mayberg MR, Zervas NT, Moskowitz MA. Trigeminal projections to supratentorial pial and dural blood vessels in cats demonstrated by horseradish peroxidase histochemistry. Journal of Comparative Neurology. 1984;**223**(1):46-56

[34] Tsao MN et al. Radiotherapeutic and surgical management for newly diagnosed brain metastasis(es): An American Society for Radiation Oncology evidence-based guideline. Practical Radiation Oncology. 2012;**2**(3):210-225

[35] Schwarz LA, Luo L. Organization of the locus coeruleus-norepinephrine system. Current Biology. 2015;**25**(21):R1051-R1056

[36] Hornung J-P. The human raphe nuclei and the serotonergic system.

Journal of Chemical Neuroanatomy. 2003;**26**(4):331-343

[37] Xie J-F et al. Inactivation of the tuberomammillary nucleus by GABAA receptor agonist promotes slow wave sleep in freely moving rats and histamine-treated rats. Neurochemical Research. 2017;**42**(8):2314-2325

[38] Vincent SR. The ascending reticular activating system—from aminergic neurons to nitric oxide. Journal of Chemical Neuroanatomy. 2000;**18**(1-2):23-30

[39] Nishino S. Hypothalamus, hypocretins/orexin, and vigilance control. Handbook of Clinical Neurology. 2011;**99**:765-782

[40] Norden AD, Wen PY, Kesari S. Brain metastases. Current Opinion in Neurology. 2005;**18**(6):654-661

[41] Weltman E et al. Radiosurgery for brain metastases: A score index for predicting prognosis. International Journal of Radiation Oncology* Biology* Physics. 2000;**46**(5):1155-1161

[42] Lorenzoni J et al. Radiosurgery for treatment of brain metastases: Estimation of patient eligibility using three stratification systems. International Journal of Radiation Oncology* Biology* Physics. 2004;**60**(1):218-224

[43] Dietrich J et al. Corticosteroids in brain cancer patients: Benefits and pitfalls. Expert Review of Clinical Pharmacology. 2011;**4**(2):233-242

[44] Roth P, Happold C, Weller M. Corticosteroid use in neuro-oncology: An update. Neuro-oncology Practice. 2015;**2**(1):6-12

[45] Salvador E, Shityakov S, Förster C. Glucocorticoids and endothelial cell barrier function. Cell and Tissue Research. 2014;**355**(3):597-605

[46] Weissman DE et al. Twice-daily tapering dexamethasone treatment during cranial radiation for newly diagnosed brain metastases. Journal of Neuro-Oncology. 1991;**11**(3):235-239

[47] Richards GM, Khuntia D, Mehta MP. Therapeutic management of metastatic brain tumors. Critical Reviews in Oncology/Hematology. 2007;**61**(1):70-78

[48] Vecht CJ et al. Dose-effect relationship of dexamethasone on Karnofsky performance in metastatic brain tumors: A randomized study of doses of 4, 8, and 16 mg per day. Neurology. 1994;**44**(4):675-675

[49] Conn H, Poynard T. Corticosteroids and peptic ulcer: Meta-analysis of adverse events during steroid therapy. Journal of Internal Medicine. 1994;**236**(6):619-632

[50] Caplan A et al. Prevention and management of glucocorticoid-induced side effects: A comprehensive review: A review of glucocorticoid pharmacology and bone health. Journal of the American Academy of Dermatology. 2017;**76**(1):1-9

[51] Patchell RA et al. A randomized trial of surgery in the treatment of single metastases to the brain. New England Journal of Medicine. 1990;**322**(8):494-500

[52] Noordijk EM et al. The choice of treatment of single brain metastasis should be based on extracranial tumor activity and age. International Journal of Radiation Oncology* Biology* Physics. 1994;**29**(4):711-717

[53] Johans SJ et al. Identification of preoperative and intraoperative risk

factors for complications in the elderly undergoing elective craniotomy. World Neurosurgery. 2017;**107**:216-225

[54] Brown PD et al. Memantine for the prevention of cognitive dysfunction in patients receiving whole-brain radiotherapy: A randomized, double-blind, placebo-controlled trial. Neuro-Oncology. 2013;**15**(10):1429-1437

[55] Proescholdt M et al. Brain metastases in elderly patients—The role of surgery in the context of systemic treatment. Brain Sciences. 2021;**11**(1):123

[56] Bochev P et al. Brain metastases detectability of routine whole body (18) F-FDG PET and low dose CT scanning in 2502 asymptomatic patients with solid extracranial tumors. Hellenic Journal of Nuclear Medicine. 2012;**15**(2):125-129

[57] Bindal RK et al. Surgical treatment of multiple brain metastases. Journal of Neurosurgery. 1993;**79**(2):210-216

[58] Lamba N et al. Neurosurgical resection and stereotactic radiation versus stereotactic radiation alone in patients with a single or solitary brain metastasis. World Neurosurgery. 2019;**122**:e1557-e1561

[59] Paek SH et al. Reevaluation of surgery for the treatment of brain metastases: Review of 208 patients with single or multiple brain metastases treated at one institution with modern neurosurgical techniques. Neurosurgery. 2005;**56**(5):1021-1034

[60] Nieder C et al. Prognostic factors in brain metastases: Should patients be selected for aggressive treatment according to recursive partitioning analysis (RPA) classes? International Journal of Radiation Oncology* Biology* Physics. 2000;**46**(2):297-302

[61] Schödel P et al. Surgical resection of symptomatic brain metastases improves the clinical status and facilitates further treatment. Cancer Medicine. 2020;**9**(20):7503-7510

[62] Haar F, Patterson RH Jr. Surgery for metastatic intracranial neoplasm. Cancer. 1972;**30**(5):1241-1245

[63] Sundaresan N, Galicich JH. Surgical treatment of brain metastases. Clinical and computerized tomography evaluation of the results of treatment. Cancer. 1985;**55**(6):1382-1388

[64] Pintea B et al. Early motor function after local treatment of brain metastases in the motor cortex region with stereotactic radiotherapy/radiosurgery or microsurgical resection: A retrospective study of two consecutive cohorts. Radiation Oncology. 2017;**12**(1):1-9

[65] Patel CK et al. Trends in peri-operative performance status following resection of high grade glioma and brain metastases: The impact on survival. Clinical Neurology and Neurosurgery. 2018;**164**:67-71

[66] Hatiboglu MA, Akdur K, Sawaya R. Neurosurgical management of patients with brain metastasis. Neurosurgical Review. 2020;**43**(2):483-495

[67] Pan PC, Donovan LE, Magge RS. Supportive Medical Management of Brain Metastases Patients Including Treatment Complications. Berlin, Heidelberg, Germany: Springer International Publishing; 2020. pp. 31-51

Section 3

Childhood Central Nervous System Tumors

Chapter 7

Clinical Profile, Patterns of Care and Outcomes of Childhood CNS Tumours in India

Sujith Kumar Mullapally, Vidyasagar Dusi and Raghunadharao Digumarti

Abstract

Paediatric CNS tumours are the third most common childhood malignancy in India. They account for 14% of all cancers in the 1–14 years age group. There is dearth of adequate prospective or retrospective studies about patterns of care and outcomes. There is male preponderance. Primitive Neuro-ectodermal tumours (PNET) are the most common histology followed by astrocytoma and other gliomas among children from 0 to 19 years. Surgery, radiotherapy, and chemotherapy are the main modalities of treatment. Available data points to underutilisation of radiotherapy in clinical practice due to the fear of non-compliance. Paediatric CNS tumours outcomes are different from adult brain tumours due to their aggressive histology, variable clinical presentations, delay in diagnosis, etc. There is also shortage of adequate multidisciplinary paediatric neuro-oncology units in the country. Future directions include setting up more dedicated paediatric neuro-oncology units, implementation of new 2022 WHO classification by adopting molecular testing across different histology's, use of better radiation technology to prevent long term neurocognitive and other late effects and survivorship clinics to monitor for late effects and rehabilitate the childhood cancer survivors and, perhaps a registry. These issues are discussed in detail in this chapter.

Keywords: CNS, paediatric, brain tumours, clinical profile, multidisciplinary

1. Introduction

Paediatric CNS tumours are defined as tumours of brain, spinal cord, and meninges. Brain tumours form the largest group. Histology and clinical behaviour varies between different brain tumour types and they play a pivotal role in deciding specific treatment plan as per each tumour subtype [1]. Paediatric CNS tumours are among the most common paediatric cancers worldwide after leukaemia. As per GLOBOCAN estimates, there were 30,766 new cases of primary brain and other CNS tumours in children and adolescents aged 0–19 years in 2020, 24,388 of which were in children 0–14 years age.

Also, it was estimated that there were 15,337 deaths due to primary brain and other CNS tumours in children and adolescents age 0–19 years in 2020, 11,889 of which were in children 0–14 years old [2]. Recently, the revised 2021 WHO classification of Tumours of Central Nervous System has reinforced the adoption of molecular subtyping of medulloblastoma and newer paediatric diffuse gliomas have been added to the classification [3].

In India, as per the report of National Cancer Registry Programme (NCRP) 2012–2016 for age group 1–14 yrs., paediatric CNS tumours constitute 6.4% and 7.1% of childhood cancers in boys and girls respectively. Leukaemia and lymphomas constitute 60% of all childhood cancers. Paediatric CNS tumours are the second most common solid tumour in this age group after the bone tumours. Among all CNS childhood tumours 0–19 yrs., Primitive Neuroectodermal tumours (PNET) (37%) are most common followed by astrocytoma (20%) and other gliomas (20%) among both sexes [4].

A 55–120% increase in incidence of childhood brain tumours has been reported in both the sexes in India over the past 25 years from 1978 to 2002. This is most likely due to better neuroimaging facilities [5].

In this chapter, we discuss the clinical profile, patterns of care and clinical outcomes of paediatric CNS tumours in India based on the existing literature. Understanding these salient features will help us to know the current disease burden, treatment practices and in future, to plan prospective studies to improve the care of these childhood tumours.

2. Clinical profile

Multiple retrospective studies and few prospective studies are available regarding clinical profile of paediatric brain tumours. Institutions in the different zones of the country has reported their clinical profiles of paediatric brain tumours which are very much similar [6–10].

Most common symptoms reported are headache (55–90%) often associated with vomiting (35–50%), visual disturbances (35–60%), ataxia, etc., and other symptoms of raised intracranial pressure. Seizures have also been reported as presenting complaint [7, 11].

Increase in intracranial pressure can cause drowsiness, confusion, nausea, sixth nerve palsy, papilledema, generalised seizures, cognitive impairment, etc. There can be symptoms related to impairment of neurohormonal axis at the onset of disease; shortly after surgery or several months to years later following radiotherapy in children with brain tumours. The degree of neurohormonal axis involvement is related to the location of the tumour. The true prevalence of neuroendocrine dysfunction in patients is underestimated as a significant portion of the patient can be asymptomatic for a long time. Due to the radiosensitive nature of hypothalamus and pituitary, there is a higher risk of developing neuroendocrine disorders in patients undergoing RT. Involvement of the hypothalamus can cause hypothalamic syndrome characterised by thirst disorders, increase in appetite, sleep disturbances, impaired temperature regulations etc. Focal signs and symptoms when present reflect the involvement of specific structures directly by tumour or by compression [12]. The other common neuroendocrine disorders seen in children with CNS tumours are Growth hormone deficiency, precocious puberty and diabetes insipidus.

There is a slight male preponderance in all the studies reported as shown in **Table 1**.

Tables 2 and **3** shows the age distribution and clinical presentation reported in various studies.

The most common tumours in paediatric brain tumours are supratentorial tumours in the age group (1–14 years) and among children up to 5 years, infratentorial tumours are the commonest. Though the NCRP data is suggestive of PNET as the most common histology, in different case series, astrocytoma is the most common single histology followed by medulloblastoma and there are variations in the different subsets based on the age groups like 1–5 years, 6–10 years and 11–14 years, etc.

Tables 4 and **5** is a compilation of the location and different frequencies of various histological types of paediatric brain tumours as seen in the published studies respectively.

Table 6 represents the most common types of astrocytoma.

Characteristics	Divya Sree et al. [13]	Govindan et al. [14]	Trivedi et al. [7]	Dwivedi et al. [15]	Madhavan et al. [8]
No. of patients	147	71	50	64	250
Duration of study (In years)	25	5	2	7	5
Mean age (In years)	11.06	8.3	8	13.2	Not specified
M: F ratio	1.1: 1	1: 0.9	1.2: 1	0.7: 1	Not specified

Table 1.
Male: Female ratio of paediatric CNS tumours in various Indian studies.

Age distribution in years	Trivedi et al. [7]	Govindan et al. [14]	Divya Sree et al. [13]	Dwivedi et al. [15]	Madhavan et al. [8]	Total
0–5	15	27	29	8	52	131
6–10	25	21	38	9	91	184
11–18	10	23	80	47	107	267

Table 2.
Age distribution of paediatric CNS tumours in various Indian studies.

Clinical symptom	Madhavan et al. [8]	Dwivedi et al. [15]	Suresh et al. [16]
Headache	61.2%	92.3%	37.5%
Vomiting	53.1%	23.1%	62.5%
Hemiparesis	51%	28.8%	20%
Impaired vision	28.6%	42.3%	35%
Seizures	20.4%	11.5%	2.5%
Incontinence	8.2%	3.8%	5%

Table 3.
Clinical presentation of paediatric CNS tumours in various Indian studies.

Primary site of disease	Study author details			
Location	Divya Sree et al. [13]	Trivedi et al. [7]	Dwivedi et al. [15]	Govindan et al. [14]
	No. of patients	No. of patients	No. of patients	No. of patients
Brain				
Supratentorial				40
Cerebrum	85	09	13	
Ventricles	02	15	02	
Sellar region	03	07	10	
Cranial nerves	0	0	04	
Infratentorial		18		31
Cerebellum	19		14	
Brain stem	03		04	
Spinal Cord		01	10	
Cervical	29			
Thoracic	02			
Lumbar	02			
Sacral	02			

Table 4.
Sites of paediatric CNS tumours in various Indian studies.

Study author	Three most common paediatric CNS tumours		
	1	2	3
Divya Sree et al. [13]	Juvenile pilocytic astrocytoma (37.5%)	Nerve sheath tumours (37.1%)	Embryonal tumours (21.4%)
Govindan et al. [14]	Medulloblastoma (22.5%)	Ependymoma (15.5%)	Pilocytic astrocytoma (14.1%)
Trivedi et al. [7]	Astrocytoma (28%)	Medulloblastoma (26%)	Ependymoma (16%)
Jain et al. [17]	Astrocytoma (34.7%)	Embryonal tumours (22.4%)	Craniopharyngioma (10.2%)
Shah et al. [18]	Astrocytoma (40.8%)	Embryonal tumours (29%)	Craniopharyngioma (11.8%)

Table 5.
Most common paediatric CNS tumours in various Indian studies.

There is sparse date from India on the use of molecular studies for diagnosis of paediatric brain tumours as proposed in the 2016 WHO classification of CNS tumours and recently by 5th edition (WHOCNS5) [19]. A few studies reported the adoption of the molecular subtyping especially in medulloblastoma [20].

Astrocytoma subtype	Jain et al. [17]	Divya Sree et al. [13]	Trivedi et al. [7]	Govindan et al. [14]
Pilocytic	23%	19.2%	35%	14.1%
Diffuse	5.1%	33.3%	28.5%	Not specified
Anaplastic	2.1%	1.2%	14.2%	Not specified
GBM	4.4%	19.2%	NS%	5.6%

Table 6.
Types of astrocytoma in various Indian studies on paediatric CNS tumours.

3. Patterns of care

Multidisciplinary team management in paediatric CNS tumours involves neurosurgery, radiation oncology, paediatric oncology, onco-pathology, neuroradiology, medical social workers, palliative care, and onco-nursing as depicted in the **Figure 1**.

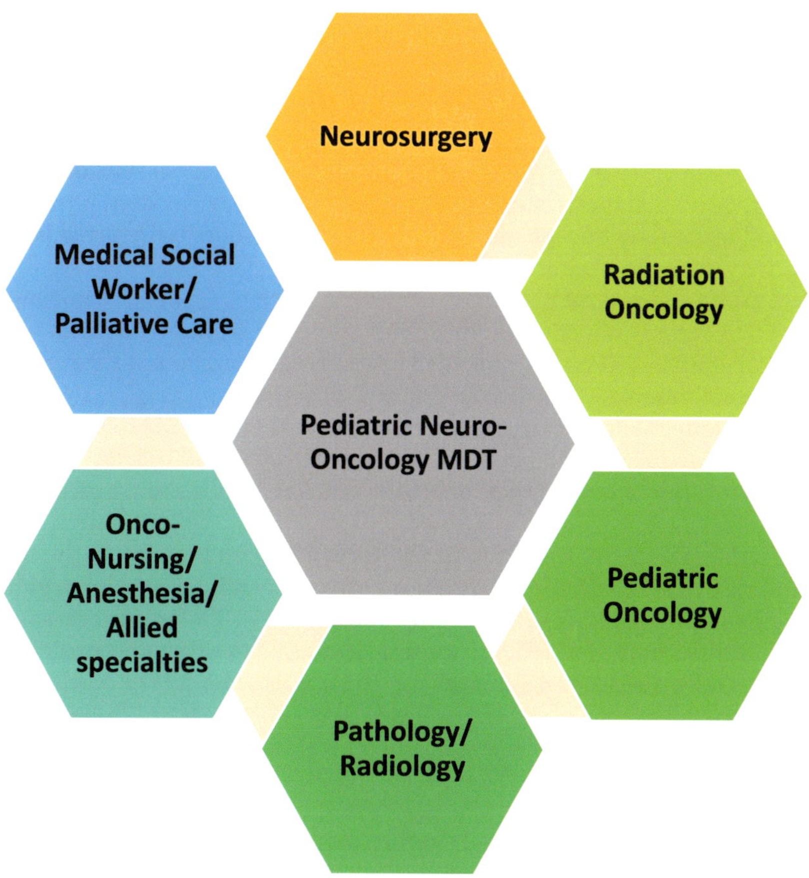

Figure 1.
Components of paediatric neuro-oncology multidisciplinary team.

3.1 Surgery

The initial treatment modality is often surgery. This provides tissue for diagnosis and also is the main curative step in multimodality management. The aim is to achieve complete tumour resection if feasible.

In low grade gliomas, the commonly used surgical approaches depend on the location. A fronto-parietal or temporal craniotomies are done for respective locations. Though the aim is to have total resection of the tumours, preservation of function is also utmost important to have the quality of life preserved. A complete surgical excision is often feasible in non-diencephalic tumours like tumours in cerebral hemispheres and cerebellum.

Brain stem gliomas are another subset of gliomas which are not amenable for surgery because of their eloquent location and their prognosis is guarded. These tumours are observed or often treated with radiotherapy.

In high grade gliomas also, the anatomical location and the likely functional morbidity post-surgery plays an important role in the extent of surgical resection and in all cases, adjuvant radiation therapy preferably with highly precision radiation techniques is used.

PNETs are usually large lesions but can resected most of the times as the plane of cleavage from the surrounding normal structures is good. Blood loss during the resections becomes important and needs to be addressed concomitantly.

Medulloblastomas are located predominantly in the 4th ventricle and there are guidelines regarding the extent of resection. Midline suboccipital craniotomy, transvermian approach is the most common approach used. It is very well known that post-surgery macroscopic residual disease is a poor prognostic factor despite of adjuvant chemotherapy and radiation therapy. In patient presenting with raised intracranial pressure and marked hydrocephalus, CSF diversion procedure is preferred however preoperative ventriculo-peritoneal shunt is generally avoided to prevent seeding of peritoneal cavity and reverse herniation of superior vermis. Optimal maximally safe resection is the surgery of choice for medulloblastoma. Within 24–48 hrs of resection, a postoperative MRI is recommended to assess completeness of the surgery and residual tumour volume.

Newer techniques like endoscopy, stereotaxy have their specific roles in intraventricular lesions such as choroid plexus tumours and deep seated lesions.

Table 7 has the details of surgical approach practiced in different case series from tbe country.

Tumour debulking and diversion of CSF depending on location of the tumour, grade, and risk of dissemination is also used often. Overall, surgical morbidity rates vary from 10 to 54% as per available literature [21]. The role for re-surgery is not well defined in case of recurrent brain tumours but often are considered when there is long disease free interval and there is less chances of morbidity post-surgery.

3.2 Radiation therapy

Radiotherapy is an important modality in paediatric brain tumours. It is used mostly as adjuvant to surgery. It influences the local recurrence and overall survival especially in medulloblastoma and other embryonal tumours. Highly conformal radiation techniques as stereotactic radiotherapy has shown to decrease the incidence of neurocognitive and neuroendocrine side effects.

Indian study	Year of study publication	Total	Surgery	Radiation therapy	Chemotherapy
Dattatraya [31]	2011	209-Medulloblastoma	99.2% resection (53% total, 28,6% near total, 17.6% partial)	67.3%-Craniospinal Irradiation (35 Gy to craniospinal axis and 20G to posterior fossa)	32.7% (6.6% exclusively chemotherapy as below 3 yrs)
Madhavan [8]	2017	250-mostly Astrocytoma	92% resection (16% total, 46% partial, 20% biopsy)	74% offered RT, only 42% received (32% defaulted)	16%
Supriya [16]	2017	52	69% (53%-total, 38%-subtotal) biopsy-6%	54%	50%
Nair [6]	2018	375	76.5% Surgery (88%- total/ subtotal), 12%- Biopsy)	58%	26%
Chilkuri [25]	2020	27	96% (total-57%, 40%-partial, 3%-biopsy)	100% (proton) Median dose –54.8 cGy equivalent	22%-adjuvant chemotherapy, 30% concurrent chemotherapy

Table 7.
Enumerates the patterns of care of paediatric brain tumours reported in Indian studies.

Neurocognitive dysfunction is the most common long term side effect in paediatric age group and 20–70% patients suffer from neurocognitive deficit as a long term sequelae of radiotherapy [22]. Half of patients treated with conventional radiotherapy were found to have new neuroendocrine dysfunctions over 5 years follow up period. Newer radiation therapy like stereotactic conformal radiotherapy (SCRT) is useful in this context. Other late radiation-related adverse events include growth retardation, hearing impairment, vascular disorders, social and cognitive problems as well as secondary cancer incidence, which is described in various retrospective series as 9.3 to 19% at 30 years [23].

Proton therapy for paediatric cancers provide an innovative and conformal type of RT and is being increasingly used in treatment of childhood tumours as immature, growing tissue of children makes them particularly vulnerable to risk of secondary tumours and late radiation injury. This is possible due to superior dose conformity and lower normal tissue dose, offering better Quality of Life (QoL) for childhood cancer patients and survivors [24]. Chilkuri et al. demonstrated a low incidence of grade 3 acute toxicities despite a median dose of 54 CGE for CNS tumours with overall, 62%, 26%, and 0% of patients having grade 1, grade 2, and grade 3 fatigue, respectively [25].

Especially in craniospinal irradiation for medulloblastoma, multiple prospective and retrospective studies confirm this benefit though the patterns of failure and overall survival is similar between photon and proton therapy. Proton beam therapy conferred better dose sparing for the lens (Dmax < 10 Gy, thyroid (Dmean < 6 Gy and heart (Dmean <3.5G) and also significantly superior results for dose constraints of the hippocampus, normal brain, and brainstem when compared to photon therapy [26].

In non-medulloblastoma paediatric CNS tumours also, better use of intensity modulated radiotherapy and also proton therapy if feasible should be considered as there is evidence for lesser decline of neurocognitive functions in patients who received stereotactic radiation when compared to conventional radiation [27].

3.3 Chemotherapy

The role of chemotherapy in paediatric brain tumours is mainly as an adjuvant therapy to surgery and radiation therapy. Especially in embryonal tumours like medulloblastoma, chemotherapy given as concurrent with radiation therapy and as adjuvant results in better overall survival and disease control. In paediatric glioblastoma, the role of addition of temozolomide as concurrent and adjuvant therapy was studied by Mallick et al. and found to have superior overall survival rates with adjuvant temozolamide when compared to concurrent temozolamide alone.

In a retrospective analysis of 23 paediatric glioblastoma patients, the estimated median OS was 41.9 months at a median follow-up of 18 months (range: 2.1–126 months). For patients receiving concurrent and adjuvant TMZ, median OS was 41.9 months ($P = 0.081$) when compared to only concurrent TMZ which was 8 months. Estimated median OS for patients who did not complete six cycles of adjuvant TMZ was 9.5 months versus not reached for those who completed at least six cycles ($P = 0.0005$) [28].

3.4 Proton therapy

Since 2020, proton therapy is available in the Indian subcontinent. There are published literature from India on initial experience regarding the clinical profile and acute tolerance of proton therapy in childhood CNS tumours. Of total 39 patients in the 1–18 yrs. age group, 48% were CNS tumours. Majority of them received CSI (44%) followed by focal supratentorial or infratentorial radiation. Fatigue with radiation was seen as grade 1 (62%), grade 2 (26%), and none of patients had grade 3 fatigue. The various CNS tumours treated with proton therapy in this Indian study included medulloblastoma esp. craniospinal irradiation, glioma, ependymoma, craniopharyngioma, germ cell tumours, pinealoblastoma [25]. Globally, most of the paediatric oncologists prefer to use proton therapy in paediatric CNS tumours in view of the long term benefits previously discussed in this chapter.

3.5 Multidisciplinary treatment

Current practice of paediatric neuro-oncology depends precisely on the multidisciplinary team including neurosurgeon, radiation oncologist, paediatric oncologist, neuroradiologist etc. [29]. Detailed review of the various multimodality treatment protocols in paediatric neuro-oncology are out of the scope of this chapter [30].

Medulloblastoma is a classic example of multidisciplinary treatment. Post-surgery, for average risk the standard of care remains CSI to a dose equivalent to 23.4 Gy in 11 fractions followed by boost to the tumour bed up to a dose of 54–55 Gy along with vincristine used concomitantly on weekly basis. This is followed by adjuvant chemotherapy of 6 cycles using vincristine, cyclophosphamide, and cisplatin-based chemotherapy. High-risk patients are treated with standard dose CSI (35 Gy) delivered concurrently with carboplatin for first 15 fractions and the entire posterior fossa is boosted up to 54–55 Gy. Boost is also considered for areas with gross disease. This is followed by adjuvant chemotherapy follows same protocol as in standard-risk. A large series on medulloblastoma by Mazumdar et al. has described the pattern of care in about 365 patients from 1985 to 2010 [31]. **Table 7** illustrates the role of multidisciplinary tumour boards as reported in various Indian studies.

4. Outcomes

There is lack of enough randomised controlled studies or prospective data on the outcomes from the lower- and middle-income countries (LMIC). Cure rates in children with brain tumours are seen to be lower in LMICs.

The improvement in survival for children with brain tumours noted in high income countries over last few decades are not seen in LMICs because of under-diagnosis, incorrect clinical assessment, and lack of availability of appropriate services like neurosurgical, radiotherapy and radiology [1].

Multidisciplinary team management in tertiary cancer centres is recommended to treat childhood CNS tumours because of the complexity and rarity of these cancers. Aggressive tumour subtypes with high histological grades, younger age, difficult localization with inoperability, and as often seen in LMICs, delays in diagnosis and treatment can contribute to dismal outcomes [28, 29].

Coordinated paediatric neuro-oncology units are available only in few centres in India. Comprehensive multidisciplinary treatment in a co-ordinated manner, study of the epidemiology of paediatric brain tumours, reduction of treatment abandonment, and improvement in the follow-up of paediatric brain tumour patients has been reported when such programs are started [6].

Prospective studies on neurocognitive function of young brain tumour patients who received SCRT revealed young age (<13 y) and left hippocampus dose predicted for clinically relevant decline in certain neurocognitive domains on multivariate analysis. A mean dose of ≤30 Gy to the left hippocampus as a dose constraint for preserving intelligence quotient was suggested by the authors [30].

Dattatraya et al. [31] reported 5-year PFS of 73% and 10 yr. PFS of 41% in their series of medulloblastoma patients for average risk. In case of high risk, the 5 yr. PFS was only 34%. They also reported a 10-year overall survival rate of 15% only in the patients who were treated from 1985 to 2000. The 5-year survival rate was found to be 33.2% (44 patients). 11.9% (29 patients) were recurrence-free at 5 years. Local recurrence was seen in 13.9% patients and all of which were re-explored. 5 were operated for spinal metastasis. Supratentorial metastasis was seen in 4.9% (10 cases) and 6.4% had spinal metastases.

A study on 200 young patients with low grade brain tumours (cerebral and cerebellar astrocytoma, optic pathway glioma, craniopharyngioma, ependymoma) from Tata memorial hospital by Jalali et al. [22] reported 5-year tumour control rate for the Stereotactic Conformal RT (SCRT) arm as 93% (95% CI, 84–98%) and 92% (95% CI, 83–96%) for the Conventional RT arm ($P = 0.49$). At the time of progression, patients were managed with a range of attempted salvage therapies including re-excision, chemotherapy, and supportive care only; 6 of these patients in the SCRT arm and 5 in the Conventional RT arm experienced disease progression. There were 14 and 11 deaths in the SCRT and Conventional RT arms, respectively. For the entire cohort of 200 patients, as per intent-to-treat analysis, 5-year rate of overall survival in the SCRT arm was 86% (95% CI, 76–92%) and 91% (95% CI, 83–95%) for the Conventional RT arm ($P = 0.54$).

Supriya et al. [16] reported outcomes in their series of 52 paediatric CNS tumours patients treated with multimodality treatment. Eight (15.3%) died due to the progression of disease, but of more concern was that 44% abandoned treatment due to the progression/recurrence of disease. This happened mostly among the high-risk groups with poor prognosis such as medulloblastoma (high risk), pontine glioma and primitive neuroectodermal tumour.

In this same context, Nair et al. [6] published their experience on establishment of dedicated paediatric neuro-oncology unit and reported that patient follow-up rates improved from 37.2 to 82.6% and treatment abandonment decreased from 35.8% to 14.8% over the years of implementation of the paediatric neuro-oncology clinic.

In case of non medulloblastoma tumours like astrocytoma and ependymoma, there is no published literature regarding survival rates from the Indian subcontinent. This points to the need for developing a prospective national database for these cancers.

5. Future directions

Paediatric CNS tumours management depends precisely on multimodality approach starting from the diagnosis with latest neuroimaging tools, molecular pathology, neurosurgical interventions, higher radiation techniques including proton therapy wherever feasible, combination chemotherapy regimens and paediatric survivorship clinics for optimum rehabilitation of the children who get cured. This mandates dedicated paediatric neuro-oncology clinics in the institutions where they are being treated. There is substantial evidence to show that such integrated approaches can improve patient outcomes and decrease the treatment abandonment rates [6]. This is an important step in the future direction for paediatric CNS tumour management.

There is very scarce data on the patterns of care and clinical outcomes of paediatric CNS tumours treated in our country and other low- and middle-income countries [1]. There is improvement in overall survival in high income countries during the last few decades, but such information is lacking due to absence of a prospective national database on paediatric CNS tumours [32]. This data assumes importance for both the clinicians and administrative services to plan for improvement in tertiary oncology care for these patients and to establish adequate treatment support like financial and logistics to enable completion of planned treatment and to prevent abandonment of treatment. Also, as the cure rates improve, there is need for better rehabilitation of survivors into the mainstream. There are multiple studies on the paediatric brain tumour survivorship which recommend a multipronged approach to solve the issue [33].

The other challenge that current and future paediatric neuro-oncology management in LMICs face is the increasing incorporation of molecular classification into routine practice. There is more focus on the molecular subtyping in other paediatric CNS tumours apart from medulloblastoma where it has established as the standard practice.

In the current WHO classification of Gliomas, Glioneuronal Tumours, and Neuronal Tumours, 14 new types are added and nearly all of these newly recognised types can be diagnosed on the basis of standard histological, immunohistochemical, and molecular analyses [3]. The critical concern in this regard is the lack of adequate infrastructure to support these advancements and guidelines for classification in LMICs where the basic facilities for integrated paediatric neuro0oncology care itself is limited.

There is need for region specific consensus guidelines regarding the implementation of new WHO classification in India and other LMICs as developed in medulloblastoma [34]. Adequate networking between health care teams from each specialised centre would ensure exchange of advances in diagnosis, treatment nuances and promote pooled data for measuring outcomes.

Conflict of interest

The authors report no conflict of interests.

Author details

Sujith Kumar Mullapally[1], Vidyasagar Dusi[2] and Raghunadharao Digumarti[3]*

1 Apollo Proton Cancer Centre, Chennai, India

2 Omega Hospitals, Visakhapatnam, India

3 Medical Oncology, GSL Medical College, Rajahmundry, India

*Address all correspondence to: rdigumarti@gmail.com

References

[1] Girardi F, Allemani C, Coleman MP. Worldwide trends in survival from common childhood brain Tumors: A systematic review. JCO Global Oncology. Oct 2019;**5**:1-25. DOI: 10.1200/JGO.19.00140. PMID: 31682549; PMCID: PMC6882508

[2] Sung H, Ferlay J, Siegel RL, Laversanne M, Soerjomataram I, Jemal A, et al. Global Cancer statistics 2020: GLOBOCAN estimates of incidence and mortality worldwide for 36 cancers in 185 countries. CA: a Cancer Journal for Clinicians. 2021;**71**(3):209-249

[3] Louis DN, Perry A, Wesseling P, Brat DJ, Cree IA, Figarella-Branger D, et al. The 2021 WHO classification of Tumors of the central nervous system: A summary. Neuro-Oncology. 2021;**23**(8):1231-1251

[4] Chapter4ChildhoodCancers. Pdf. [cited 2022 Jul 16]. Available from: https://ncdirindia.org/All_Reports/Report_2020/resources/Chapter4ChildhoodCancers.pdf

[5] Arora RS, Eden TOB, Kapoor G. Epidemiology of childhood cancer in India. Indian Journal of Cancer. 2009;**46**(4):264

[6] Nair M, Raghavan RK, Prahladan A, Mathews A, Parukkutty K. Building a neuro-oncology program and epidemiological profiling of Pediatric brain Tumors in a tertiary Cancer Care Center in India. Middle East Journal of Cancer. 2018;**9**(3):228-234

[7] Trivedi PP, Goel DK, Mehta SP, Jetly DH. An epidemiological study of paediatric central nervous system (CNS) tumours in Gujarat cancer research institute, Ahmedabad. IJPO-Indian Journal of Pathology and Oncology. 2019;**6**(4):642-646

[8] Madhavan R, Kannabiran BP, Nithya AM, Kani J, Balasubramaniam P, Shanmugakumar S. Pediatric brain tumors: An analysis of 5 years of data from a tertiary cancer care center, India. Indian Journal of Cancer. 2016;**53**(4):562-565

[9] Paul M, Bhattacharyya M, Hazarika M, Kalita AK, Baishya N, Kalita MK. Primary brain tumours in Pediatric age group and the patterns of care in patients of the north-eastern region of India : A hospital based retrospective analysis. National Journal of Medical Research. 2020;**10**(2):60-63

[10] Gupta A. Morphological Spectrum of Pediatric central nervous system Tumors - a seven year study from Central India. Journal of Medical Science And Clinical Research. February 2019;7(2):1121-1126

[11] Shirazi N, Gupta M, Bhat NK, Kalra BP, Kumar R, Saini M. Profile of primary Pediatric brain and spinal cord Tumors from North India. Indian Journal of Medical and Paediatric Oncology. 2017;**38**(01):10-14

[12] Alomar SA. Clinical manifestation of central nervous system tumor. Seminars in Diagnostic Pathology. 2010;**27**(2):97-104

[13] Udayagiri DS, Chowhan AK, Nandyala R, Prayaga AK, Lakshmi A, Venkata PB, et al. Primary paediatric CNS tumours: A 25 years analysis at a tertiary referral Centre in Southern India. Journal of Clinical and Diagnostic Research. May 2020;**14**(5):EC01-EC05. Available from: https://jcdr.net/

article_fulltext.asp?issn=0973-709x&year=2020&volume=14&issue=5&page=EC01&issn=0973-709x&id=13672

[14] Govindan A, Parambil RM, Alapatt JP. Pediatric intracranial tumors over a 5-year period in a tertiary care center of North Kerala, India: A retrospective analysis. Asian Journal of Neurosurgery. 2018;**13**(4):1112

[15] Dwivedi R, Sudhapriya P, Padmavathi P, Sharma V, Rameshchandra VV, Prasad BCM, et al. Epidemiological analysis of central nervous system tumors in pediatric patients from a tertiary care Centre in India. International Journal of Contemporary Pediatrics. 2019;**6**(6):2497-2503

[16] Suresh SG, Srinivasan A, Scott JX, Rao SM, Chidambaram B, Chandrasekar S. Profile and outcome of Pediatric brain Tumors – Experience from a tertiary care Pediatric oncology unit in South India. Journal of Pediatric Neurosciences. 2017;**12**(3):237-244

[17] Jain A, Sharma MC, Suri V, Kale SS, Mahapatra AK, Tatke M, et al. Spectrum of pediatric brain tumors in India: A multi-institutional study. Neurology India. 2011;**59**(2):208

[18] Shah HC, Ubhale BP, Shah JK. Demographic and histopathologic profile of pediatric brain tumors: A hospital-based study. South Asian Journal of Cancer. 2015;**04**(03):146-148

[19] Mahajan S, Suri V, Sahu S, Sharma MC, Sarkar C. World Health Organization classification of Tumors of the central nervous system 5th edition (WHO CNS5): What's new? Indian Journal of Pathology & Microbiology. 2022;**65**(5):5

[20] Dasgupta A, Gupta T, Jalali R. Indian data on central nervous tumors: A summary of published work. South Asian Journal of Cancer. 2016;**5**(3):147-153

[21] Sandri A, Sardi N, Genitori L, Giordano F, Peretta P, Basso ME, et al. Diffuse and focal brain stem tumors in childhood: Prognostic factors and surgical outcome. Experience in a single institution. Childs Nerv Syst ChNS off J Int Soc. Pediatric Neurosurgery. 2006;**22**(9):1127-1135

[22] Jalali R, Gupta T, Goda JS, Goswami S, Shah N, Dutta D, et al. Efficacy of stereotactic conformal radiotherapy vs conventional radiotherapy on benign and low-grade brain Tumors: A randomized clinical trial. JAMA Oncology. 2017;**3**(10):1368-1376

[23] Eaton BR, MacDonald SM, Yock TI, Tarbell NJ. Secondary malignancy risk following proton radiation therapy. Frontiers in Oncology. 2015;**5**:261. DOI: 10.3389/fonc.2015.00261

[24] Thomas H, Timmermann B. Paediatric proton therapy. The British Journal of Radiology. 2020;**93**(1107):20190601

[25] Chilukuri S, Burela N, Uppuluri R, Indumathi D, Nangia S, Panda PK, et al. Preliminary experience of treating children and young adults with image-guided proton beam therapy in India. Journal of Global Oncology. 2020;**6**:GO.20.00319

[26] Carbonara R, Di Rito A, Monti A, Rubini G, Sardaro A. Proton versus photon radiotherapy for Pediatric central nervous system malignancies: A systematic review and Meta-analysis of Dosimetric comparison studies. Journal of Oncology. 2019;**2019**:e5879723

[27] Goda JS, Dutta D, Krishna U, Goswami S, Kothavade V, Kannan S,

et al. Hippocampal radiotherapy dose constraints for predicting long-term neurocognitive outcomes: Mature data from a prospective trial in young patients with brain tumors. Neuro-Oncology. 2020;**22**(11):1677-1685

[28] Mallick S, Gandhi AK, Joshi NP, Kumar A, Puri T, Sharma DN, et al. Outcomes of pediatric glioblastoma treated with adjuvant chemoradiation with temozolomide and correlation with prognostic factors. The Indian Journal of Medical and Paediatric Oncology. 2015;**36**(2):99-104

[29] Pollack IF. Multidisciplinary management of childhood brain tumors: A review of outcomes, recent advances, and challenges: A review. Journal of Neurosurgery. Pediatrics. 2011;**8**(2):135-148

[30] Bennett J, Erker C, Lafay-Cousin L, Ramaswamy V, Hukin J, Vanan MI, et al. Canadian Pediatric neuro-oncology Standards of Practice. Frontiers in Oncology. 2020;**10**:593192. doi: 10.3389/fonc.2020.593192

[31] Muzumdar D, Deshpande A, Kumar R, Sharma A, Goel N, Dange N, et al. Medulloblastoma in childhood-king Edward memorial hospital surgical experience and review: Comparative analysis of the case series of 365 patients. Journal of Pediatric Neurosciences. 2011;**6**(Suppl. 1):S78-S85

[32] CBTRUS Fact Sheet for Pediatric Brain Tumors.Pdf. [cited 2022 Jul 16]. Available from: https://www.soc-neuro-onc.org/UploadedFiles/CBTRUS%20Fact%20Sheet%20for%20Pediatric%20Brain%20Tumors.pdf

[33] Stavinoha PL, Trinh-Wong T, Rodriguez LN, Stewart CM, Frost K. Educational pain points for Pediatric brain tumor survivors: Review of risks and remedies. Children (Basel, Switzerland). 2021;**8**(12):1125

[34] Gupta T, Sarkar C, Rajshekhar V, Chatterjee S, Shirsat N, Muzumdar D, et al. Indian Society of Neuro-Oncology consensus guidelines for the contemporary management of medulloblastoma. Neurology India. 2017;**65**(2):315-332

Section 4

Diagnosis of the Central Nervous System Tumors

Chapter 8

Multistage Classification and Segmentation of Brain MR Image Using Modified Soft Computing Techniques

G. Sethuram Rao and D. Vydeki

Abstract

Recent studies indicate that brain tumor is one of the major causes of human casualties. Timely and accurate diagnosis of this life taking disease could reduce the casualty rate and extend the life of a person. In this research paper, techniques for brain tumor detection from MR Images with malignancy using modified soft computing approaches are presented and analyzed. An automated tumor detection system using artificial neural network (ANN) is proposed to classify the images as any of the four classes: Glioblastoma multiforme, Meningioma, secondary tumor-Metastasis and No Tumor. The classified image undergoes a segmentation process that predicts the size of the tumor in terms of pixels. Traditionally, conventional self-organizing map (CSOM) and Conventional back Propagation network (CBPN) are used for classification and segmentation respectively. However, these methods provide less accurate results in addition to high computational complexity. Moreover, due to unstable target weights, the number of iterations is large. These drawbacks are overcome in the proposed technique by developing a modified SOM (MSOM) for classification of images and modified BPN (MBPN) for segmentation. Simulated results show that the proposed modifications minimize the computational complexity without compromising on the accuracy. It is shown that MSOM increases the accuracy of classification by 10% compared to its conventional counterpart. Similarly segmentation accuracy is improved by 8% using MBPN.

Keywords: brain MR images, feature extraction, neural network, BPN, SOM, image classification, segmentation

1. Introduction

Medical image analysis helps in wide variety of healthcare applications and aid the diagnosis and treatment of ailing patients. Out of several techniques artificial neural networks lead in medical imaging applications, especially in brain tumor detection and classification. One of the main methods among ANN approaches is self-organizing map (SOM) and back propagation networks (BPN). Although SOM and BPN provide high accuracy, it requires huge computational complexity due to existence of many hidden layers between input neuron and output neuron. Thus for any system to be efficient in terms of performance, it must achieve high accuracy at low level of computational complexity. Extensive literature survey reveals that neural network based brain tumor detection and classification is a promising research field.

This proposed work presents a modified Self-Organizing Map (MSOM) for classification of brain tumor into different classes and a modified Back Propagation Network (MBPN) for segmentation of brain tumor, so that abnormal portion is extracted from any MR brain image.

The major contributions of this research work are as follows:

i. The accuracy of the MSOM is higher, since the weights obtained are more stabilized than CSOM.

ii. As the algorithm is free from iterations the convergence rate is also improved. The computation time required is less than 1 CPU seconds.

iii. Independent nature of MBPN on iterations makes it immune to local minima.

Rest of the paper is organized as follows. Section 2 contributes to analysis and study of associated research papers. The proposed research work is narrated in Section 3. Section 4 deals with feature extraction method for both classification and segmentation. Section 5 to 7 gives the relative analysis of proposed method in comparison with the existing methods. The simulated results and its respective analysis are presented in subsequent sections. Section 8 gives the conclusion and future scope of the research work.

2. Literature survey

DNN based MR brain tumor image classification is explored by Heba M [1]. Three classes of brain tumor benign, malignant and no tumor are described in this work. Conventional training method is adapted to exploit the three tumors in brain MR image. The works by El-Dahsan, Hosny T [2] used DWT for feature extraction and reduction with one of the main techniques as principal component analysis. This paper achieves up to 97% accuracy using feed forward back propagation neural network (BPNN) and k-nearest neighbor (KNN) classifiers respectively. Zarchari [3] used GLCM, Gabor, intensity, shape and statistical feature extraction techniques to develop multiclass classification of brain tumors by extracting 100 features. Eli et al. [4] proposed algorithm for medical image processing using deep learning techniques. The prime focus is based on open-source software available for brain tumor segmentation and classification. Michael S [5] developed human visual perception using deep learning approach for image classification. The limitations and suggestions of conventional methods used in neural networks are available in this work. Ling-Li Z [6] worked on auto encoder neural network based MRI and f-MRI brain image classification. Another survey by Chensi C [7] on deep learning algorithms for bio medical applications is available. Yazhou K [8] proposed classification using deep neural network. The limitation of this paper is only two level classification can be achieved to determine whether a tissue is normal or abnormal.

Hongmin L [9] proposed modified DCNN. This algorithm is designed such that it uses a reduced amount of data set for training and testing. The limitation is very poor accuracy in classifying right tumor. Usman and Rajpoot [10] have presented a paper on brain tumor categorization from multi-modality MRI by means of wavelets and machine learning. Random forest method is used to find the tumor class. This method gives the accuracy of 88% in categorization compared to ground truth images. Papers from [11–14] is used to explore segmentation techniques. These papers exploit the techniques used to separate tumor portions from properties such as color, contrast, brightness and gray level. The tumor portions are then evaluated for tissues, such as white matter-WM, gray matter-GM and cerebrospinal fluid-CSF. Youyong et al. [15] proposed a approach on segmentation, primarily positioned on information theoretic learning. This concept mainly practices feature selection data clustering of brain tumor at supervoxel-level. Both the method requires iterative tuning to achieve superior segmentation results. Hence this method consumes large duration to obtain better segmentation results. Damodharan and Raghavan [16] have developed a method for brain tumor analysis using neural network. This paper uses k-nearest neighbors (K-NN) and Bayesian algorithm. This method produces an accuracy result of 83%.In all these proposals mentioned above, image processing techniques such as pre-processing, feature extraction, segmentation and classification play a vital role. The primary idea from all these literature survey using computer aided diagnosis (CAD) systems is to produce highest level of accuracy with minimum computation time. Although many approaches are available, robust and efficient brain tumor classification is still an important and challenging task.

3. Proposed system

Figure 1 provides the mainstream block diagram for the proposed system. Image data sets used in the proposed system are MR brain images. The images as a whole are used for image classification and pixels within a single image are used for image segmentation. All the images used in the framework are of 256 × 256 dimension. The major steps in the proposed system include image pre-processing of MR brain images

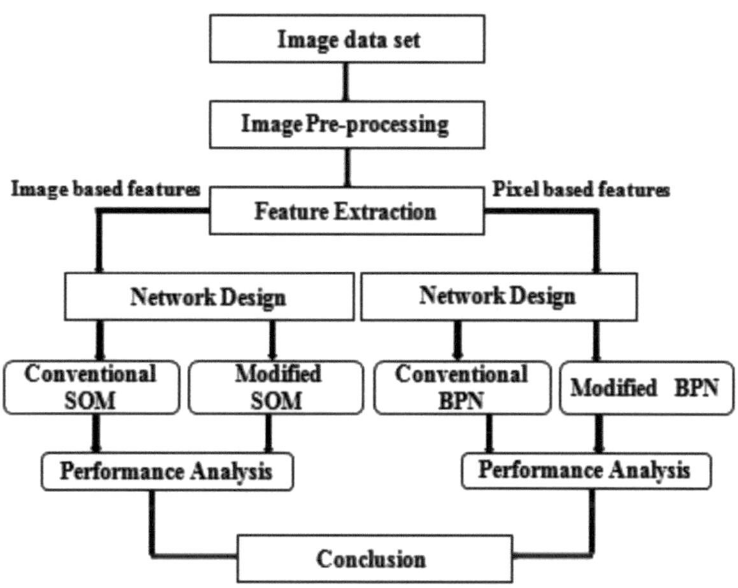

Figure 1.
Block diagram of proposed system.

followed by image-based and pixel-based extraction of features. The brain MR images are classified as any one of the four classes' Glioblastoma multiforme (GBM), Meningioma (MEN), secondary tumor-Metastasis (MET) and no Tumor (NT) using both conventional SOM and modified SOM. Similarly, image segmentation is done using conventional BPN and modified BPN to extract abnormal portion on a single MR brain image. Finally, performance estimation and comparison analysis are done through training and testing with both conventional and modified methods.

3.1 MR image dataset

In the proposed system 59 patients dataset constituting of 125 Glioblastoma (GBM), 120 Meningioma (MEN), 135 Metastasis (MET), and 430 are No tumor (NT). For each patient data, T1,T2, FLAIR and post gadolinium is available. The MR images used in this proposal are simulated images collected from Centre for Diagnostic Imaging, Tirupathi, Andhra Pradesh, India over a time period of August 2018 to November 2019. Ground truth images of WM, GM, CSF and tumor are also provided by the diagnostic centre. The equipment used for acquiring MRI are Siemens verio, Erlangen, Germany, 3 tesla MR scanner. The number of no tumor region MR image is taken significantly larger than the malignant regions to well recognize highly varying anatomical regions. The MR images are ground truth images certified by neurological surgeon Dr.D.Jagadeeswara Reddy, MBBS, MCh. (NIMS). In total 810 brain MRI data set as shown in **Table 1** constitutes simulated, ground truth and real time images. 60% of the dataset is used for training 40% of dataset used for testing in this proposal.

3.2 Software implementation

Proposed method is implemented using MATLAB 8.0 and is trained for brain tumor MR images of size 256 × 256. The research is done on personal computer having Intel™ Core 2 Duo 2.0 GHz processor with 3 GB RAM.

3.3 Image pre-processing

Magnetic resonance imaging (MRI) used for brain analysis is a safe and painless test. MRI uses radio waves generated due to magnetic field to produce detailed brain image. MR brain image can detect variety of conditions like tumors, swelling, bleeding and other brain abnormalities. The obtained MR brain image is given as input to the initial pre-processing step. **Figure 2** gives the flow diagram of image pre-processing. The input MR image is in the form of raw quality which needs enhancement to make it appropriate for the proposed application. Moreover pre-processing improves

Category	Training Image	Testing Image
Glioblastoma	75	50
Meningioma	72	48
Metastasis	81	54
No tumor	258	172

Table 1.
Brain MR image database.

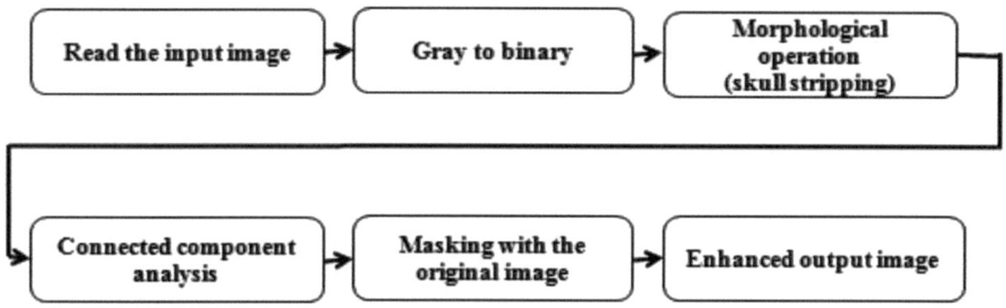

Figure 2.
Flow diagram of pre-processing.

parameters of MR brain image like smoothing, preserving edges, signal to noise ratio, redundant information, unrelated noise and unwanted background information.

3.3.1 Gray to binary image conversion

Initially, MR brain image which is in the form of a gray image is converted to a binary image as shown in **Figure 2**. A gray scale image that has gray values from 0 to 255 is subjected to suitable threshold, to make the image binary. The threshold value selected in this proposal is 45; if the pixel value is above 45 then these pixels are made equal to 255. If the pixel value is less than 45 then those pixels are made equal to 0. Thus all the pixel value of MR brain image drops to either 0 or 255.

3.3.2 Skull stripping

Additional tissues in brain MR image such as fat, skin and skull affect the segmentation results. Hence to remove this unwanted information, skull stripping is done based on morphological operation. Morphological operation removes the pixels on object boundaries. Erosion operation uses a specified neighborhood technique to darken tiny bright areas such as scull boundary over brain tissue.

3.3.3 Connected component analysis

Connected component analysis is used to detect connected regions in MR brain images. This technique works by labelling the vertices based on the connectivity, for example 4-connected or 8-connected neighborhood. Thus this process helps to create objects in an image disappear as they are replaced with values that blend in with the background area.

3.3.4 Masking

Masking is needed to change the pixel values from 0 to 255 to 0–1. It is implemented by performing a product function between an original image and the mask. Thus the output images shown in **Figure 3** are free from extra cranial tissues.

In **Figure 3**, experimental results on MR brain image for pre-processing steps are shown. The MR images shown in **Figure 3** (a) are the images given as input to the preprocessing stage. **Figure 3** (b) shows the eroded images where the outer layer skull is mostly disappeared from the brain tissue. In **Figure 3** (c) gray images are converted to

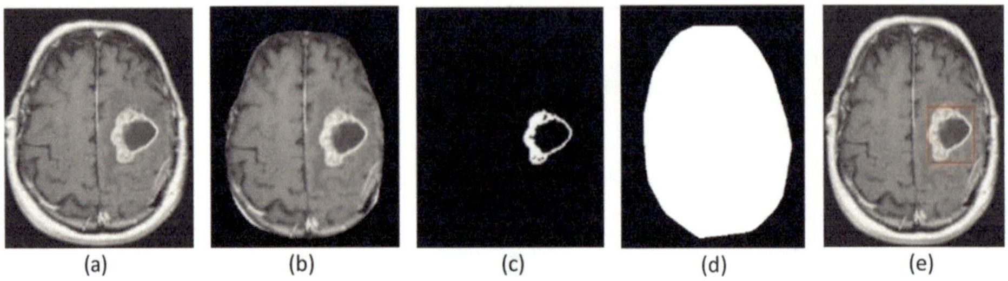

Figure 3.
Pre-processed sample images (a) input images (b) eroded images (c) images after thresholding (d) images after connected component analysis (e) enhanced output images.

binary by setting a threshold value of 45, resulting in only 0 or 1 pixel value. In **Figure 3** (d), a mask is obtained using connected component analysis and this mask is multiplied with the input image. Each pixel of input image from (a) is multiplied with each pixel of the image in (0 or 1) (d), Hence, only the white portion which is equal to 1 will appear in output while the black portion which is equal to zero does not appear in output. Finally **Figure 3** (d) presents the original images without the portion of the skull.

4. Feature extraction

Feature extraction is one of the widely used techniques to reduce the complexity of the classifier by knowing the characteristics of the image in terms of color, texture size and edges of the body. In this proposal, two types of features: image-based and pixel-based textual features are used for classification and segmentation respectively. In image-based textual features, classification of four set of tumor classes Glioblastoma multiforme (GBM), Meningioma (MEN) secondary tumor-Metastasis (MET) and No Tumor (NT) are done on MR images as shown in **Figure 4**. Similarly, in pixel-based textual features image segmentation is done to determine non-tumorous and tumorous regions.

4.1 Image classification

Image based textual features of brain MR images are used to classify the given image belonging to any one of the four classes: secondary tumor-Metastasis (MET), Glioblastoma multiforme (GBM), Meningioma (MEN) secondary tumor-Metastasis (MET) and No Tumor (NT). These features represent the characteristics of the input image which aid in distinguishing the different types of image. The eight textual

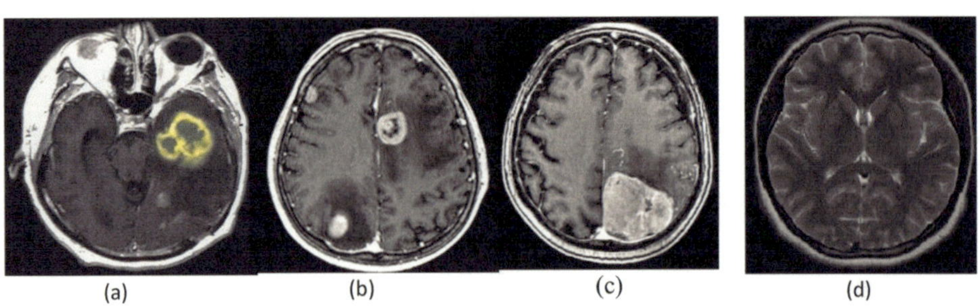

Figure 4.
(a). Class I-glioblastoma (b). Class II-meningioma (c). Class III-metastasis (d). Class IV-No tumor.

features that are used in this proposal are i). Angular second moment ii). Contrast iii). Correlation iv). Variance v). Inverse difference moment vi). Entropy vii). Skewness and viii). Kurtosis. The following expressions are used in the formulae.

p(i, j) = Size of the MR image 256 × 256.

p_x = vector elements along horizontal summation p(i, j); size(256 × 1).

p_y = vector elements along vertical summation p(i, j); size(1 × 256).

i. Angular second moment (ASM): It is measure of textural uniformity of an image. Energy reaches to highest value when gray level values of image reaches to constant or periodic form.

For a MR image p(i, j) of size 256 × 256

$$f_1 = \sum_i \sum_j \{p(i,j)\}^2 \quad (1)$$

where i = 1,2, … .256; j = 1,2, … .256;

ii. Contrast: Degree of difference between pixel to pixel in an image.

$$f_2 = \sum_{n=0}^{Ng-1} n^2 \left(\sum_{i=1}^{Ng} \sum_{j=1}^{Ng} p(i,j) \right)^2 \quad (2)$$

where i = 1, 2, … .256; j = 1, 2, … .256;

iii. Correlation: Process of establishing relationship by finding the connection between the two pixels.

$$f_3 = -\frac{\sum_i \sum_j (i,j) p(i,j) - \mu_x \mu_y}{\sigma_x \sigma_y} \quad (3)$$

where π_x, π_y, σ_x and σ_y denote the means and standard deviations.

iv. Variance: Quality of being different, divergent or inconsistent

$$f_4 = \sum_i \sum_j (i-\mu)^2 p(i,j) \quad (4)$$

v. Inverse difference moment (IDM): It is a measure of image homogeneity.

$$f_5 = \sum_i \sum_j \frac{1}{1+(i-j)^2} p(i,j) \quad (5)$$

vi. Entropy: It is a measure of randomness in the information being processed.

$$f_6 = \sum_i \sum_j p(i,j) \log(p(i,j)) \quad (6)$$

vii. Skewness: Gives a measure of which the given distribution differs from normal distribution.

$$f_7 = \frac{1}{\sigma^3} \sum_i \sum_j (p(i,j) - \mu)^3 \tag{7}$$

viii. Kurtosis: It is a statistical measure to show how deeply the tails of the distribution differ from the tails of normal distribution.

$$f_8 = \frac{1}{\sigma^4} \sum_i \sum_j (p(i,j) - \mu)^4 - 3 \tag{8}$$

The above 8 features are extracted from brain MR image and given as input to neural network for further classification.

4.2 Feature values for image classification

Eight features mentioned in Section 4.1 are extracted from the brain MR images. The MR images used are ground truth images. The values shown in **Table 2** are the average values of the entire image dataset. Close inspection of the values in this table reveals that each category of No Tumor, Glioblastoma, Meningioma, and Metastasis are having clear divergent values. These values make the classification process easier.

4.3 Feature values for image segmentation

Similar to classification, image segmentation is carried out to differentiate a non-tumorous region and a tumor region with the help of the eight features mentioned in Section 4.1. Here, only the pixels within a single image are used for image segmentation. Hence, the data required for image segmentation does not depend on the number of images but depends on number of pixels. The values shown in **Table 3** are average values of entire image data set. Only bi-level segmentation is performed on real-time images due to availability of ground truth images only for the tumor region.

Features	No Tumor	Glioblastoma	Meningioma	Metastasis
ASM (f_1)	1.0022	223,000,562	604,422,470	384,652,269
Contrast(f_2)	8,763,785	2,177,180	6,457,236	3,700,147
Correlation(f_3)	3.2290	2.0014	4.2467	1.6320
Variance(f_4)	4.5537	2.3593	3.8371	2.1467
IDM(f_5)	6.5250	3.7115	4.2941	2.1614
Entropy(f_6)	3.1745	8.5147	1.3335	2.8693
Skewness(f_7)	3.9760	9.5895	2.7925	1.6630
Kurtosis(f_8)	5.5760	1.3690	2.7647	4.7109

Table 2.
Image based feature values for image classification.

Features	Non-tumorous region	Tumor region
ASM (f_1)	132,975	202
Contrast(f_2)	59,454,525	2,210,850
Correlation(f_3)	−457	3
Variance(f_4)	3,786,322	117
IDM(f_5)	547	20
Entropy(f_6)	1268	−160
Skewness(f_7)	4443	60
Kurtosis(f_8)	596	2.7022

Table 3.
Pixel based feature values for image segmentation.

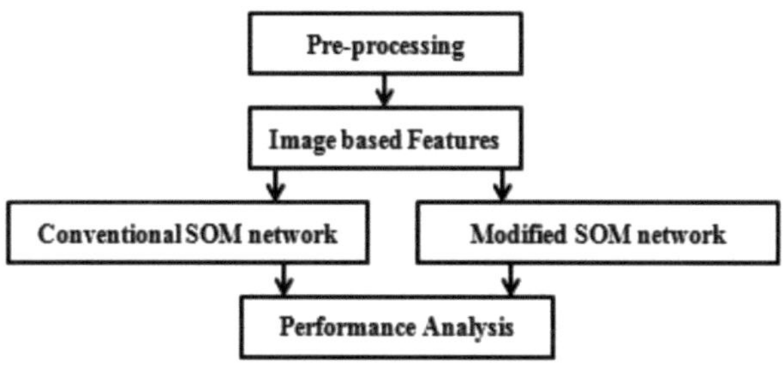

Figure 5.
Proposed methodology for image classification.

The various features provided in the **Tables 1** and **2** have yielded sufficiently diversified values which ultimately guarantee the success of the classification and segmentation process in detecting the brain tumor.

5. Proposed methodology for image classification using SOM

In this paper, brain MR image classification is done with a modified self-organizing map (MSOM) network and the results are compared with existing conventional self-Organizing map network (CSOM). Four categories Glioblastoma, Meningioma, Metastasis, and no tumor, are detected using both CSOM and MSOM. The performance of both methods is estimated in terms of classification accuracy, sensitivity, computational complexity and convergence rate. **Figure 5** shows the proposed methodology for image classification.

5.1 Conventional self-organizing map (CSOM) network based classification

Figure 6 shows the conventional self-organizing map network in a single layered ANN. The architecture is associated with one set of weight matrix (w). The training algorithm involves the concept of unsupervised training methodology. Basically, the architecture involves eight neurons in the input layer. The reason for selecting eight input neurons is based on eight features ASM (f_1), Contrast (f_2), Correlation (f_3), Variance (f_4), IDM (f_5), Entropy (f_6), Skewness (f_7), Kurtosis (f_8) which are considered as

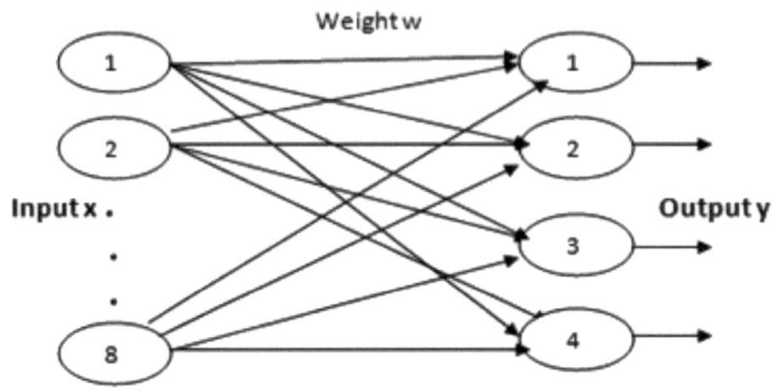

Figure 6.
Architecture of CSOM with 8 input and 4 output classes.

input to ANN architecture. Stabilized weight matrices (w) will decide the main objective of training. The following are the steps involved to train the algorithm.

5.2 Training algorithm of CSOM

Step 1: Initialization done randomly on weight vectors.
Step 2: Still stopping condition becomes false, steps 3 to 6 will be repeated.
Step 3: The Euclidean distance is computed for each output layer neurons 'j'.

$$D(j) = \sum_i (w_{ij} - x_i)^2 \tag{9}$$

Step 4: Value of index 'j' is computed till it becomes minimum.
Step 5: Winner neuron's weight which is updated one is used by implementing the rule.

$$w_{ij}(new) = w_{ij}(old) + \alpha(x_i - w_{ij}(old)) \tag{10}$$

'x_i' determines the intensity values obtained from input data set,'α' determines the learning rate.

Step 6: Maximum number of iterations will decide to determine the test for stopping condition.

5.3 Performance measure of tumor segmentation using CSOM

See (**Table 4**).

Performance Measure	Description
Sensitivity	TP/TP + FN
Specificity	TN/ TN + FP
Classification Accuracy	TP+ TN/TP + FP + TN + FN
WhereTP, TN, FP and FN are true positive, true negative, false positive and false negative respectively.	

Table 4.
Sensitivity, specificity and classification accuracy.

5.4 Result analysis of CSOM

Table 5 clearly shows that classification accuracy is very low. The main reason for low accuracy is the lack of standard convergence condition. Since the weight vector is randomly initialized, more number of iterations is required to stabilize the weight matrix. Thus, for single layer CSOM, the computational complexity in the training algorithm is as below:

a. Euclidean distance calculation

Mathematical operations = 1 subtraction and 1 multiplication.

Total no of operations = 2ap, where 'a' input neurons and 'p' output neurons

b. Weight calculation between input layer and output layer

Mathematical operations = 1 sub, 2 mull and 1 add.

Total no of operations = 4ap, where 'a' input neurons and 'p' output neurons

c. Total Mathematical operations (a) and (b) put together = 6ap

d. Convergence rate for CSOM for the above computation is 650 CPU seconds.

Thus, from the above analysis, it could be inferred that though CSOM is computationally effective the accuracy produced is low. As accuracy is the critical performance parameter, a low value of it could not be accepted. Hence, this paper proposes a Modified Self-Organizing Map to improve the accuracy.

5.5 Modified self-organizing map (MSOM) network

The main objective of MSOM is to reduce the number of iterations required for stabilizing the weight matrix. Moreover, as mentioned in **Table 5**, classification accuracy for CSOM is around 85% only. Hence, without changing the architecture of CSOM, the algorithm is modified to reduce the computational complexity and to increase the classification accuracy.

5.6 Modified training algorithm of MSOM

Instead of randomly initializing weights, the weight matrix is closely matched to the input vector. Hence the weights are determined using the following modified equations.

	Class I	Class II	Class III	Class IV
Class I	59	9	8	7
Class II	7	51	8	9
Class III	7	7	45	6
Class IV	8	6	6	59

Table 5.
Confusion matrix of CSOM.

	TP	TN	FP	FN	sensitivity	specificity	classification accuracy
Glioblastoma	59	197	23	23	0.719	0.895	84.7
Meningioma	51	203	23	23	0.689	0.898	84.6
Metastasis	45	215	23	21	0.681	0.903	85.5
no tumor	59	199	23	21	0.74	0.896	85.4
Average value					0.707	0.898	85

Table 6.
Performance metrics for sensitivity, specificity and classification accuracy.

	Class I	Class II	Class III	Class IV
Class I	76	2	2	3
Class II	2	69	3	3
Class III	3	2	58	2
Class IV	2	2	4	71

Table 7.
Confusion matrix of MSOM.

$$\|X - W\| = 0 \tag{11}$$

$$\|X - W\| = 0$$

X = W where X is input vector and W is the weight matrix.

Thus, the minimum value can be obtained by making X = W and by doing this, the weights can be stabilized with the minimum number of iterations. The closest match is determined by finding the weight vector which gives the minimum distance value between them. Another modification done is the normalization of input vectors. Normalization helps to reduce measurements to a neutral or standard scale. Hence the normalized values only change in magnitude in the range [0, 1]. Apart from this modification, all other steps mentioned in Section 4.1 of CSOM training algorithm remain same. The testing process is same as that of the conventional SOM. The testing input is selected to the class for which the corresponding output neuron value is minimum (**Table 6**).

5.7 Performance measure of tumor segmentation using MSOM

From the **Tables 7** and **8** it is clear that the accuracy of the modified SOM is higher than the conventional SOM (96%). The reason for the improvement is weights

	TP	TN	FP	FN	Sensitivity	Specificity	Classification Accuracy
Glioblastoma	76	210	6	6	0.926	0.972	96
Meningioma	69	217	5	7	0.907	0.977	96
Metastasis	58	226	8	6	0.906	0.965	95
No Tumor	71	213	7	7	0.906	0.968	96
Average value					0.912	0.970	96

Table 8.
Performance metrics for sensitivity, specificity and accuracy using MSOM.

obtained using MSOM are more stabilized than the CSOM. Also the time requirement for MSOM reduced from 650 CPU to 1 CPU second. The main reason for improvement in convergence rate is the algorithm is free from iterations.

6. Proposed methodology for image segmentation using BPN

Figure 7 shows the proposed methodology for image segmentation. Back propagation network (BPN) based image segmentation is used to extract abnormal portion of brain tumor from any MR brain image. This method is mainly used for volumetric analysis, such as finding size and area of the tumor. With the help of this analysis after-effect of the treatment can be determined. In this paper conventional back propagation network (CBPN) results are compared with modified back propagation network (MBPN) by testing both simulated images and real-time images. The performance is measured by calculating segmentation efficiency (SE), correspondence ratio (CR) and convergence rate.

6.1 Conventional back propagation network (CBPN)

Features obtained in **Table 2** are used for image segmentation to discover non-tumorous and tumorous regions. In this method, input pixels (256x256) are divided into training data set and testing data set. Training dataset contains pixels from GM, WM, CSF and tumor region. Ground truth (GT) images are used randomly for training purposes. BPN is trained with training pixels, each pixel is represented by 8 features given in **Table 2** and target vectors. Thus BPN is trained with the training algorithm to determine the stabilized set of weights. Finally the network is tested with the testing data and categories of all the pixels are determined. And the category of interest is assigned a value of '255' and the other category is assigned a value of '0'.

BPN comes under supervised feed forward neural network type and the training comes under gradient descent rule. Input vectors and corresponding target vectors are used to train the network until it classifies input vectors as GM, WM, CSF and tumor region as proposed in this paper. **Figure 8** shows the architecture of CBPN. The network used is an 8–12-4 layered network. The target vector is supplied to the output layer. The target representation for each class GM, WM, CSF and tumor region is given as [1 0 0 0; 0 1 0 0; 0 0 1 0; 0 0 0 1] respectively. Two sets of weight matrices are determined at the end of the training procedure **Figures 9** and **10** shows the sample results of Conventional Back Propagation Network (CBPN).

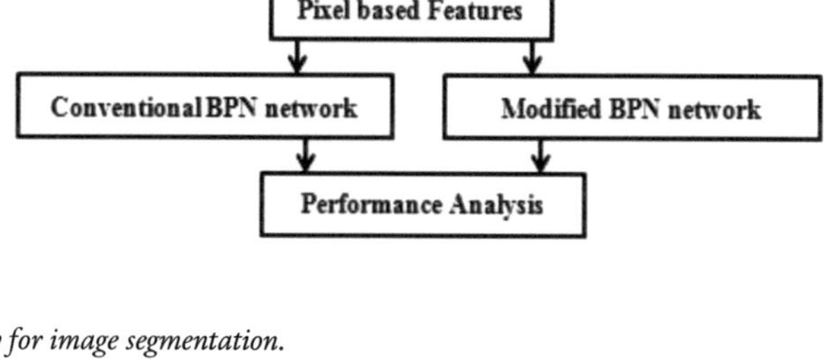

Figure 7.
Proposed methodology for image segmentation.

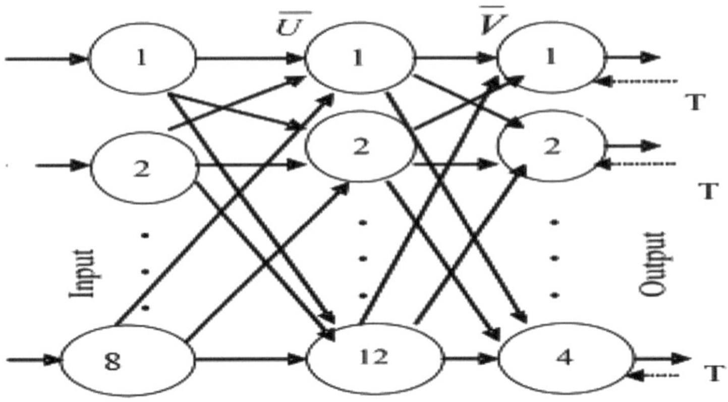

Figure 8.
Architecture of CBPN with 8 input and 4 output classes.

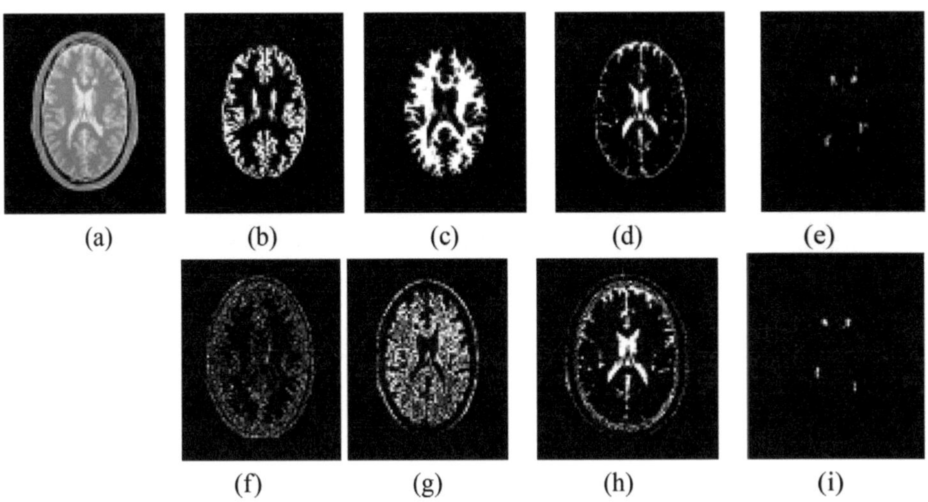

Figure 9.
Sample results of CBPN (a) original image (b) gray matter (GM) phantom (c) white matter (WM) phantom (d) CSF phantom (e) tumor phantom (f) GM segment (g) WM segment (h) CSF segment (i) tumor segment.

6.2 Training algorithm of CBPN

The training algorithm of CBPN involves three stages. Feed forward of the input signals, back propagation of the associated error and the adjustment of weights. The algorithm for training is given as follows.

Step 1: Initialize the weights U_{ij} and V_{jk}.

Step 2: Repeat steps 3–9 for each training pair.

Feed forward:

Step 3: Each input unit receives the input signal and transmits the signals to the hidden layer neurons.

Step 4: Each hidden unit sums its weighted input signals.

$$z\_in_j = \sum x_i.u_{ij} \tag{12}$$

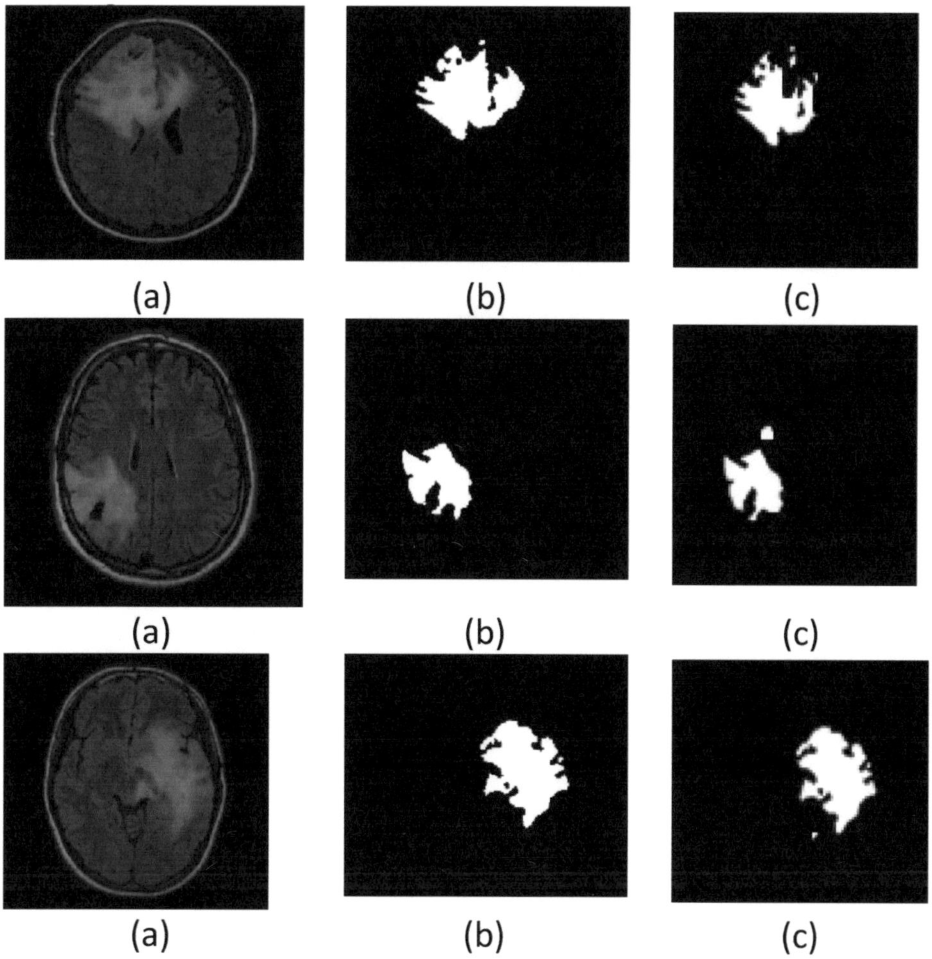

Figure 10.
Sample results of CBPN (a) input image (b) tumor segment (c) tumor phantom.

The above equation activation function z_in_j, is applied to compute its output signal z_j

$$z_j = f\left(z_{inj}\right) \quad (13)$$

The activation function used in this work is sigmoid function. The output signal is fed to the output layer neurons.

Step 5: Each output unit sums its weighted input signals.

$$y\_in_k = \sum z_j.v_{jk} \quad (14)$$

The above equation activation function y_in_k, is applied to compute its output signal y_k

$$y_k = f(y\_in_k) \quad (15)$$

Back propagation of error

Step 6: Each output unit receives a target pattern (t_k) and compute its error information term

$$\delta_k = (t_k - y_k).f(y\_in_k) \tag{16}$$

From δ_k weight correction term is calculated as follows

$$\nabla v_{jk} = \alpha.\delta_k.z_j \tag{17}$$

Step 7: Each hidden unit compute its error information term

$$\delta_j = \sum \delta_k v_{jk}.f(z\_in_j) \tag{18}$$

From the above equation weight correction is calculated as follows

$$\nabla u_{ij} = \alpha.\delta_j.x_i \tag{19}$$

Update weights.
Step 8: Each output unit updates its weight by

$$v_{jk}(new) = v_{jk}(old) + \nabla v_{jk} \tag{20}$$

Each hidden unit updates its weight by

$$u_{ij}(new) = u_{ij}(old) + \nabla u_{ij} \tag{21}$$

Step 9: The training stops when the weight correction terms are equal to zero or when it reaches to predefine minimum value.

6.3 Quantitative analysis of CBPN

6.4 Result analysis of CBPN

The analysis presented in the **Tables 9–11** indicates that the requirement for convergence time is significantly high i.e. 1650 CPU seconds using personal computer having Intel™ Core 2 Duo 2.0 GHz processor with 3 GB RAM (32-bit version). MATLAB 8.0 software is used for brain tumor MR images of size 256 × 256. The dependent nature of

Input	Category	GT	TP	FP	SE = TP/GT(%)	CR = [TP-0.5xFP)]/GT
Severe stage image	WM	11,778	9259	1570	78.61	0.719
	GM	10,944	3173	1286	28.99	0.231
	CSF	6505	3469	1918	53.32	0.385
Moderate stage image	WM	11,768	8850	1099	75.20	0.705
	GM	17,940	5452	663	30.39	0.285
	CSF	6501	3249	1047	49.97	0.419
Mild stage image	WM	11,775	10,497	2274	89.14	0.794
	GM	10,941	2772	1346	25.33	0.191
	CSF	6501	3308	2025	50.88	0.353

Table 9.
Simulated images (for non-tumorous region).

Input image	GT pixels	TP pixels	FP pixels	SE (%)	CR
Severe stage image	297	277	90	93	0.78
Moderate stage image	86	69	31	80	0.62
Mild stage image	21	9	9	43	0.22

Table 10.
Simulated images (tumorous region).

Input image	GT pixels	TP pixels	FP pixels	SE (%)	CR
Image 1	1598	1338	41	83.7	0.824
Image 2	3840	3259	522	84.8	0.780
Image 3	5409	4536	531	83.8	0.789

Table 11.
Real-time images: (for tumorous region).

CBPN on iterations is also one of the drawbacks since it leads to local minima. Also for real time images the segmentation efficiency is low around 83–85% and convergence rate is low around 0.79 to 0.82. Hence there is scope for improvement in convergence rate, accuracy to increases the efficiency of the entire system. These limitations of CBPN can prevail over using Modified Back Propagation network (MBPN).

6.5 Modified back propagation network (MBPN)

The modified BPN is framed to overcome the drawbacks of computational complexity of CBPN without compromising the accuracy. The modification done in MBPN architecture is target vector is also given to the hidden layer with different representation. The algorithm proceeds with fixed error value. This reduces the number of iterations required to calculate the weights. Here weight estimation is first done for the hidden layer weights and then performed for the output layer weights. With fixed error value, the output values of the hidden layer are determined. Using the output values, the net value is determined by the inverse operation of sigmoid function. Further, the weights are determined using the input and net value of the hidden layer.

Figure 11 shows the architecture of MBPN with 8–12-4 layered network. As mentioned above, target is supplied both to hidden layer and output layer. Target representation for hidden layer is: [1 1 1 0 0 0 0 0 0 0 0 0; 0 0 0 1 1 1 0 0 0 0 0 0; 0 0 0 0 0 0 1 1 1 0 0 0; 0 0 0 0 0 0 0 0 0 1 1 1]. Two set of weight matrices are determined at the end of the training procedure. The weight values are obtained when the error value i.e. target output is equal to zero or a predefined minimum value. The error value intended for achieving the convergence in this paper is 0.01.

6.6 Weight matrix calculation between input and hidden layer

Step 1: Since target –output = 0.01 for convergence, the output of the hidden layer neurons is calculated using

$$E = target - output; z_j = t_j - 0.01 \tag{22}$$

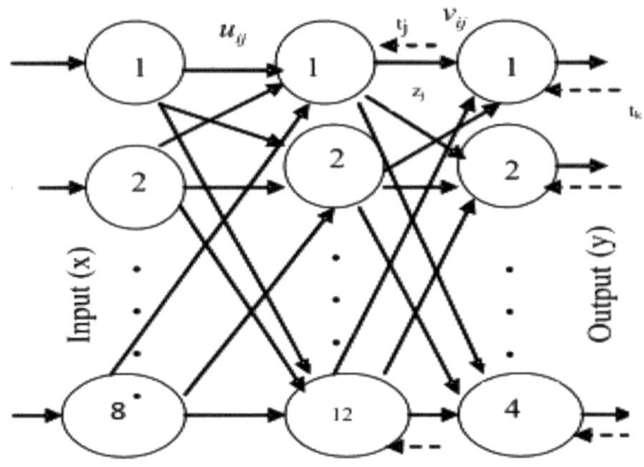

Figure 11.
Architecture of MBPN with 8 input and 4 output classes.

Step 2: Once the output value is calculated, the following equation yields the value for net value.

$$Z_j = f\ (Z_{\_inj}); Z_j = \left[1/_{1+e}\left({}^{-Z_{inj}}\right)\right] Z_{\_inj} = ln\left[Z_j/\left|1-Z_j\right|\right] \quad (23)$$

Step 3: Based on the net values, the weight matrix for the hidden layer is calculated using

$$Z_{\_inj} = \sum x_i . u_{ij} \quad (24)$$

Step 4: The following equations are used to determine the weight matrices between hidden layer and output layer

$$y_k = t_k - 0.01; y_{\_ink} = ln\left[y_k/\left|1-y_k\right|\right]; y_{\_ink} = \sum z_j . v_{jk} \quad (25)$$

Step 5: The training stops when the weight correction terms are equal to zero or when it reaches to predefine minimum value.

Input image	Category	GT	TP	FP	SE(%)	CR
Severe stage image	WM	11,778	10,501	3572	89.15	0.739
	GM	10,944	3395	1126	31.02	0.258
	CSF	6505	2918	524	44.85	0.408
Moderate stage image	WM	11,768	10,068	3186	85.55	0.7201
	GM	17,940	3979	1938	22.17	0.1677
	CSF	6501	3826	1149	58.85	0.50
Mild stage image	WM	11,775	11,058	58	93.91	0.936
	GM	10,941	4282	3084	39.13	0.250
	CSF	6501	3348	1332	51.49	0.412

Table 12.
Simulated images: (for non-tumorous region).

6.7 Quantitative analysis of MBPN

See (**Tables 12–14**).

6.8 Result analysis of MBPN

Figure 11 shows the architecture of MBPN, where the target is supplied to both hidden layer and output layer. This helps in reduction of number of iterations, since stabilized weight values are achieved much earlier than its counterpart. Hence the convergence rate of MBPN is less than 1 CPU seconds, which is far better than CBPN (650 CPU seconds). The performance measures in terms of accuracy are better than CBPN. The independent nature of MBPN on iterations makes it immune to local

Input image	GT pixels	TP pixels	FP pixels	SE(%)	CR
Severe stage image	297	288	52	96	0.88
Moderate stage image	86	75	20	87	0.75
Mild stage image	21	15	9	71	0.55

Table 13.
Simulated images (tumorous region).

Input image	GT pixels	TP pixels	FP pixels	SE (%)	CR
Image 1	1598	1416	36	88.6	0.874
Image 2	3840	3578	370	93.1	0.883
Image 3	5409	5018	465	92.7	0.884

Table 14.
Real-time images (for tumorous region).

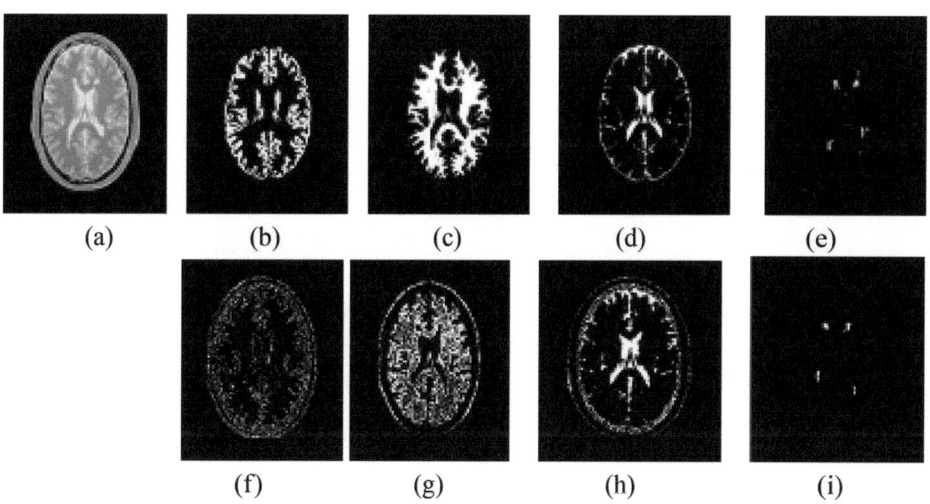

Figure 12.
Sample results of MBPN (a) original image (b) gray matter (GM) phantom (c) white matter (WM) phantom (d) CSF phantom (e) tumor phantom (f) GM segment (g) WM segment (h) CSF segment (i) tumor segment.

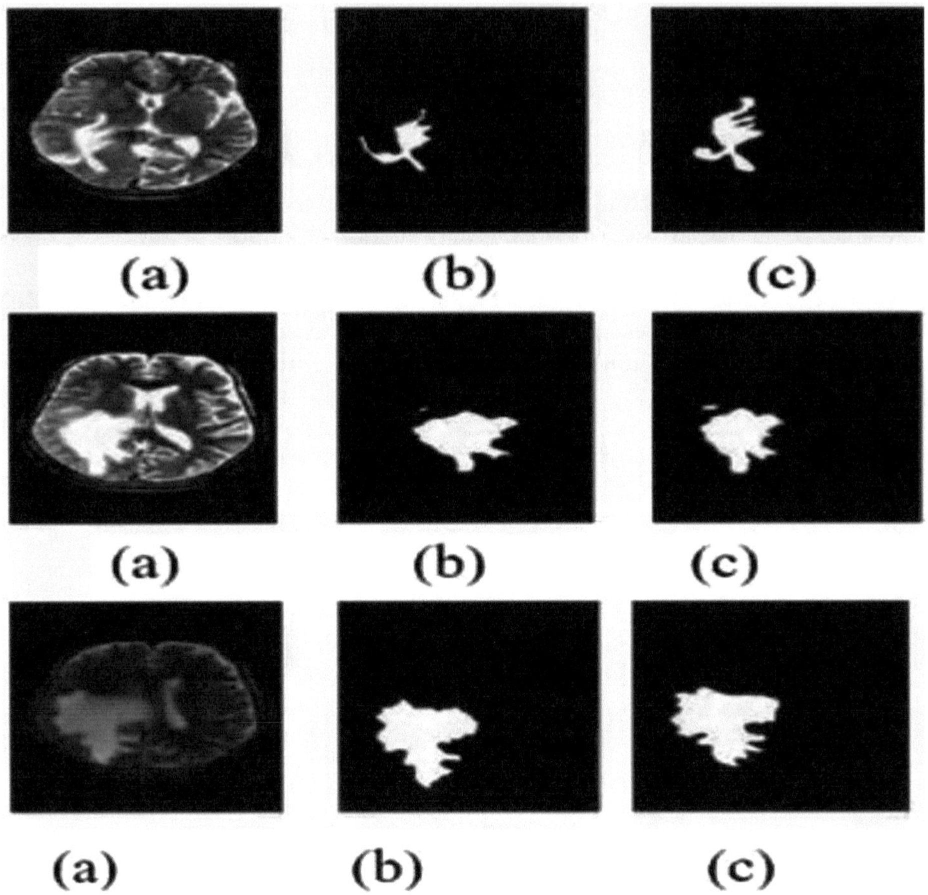

Figure 13.
Sample results of MBPN (a) input image (b) tumor segment (c) tumor phantom.

minima. CBPN has 83% and MBPN has 91% segmentation efficiency. Hence 8% increase in MBPN compared to CBPN indicates proposed network segments tumors of varying size and shape successfully. **Figures 12** and **13** gives a comprehensible improvement in finding GM, WM, CSF and tumor segment.

Class	CSOM			MSOM		
	Sensitivity	Specificity	Classification Accuracy	Sensitivity	Specificity	Classification Accuracy
Glioblastoma	0.719	0.895	84.7	0.926	0.972	96
Meningioma	0.689	0.898	84.6	0.907	0.977	96
Metastasis	0.681	0.903	85.5	0.906	0.965	95
No Tumor	0.74	0.896	85.4	0.906	0.968	96

Table 15.
Comparison of CSOM and MSOM.

Input	ground truth pixels count	CBPN		MBPN		Improvement of MBPN over CBPN
		correctly classified pixels count	Segmentation Efficiency (%)	correctly classified pixels count	Segmentation Efficiency (%)	
Severe stage image	1598	1338	83.7	1416	88.6	5
Moderate stage image	3840	3259	84.8	3578	93.1	8.3
Mild stage image	5409	4536	83.8	5018	92.7	8.9

Table 16.
Comparison of CBPN and MBPN.

Reference No	Method Used	Accuracy
[17]	Particle Swarm Optimization (PSO) feed forward neural network	95
[17]	PSO + Modified Counter Propagation neural network	89
[18]	GA + Adaptive Resonance Theory neural network	85
[19]	PSO + Kohnean neural network	86
Proposed Approach	Modified Self Organizing Map + Modified Back Propagation neural network	96

Table 17.
Comparative analysis with other methods.

7. Comparison between conventional and modified methods

From the above **Tables 15** and **16**, the advantage of the proposed work over existing neural network is visible clearly. This analysis proves that the modified approach is suitable replacement for conventional methods. Similarly, the accuracy is also improved. **Table 17** gives performance comparison to similar literature works with proposed approach. Since the images are real time collected from local diagnostic centre, these images are not used by other researchers.

8. Conclusion and future work

Design and analysis of modified self-organizing map and modified back propagation neural network on MR brain image are proposed and tested successfully in this research work. The proposed technique also eliminates the limitations of conventional SOM and conventional BPN by reducing the number of iterations required to stabilize the weights. Using modified SOM and modified BPN technique, an accuracy of 96%, which is 10%increase in tumor classification and an average efficiency of 93%, which is 8% improvement in segmentation could be achieved. The proposed technique gives superior results for tumors of different sizes and shapes. This will aid the doctors and physicians in accurately diagnosing the brain tumor and early treatment planning, to increase the survival rate of the patient. As a future work, different feature sets can be used to train the neural network and suitable modifications can be done in the architecture and algorithm to increase the accuracy of the system further. Appropriate feature selection and modifications could make this proposed work applicable in deducting other chronic diseases.

Acknowledgements

The authors would like to thank Dr.D. Jagadeeswara Reddy, MBBS, M.Ch.(NIMS) consultant Neurosurgeon, Regd. No 51723 Tirupathi, Andhra Pradesh, India for providing necessary guidance and help in the analysis of proposed work. Also would like to thank Centre for Diagnostic Imaging, Tirupathi for providing brain MR images and result validation.

Conflict of interest

The authors declare they have no potential conflict of interest with the regard to the work presented.

Informed consent

Informed consent was obtained from all the individual participants in the research.

Permissions

Permission to use the images/materials included in this study has been obtained from the institution named "Centre for Diagnostic Imaging, Tirupathi, Andhra Pradesh, India".

Author details

G. Sethuram Rao and D. Vydeki*
VIT Chennai, Chennai, Tamil Nadu, India

*Address all correspondence to: vydeki.d@vit.ac.in

References

[1] Heba M et al. Classification using deep learning neural networks for brain tumors. Future Computing and Informatics. 2018;**3**:6871

[2] EI-Dahshan E-SA, Hosny T, Salem A-BM. Hybrid intelligent techniques for MRI brain images classification. Digital Signal Processing. 2010;**20**(2):433-441

[3] Zacharaki EI, Wang S, Chawla S, Yoo DS, Wolf R, Melhem ER, et al. Classification of brain tumor type and grade using MRI texture in a machine learning technique. Magnetic Resonance in Medicine. 2009;**62**:1609-1618

[4] Eli G et al. Nifty net: A deep-learning platform for medical imaging. Computer Methods and Programs in Biomedicine. 2018;**158**:113-122

[5] Michael S, Gregory F. Using a model of human visual perception to improve deep learning. Neural Networks. 2018; **104**:40-49

[6] Ling-Li Z et al. Multi-site diagnostic classification of schizophrenia using discriminant deep learning with functional connectivity MRI. EBioMedicine. 2018;**30**:74-85

[7] Chensi C et al. Deep learning and its application in biomedicine. Genomics, Proteomics & Bioinformatics. 2018;**16**: 17-32

[8] Yazhou K et al. Classification of autism spectrum disorder by combining brain connectivity and deep neural network classifier. Neurocomputing. 2018;**26**:36-52. DOI: 10.1016/j.neucom.2018.04.080

[9] Hongmin L, Guoqi L, Xiangyang J, Luping S. Deep representation via convolutional neural network for classification ospatio temporal event streams. Neurocomputing. 2018;**299**:1-9

[10] Usman K, Rajpoot. Brain tumor classification from multi modality MRI using wavelets and machine learning. Cross Mark Pattern Analysis and Application. 2017;**20**:871-881. DOI: 10.1007/s1004-017-0597-8

[11] Aneja D, Rawat TK. Fuzzy clustering algorithms for effective image segmentation. International Journal of Intelligent Systems and Applications. 2013;**11**:55-61

[12] Zhao F, Liu H, Fan J. A multi objective spatial fuzzy clustering algorithm for image segmentation. Journal of Applied Soft Computing. 2017;**30**:48-57

[13] Kumar SS, Moorthi M, Madh M, Amutha R. An improved method of segmentation using fuzzy-neuro logic. In: Proc: Second International Conference on Computer Research and Development. Kuala Lumpur: IEEE; 2010. pp. 671-675

[14] Wang B, Yang F, Chao S. Image segmentation algorithm based on high dimension fuzzy character and restrained clustering network. IEEE Transactions System Engineering Electronics. 2014;**25**(2):298-306

[15] Kong Y, Deng Y, Dai Q. Discriminative clustering and feature selection for brain MRI segmentation. IEEE Signal Process. Letters. 2015;**22**(5): 573-577

[16] Damodharan S, Raghavan. Combining tissue segmentation and neural network for brain detection. International Arab Journal of Information Technology (IAJIT). 2015; **12**:42-52

[17] Hemanth DJ, Vijila CKS, Anitha J. Performance improved PSO based modified counter propagation neural network for abnormal MR brain image classification. International Journal of Advances in Soft Computing and its Applications. 2010;**2**(1):65-84

[18] Hemanth DJ, Selvathi D, Anitha J. Application of ART neural network for abnormal MR brain image classification. International Journal of Health Information Sciences and Informatics. 2010;**5**(1):61-75

[19] Hemanth DJ, Vallentina EB, Anitha J. Performance improved hybrid intelligent system for medical image classification. Proceedings of 7th Balken Conference on Informatics. 2015;**5**:29-45. DOI: 10.1145/2801081.280109

Section 5

Intraoperative Ultrasonography in the Brain Tumor Surgery

Chapter 9

Usefulness of Intraoperative 2D-Ultrasound in the Resection of Brain Tumors

José Luis Navarro-Olvera, Armando Armas-Salazar, Jesús Q. Beltrán, Gustavo Aguado-Carrillo, Fiacro Jiménez-Ponce, Edgar Abarca-Rojano and José Damián Carrillo-Ruiz

Abstract

The surgical approach to brain tumors often uses preoperative images to visualize the characteristics of pathology, guiding the surgical procedure. However, the usefulness of preoperative images during the surgical procedure is altered by the changes in the brain during the surgery because of craniotomy, inflammation, tumor resection, cerebrospinal fluid (CSF) drainage, among others. For this reason, there is a need to use intraoperative imaging evaluation methods that allow the surgeon to consider these changes, reflecting the real-time anatomical disposition of the brain/tumor. Intraoperative ultrasound (iUS) has allowed neurosurgeons to guide the surgical procedure without exposing the patient to ionizing radiation or interrupting the procedure. Technological advances have made it possible to improve image quality, have smaller probes, and facilitate the use of the equipment, in addition to the introduction of new imaging modalities, such as three-dimensional images, enhanced with contrast, among others, expanding the available options. In the context of these advances, the objective of this chapter was to review the current status of the usefulness and challenges of iUS for brain tumor resection through an in-depth review of the literature and the discussion of an illustrative case.

Keywords: ultrasonography, intraoperative, navigation, neurosurgery, brain tumors

1. Introduction

Usage of ultrasound (US) for the first time for brain surgery was reported by Chandler et al. describing the surgical outcomes of 21 cases (including 18 patients with brain tumors) using two-dimensional imaging (2D-US) [1], allowing real-time visualization of the underlying anatomy and pathology during surgical performance. Since that time, the use of intraoperative ultrasound (iUS) has allowed surgeons to improve the decision-making during a surgical procedure without exposure to ionizing radiation [2]. The technology has evolved with the improvement of image quality and neuroimaging modalities, introducing smaller probes and more seamless integration with neuronavigation systems. In addition, the introduction of related imaging modalities, such as three-dimensional US (3D-US), high-frequency ultrasound (HF-US), contrast-enhanced US (C-US), and ultrasound elastography (E-US), diversified options with different advantages [3]. In the context of these advances, we review the current state of the intraoperative usefulness of 2D-US in comparison with the other modalities for the resection of brain tumors and expose our perspective of the usefulness of this method through the discussion of a case.

2. Intraoperative 2D-ultrasound in brain tumor surgery

2.1 Equipment and technical considerations

The US system uses sound waves at high frequencies (approximately greater than 20 kHz), using transducers that emit pulses at a frequency of 1–20 MHz [4]. These pulses emitted by the transducers are scattered, absorbed, or reflected depending on the acoustic properties of the brain tissue. The transducers detect wave echoes and produce a two-dimensional image based on the time intervals between the emitted pulses and the received echoes. The higher the frequency, the higher the images will be with the limitation of less tissue penetration. In the neurosurgical setting, transducers are typically used at 5–10 MHz, at depths of 2–8 cm, to ensure resolution between 500 and 1000 μm [2]. It is important to consider the existence of more advanced transducers that work at frequencies of up to 10–25 MHz and require a resolution of 100–600 μm, with the limitation that they are only useful for depths between 2 and 4 cm. Some of these devices were evaluated by Moran et al. [5], where the highest resolution integrals were obtained using the Vevo 770 and 2100 scanners [5]. However, it is important to consider the optimal choice of transducer, type, and acquisition frequency, which depends on several variables, such as tumor location, properties of the tumor, craniotomy size, surrounding anatomy, as well as surgeon preference [4, 5].

Regarding the interpretation of intraoperative cerebral US images, it is important to have certain considerations. The normal brain, sulci, falx cerebri, choroid plexus, and vessel walls are shown as hyperechoic images, where the gray matter is slightly more hypoechoic relative to the white matter, while the ventricles, cysts, and other spaces filled with cerebrospinal fluid (CSF) are hypoechoic. On the other hand, tumors are often hyperechoic due to their relatively high mass density. Tumors become more difficult to identify in the presence of peritumoral edema because this causes greater echogenicity and can make it difficult to differentiate the margins between the tumor lesion and normal brain tissue. It is important to consider this because the echogenicity of the chronic edema is unpredictable, creating a confounding factor during surgical intervention [6].

In neurosurgery, US is used during tumor resection for different purposes: tumor location and characterization (1), surgical planning (2), and evaluation of the extent of resection (3). The application of US is limited to the size of the craniotomy. The probe can be applied to the dura mater or the brain parenchyma; during imaging, care must be taken not to apply too much pressure (it would cause deformation and limit the usefulness of the image). Once a resection cavity has been established, it is possible to insert a probe into the cavity [7]. However, in case the transducer is very large, the cavity can be filled with saline solution to attach the transducer (technique described by Tormod Selbekk et al. [8]). It is preferable to position the patient such that the resection surface is horizontal with respect to gravity in order to minimize trapped air within the cavity (improve image quality). Because the size of the craniotomy plays a very important role in the selection of the size of the transducer, cases have also been described where an exclusive craniotomy for the probe has been performed [2].

2.2 Artifacts and limitations

The acquisition and interpretation of US images is due to the fact that it requires experience. Training in ultrasonography through the use of simulators or animals guided by experts is recommended. An artifact is defined as an image that does not represent the actual anatomy of the structure being viewed, which arises for a variety of reasons. Bone (a tissue with high signal attenuation) can create a shadow that decreases the signal from surrounding tissues. The attenuation coefficient of saline solution, which is often used to fill the resection cavity, is lower than that of brain tissue, thus producing a brightness artifact at the brain/saline interface and potentially impairing identification of the residual tumor. Coagulated blood or hemostatic materials may produce a brightness artifact. In addition, differences in sound conduction speed between tissues can cause geometric distortion of the image in two-dimensional US (2D-US), and the presence of saline solution (which conducts sound at a slower speed than the brain) produces an error of approximately 1.5 mm at a depth greater than 10 cm. Even temperature can change the speed of sound and thus influence image quality [8].

2D-US has several limitations, for example, the resolution of US is not uniform in all directions, depending on the depth of focus and the location of the target within the frame [9]. One of the most important limitations is the interoperator variability in the performance and interpretation of the images. Because the appearance of the tissue depends on the angle and depth of the US waves, it is difficult to compare the images with other study modalities such as magnetic resonance imaging (MRI) and computed tomography (CT). The 2D-US image is constructed from the plane perpendicular to the face of the transducer, so this plane does not usually coincide with the axial, sagittal, or coronal sections with which the surgeon is used to working.

2.3 Different ultrasound imaging modalities

There are various US modalities other than 2D-US, which offer different types of advantages with their respective limitations. Among these, the 3-dimensional US (3D-US) is useful for volumetric reconstruction of images [10, 11]. Among others, the high-frequency ultrasound (HF-US) operates at frequencies up to 25 MHz to provide higher resolution images, giving the advantage of producing more reliable demarcation of tumor margins even in peritumoral edema and previous radiotherapy settings [5, 12, 13]. During brain tumor surgery, Doppler US (D-US) is used to assess tumor vascularity and guide the extent of the surgical approach, using the Doppler effect, which is a change in frequency seen when a US wave is reflected into the transducer in order to determine the direction and speed of the blood flow [14, 15]. On the other hand, US elastography (US-E) is another imaging modality that allows to evaluate the elastic properties of the brain tissue, relating the stiffness of the tissue to a force applied to it [16]. Finally, contrast-enhanced US (CE-US) allows real-time visualization of tissue vascularization, being useful for identifying highly vascularized tumors. Unlike contrast agents for CT or MRI, CE-US contrast is composed of small gaseous microbubbles that resonate when hit by US waves, lacking the side effects and toxicities associated with other contrast media [17–19]. **Table 1** summarizes the advantages and limitations of all these modalities compared to 2D-US.

2.4 Ultrasound applications in brain tumor surgery

Intraoperative navigation has become the standard practice for initial localization and evaluation of tumor margins during resection [20]. However, navigation may be limited by changes in the arrangement of brain tissue during the procedure due to inflammation, tumor resection, CSF drainage, among other factors. For this reason, there is a need to incorporate an intraoperative procedure that allows to evaluate these changes. Different solutions have been proposed, such as intraoperative MRI, cone beam computed tomography, stereoscopic cameras, fluorescence materials, and the incorporation of computer software's [21–23]. However, the use of iUS continues to be a very attractive option compared to other modalities, due to its accessibility (low cost), minimal interruption of surgery, and absence of radiation. In this context, the iUS has three applications that will be discussed in detail: (1) intraoperative navigation, (2) evaluation of extent of resection, (3) and brain-shift monitoring and compensation.

2.5 Intraoperative navigation

Using an intraoperative image allows to accurately assess the location of the tumor and identify the surrounding structures. As mentioned earlier, each of the modalities has its advantages and limitations for these applications. A study by Hammoud et al. evaluated the efficacy of iUS in locating and defining tumor borders and in assessing the extent of their resection, showing that the borders were well defined in 83.3% and moderately defined in 16%, in all patients the extent of the resection was well defined (measured by postoperative MRI) [24]. Moreover, Hammoud MA and his group observed that the extent of resection was poorly defined in the patients whose pathology showed radiation effects and recurrent tumors. Therefore, the iUS provides greater fidelity in cases of primary resection compared to recurrent tumors with previous surgery and/or radiation [25], a phenomenon possibly explained by the greater echogenicity of the edema, scar tissue (gliosis), and post-radiation necrosis [26]. On the other hand, beyond the evaluation of the borders, US has proven to be useful in demonstrating the relationship between the appearance of brain tissue on intraoperative ultrasonography and pathological grade of cerebral glioma, managing to differentiate low-grade gliomas (calcifications and hyperechoic), in contrast to high-grade gliomas that usually present changes due to necrosis [27]. If what is desired is to improve the identification of the tumor volume, US can be combined with MRI, improving the visualization beyond the margins visualized with MRI contrast (gadolinium), helping to differentiate the tumor from the edema visible on T2-weighted images [28]. In addition, US is comparable to CT in stereotactic guidance for taking brain biopsies, according to diagnostic yield rate [29].

The utility of 3D-US was first evaluated by Unsgaard et al. in a series of 28 patients for the resection of primary and metastatic brain tumors, showing that this modality gives a good delineation of metastases and the solid part of tumor (gliomas) before starting the resection. When comparing tumor identification using 3D-US versus pathologic diagnosis, biopsies taken from the edge of the tumor revealed more than 70% correlation in low-grade and anaplastic astrocytoma's,

Imaging modality	Advantages	Limitations
2D-US	• Fast image acquisition • Relatively easy to use • Equilibrium between resolution and penetration • Accessibility (low cost)	• Difficult three-dimensional interpretation of the anatomy • High variability (during the procedure) • Similar echogenicity between chronic edema and tumor mass
3D-US	• Volumetric image (avoid arbitrary planes) • Different ways of image production (asynchronous, mechanical translation, and phased array) • Flexible field of view	• Pressure applied to the brain produce artifacts • Slow acquisition of image reconstruction (phases array is comparable to that of 2D-US) • Reconstruction quality (subject to interoperator variability and highly sensitive to motion artifacts)
HF-US	• Frequency up to 25 MHz (higher resolution) • More reliable demarcation of tumor margins • Better differentiation of peritumoral edema • Small transducers (easier insertion in cavities)	• Poor depth (penetration) of view • Visualization of small regions at a time (lower intraoperative usefulness)
D-US	• Assess tumor vascularity • Different modalities (color, power and 3D) • Power D-US: less noise, less angle-dependent, higher resolution of small vessels, and no aliasing. • 3D D-US: simultaneously demonstrate arteries and veins (include small-caliber vessels).	• Poor resolution and high noise • D-US: angle-dependent (flow perpendicular to US waves = no signal) • Power D-US: less information about flow direction and velocity, vessels appear larger (visualization of small vessels of limited relevance) • Aliasing (artifact): incorrect flow magnitude
US-E	• Maps elastic properties of tissue	• Negligible acquisition and computation times • Uncertain correlation with histopathology • Brain tissue damage during assessment • High noise
CE-US	• Real-time visualization of tissue vascularity (identified tumors that recruit an avid vascular supply) • Help the surgeon to navigate around vascular structures • Image quality is unaffected by angle of insonation • Unlike D-US, CE-US can simultaneously show high- and low-flow vessels (perfusion dynamics)	• Require that image occur prior to coagulation of tumor feeding vessels (alter operative workflow) • Field of view is constant during contrast injection • No FDA-approved contrast agents for neurosurgery

2D-US: two-dimensional ultrasound; 3D-US: three-dimensional ultrasound; HF-US: high-frequency ultrasound; D-US: Doppler ultrasound; CE-US: contrast-enhanced ultrasound; US-E: ultrasound elastography; and FDA: Food and Drug Administration.

Table 1.
Comparison of the advantages and limitations between the different ultrasound (US) modalities.

glioblastomas, and metastasis. A very remarkable aspect regarding the usefulness of 3D-US is that the use of iUS to delineate the histopathological margin of the tumor has been shown to be equivalent to MRI [30]. A series of glioma resections performed by Sure et al. with the integration of US technology into neuronavigation to define the main vascular structures in preoperative images, highlight the limitations to identify these structures due to brain-shift in the use of neuronavigation [31]. On the other hand, they highlight the usefulness of the D-US to locate and guide the surgical approach considering the vasculature of the tumor and the adjacent vascular structures. Other methods such as power Doppler and CE-US have allowed intraoperative navigation around major vascular structures without relying on preoperative imaging that does not account for brain displacement [32, 33]. However, it must be considered that the magnitude of CE-US does not correlate with the degree of contrast enhancement observed on CT or MRI [34]. The utility of E-US is still in the early stages of characterization with respect to brain tumor resection. As mentioned earlier, this study is based on the use of pulsations to identify the tension/rigidity of a tissue in order to differentiate the tumor from the normal parenchyma. However, these images have not been with MRI or histopathology, so their true utility is unknown. On the other hand, it has been shown to be useful in predicting the location of dissection planes during resection. Scholz et al. evaluated brain tumors of different etiologies, showing that the E-US allows to differentiate the tumor from the normal parenchyma. Therefore, it could be said that this modality is especially useful to define the resection margin [16].

2.5.1 Assessment of extent of resection

The extent of the resection contributes to improving patient survival in the surgical management of brain tumors [35]. However, the evaluation of the resection extension is complex, and the use of the US offers a promising option due to its accessibility and real-time feedback. However, its ability to reliably identify residual tumor is limited by a variety of factors [36]. Chacko et al. published an article where brain tissue samples were taken from tumor margins (defined by iUS), showing a correlation between the histopathological study and the iUS greater than 80% [37]. A previous study of intraoperative iUS in glioma resection reported that 89% concordance with histopathology in hyperechoic areas that clearly extended into isoechogenic brain parenchyma, in contrast with a 56% concordance along the hyperechoic rim of the resection cavity [38]. Due to the concern generated by histological confirmation with imaging data, different solutions have been sought, one of them being the use of other modalities other than 2D-US, for example, the use of HF-US that offers superior intraoperative tumor detectability in primary and recurrent surgery for the study of glioblastomas. HF-US was shown to have a higher sensitivity for tumor detection (76%) [12]. On the other hand, comparison of iUS and intraoperative 1.5 T MRI in 26 patients with multiple brain tumors reliably detected residual tumor in those tumors that were larger than 1 cm. However, the usefulness of iUS is limited for smaller tumors [39].

2.5.2 Brain-shift monitoring and compensation

Surgical intervention produces changes in the anatomical arrangement of the brain due to various factors. Due to its low cost (accessibility), security, and speed, the US is a suitable candidate option to compensate for these changes in real time.

These changes can be represented in the form of a deformation field in order to update the preoperative images obtained generally by MRI. The generation of the deformation field is based on an algorithmic alignment of two images of the same anatomy (preoperative and postoperative image). There are different registration strategies for obtaining the deformation field. However, the most used are the rigid and non-rigid techniques, where the rigid maps two images with the translation and rotation of the image, compared to the non-rigid registration where the images can be obtained in a more flexible way. In general, the non-rigid records more accurately represent the observed changes, with the limitation that they require a greater calculation time [40]. Other strategies have been proposed to fuse the iUS with the preoperative anatomical record. However, these studies have been conducted in small groups of patients. These include the use of probabilistic functions that match hyperechoic structures (for rigid use) [41], Bayesian logarithmic registration incorporating local region information to improve compensation for missing tissue [42], the generation of a very similar to US from MRI [43], and D-US recording to preoperative MRI angiography [44]. Mercier et al. described a study that sought to find an intraoperative registration technique that would improve the alignment of US images taken before and after brain tumor resection. The study was performed in 16 cases using 2 different registration methods, the first one was performed with manually selected labels in pre- and post-resection US to calculate the mean distance between corresponding points in the two volumes before and after registration (rigid registration), and in the second one, the surgeon was asked to classify and rate the quality of the alignment before and after registration (nonlinear registration). The mean distance was 2.7 mm after rigid registration, and 1.7 mm after nonlinear registration. Consistent with distance and classification metrics, the nonlinear registration approach significantly improved the alignment of US images [45].

3. Illustrative case

3.1 Case presentation

A 65-year-old female patient began her condition 15 days prior to hospital admission with a throbbing holocranial headache, of variable intensity from 6 to 8 according to the visual analog pain scale, followed by nausea and vomiting, added with dysphasia, and weakness in the left hemibody. During the physical examination, within the important findings, the presence of papilledema (intracranial hypertension) was identified, as well as the finding of left hemiparesia, grade 4/5 and increase in deep tendon reflexes, ruling out the presence of dysphagia and memory loss. It was decided to perform a simple and contrast-enhanced MRI of the brain (**Figure 1**), which evidenced the presence of an intra-axial lesion of the temporo-parietal lobe with heterogeneous enhancement of the periphery. For this reason, it was decided to perform a surgical procedure to remove the tumoral lesion.

3.2 Surgical procedure and outcomes

With the patient under general anesthesia, in dorsal decubitus position and head with lateralization to the left, a Mayfield head frame was placed, fixed with elevation, lateralization to the left, and deflection. Trichotomy, asepsis, and antisepsis (with chlorhexidine) were performed, surgical fields were placed, 2% lidocaine was

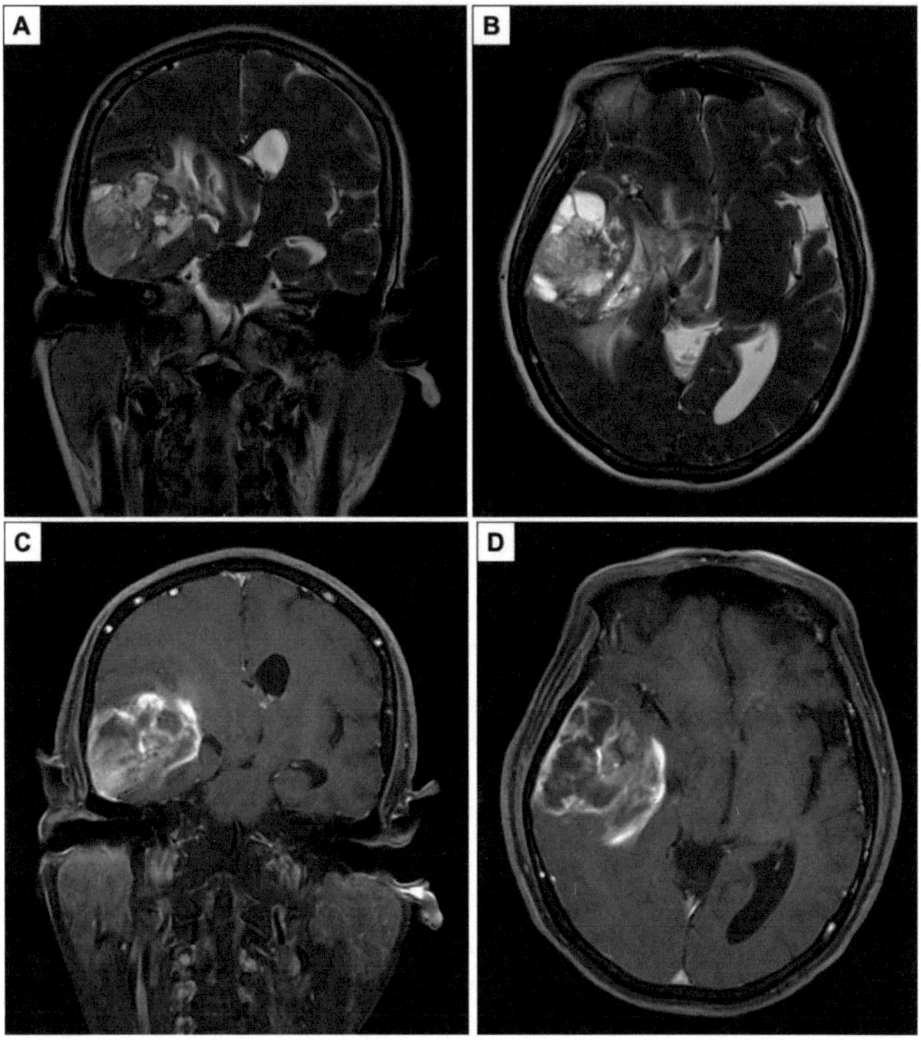

Figure 1.
Preoperative brain magnetic resonance imaging (MRI). T2-weighted MRI (A-B) A. Coronal view. B Axial view. T1. Contrast-enhanced T1-weighted MRI (C-D). C. Coronal view. D. Axial view. The images show a rounded heterogeneous cystic-appearing lesion in the right temporo-parietal region with contrast media uptake, ring enhancement, and peripheral vasogenic edema.

infiltrated, and a right Mark-type incision was made. It was incised with the scalpel in planes up to the pericranium, performing hemostasis with bipolar and preserving muscular structures. Subsequently, a pericranial dissection was performed by dissecting a skin flap and performing an interfacial dissection (displacing the muscle caudally). Afterward, a right fronto-temporal craniotomy was performed, exposing the dura mater to perform a 2D-US scan (Samsung HM70 EVO) (**Figure 2**), identifying the dissection plane from which to start the resection (**Figure 3A–E**), a complete dissection of the tumor mass identified by US in all its limits, as well as the tissue direct visualized with gliosis.

The temporal lobe dissection was performed until the skull base and tentorium were identified. A new US scan was performed to corroborate the complete resection

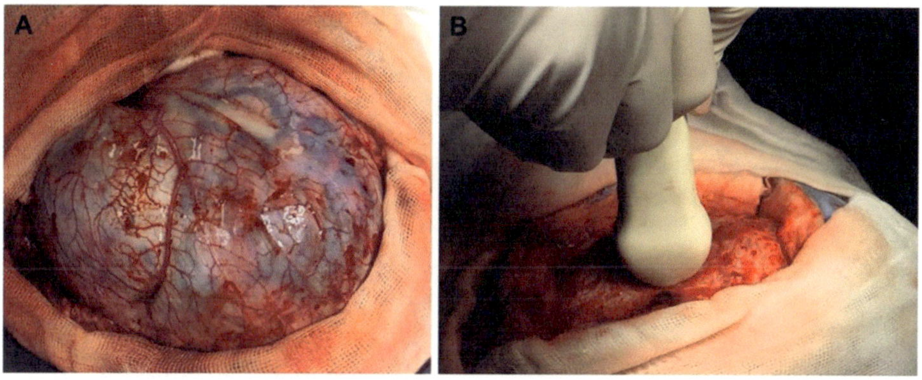

Figure 2.
Surgical approach. A. Fronto-temporal craniotomy. B. Ultrasound scan.

(**Figure 3F**). Subsequently, hemostasis was performed with surgicel and gelfoam, ending the microsurgical time, proceeding to primary closure and plasty of the dura mater with pericranial tissue. Hermetic closure was verified, and bone was placed, then a subgaleal drainage was placed closing the galea, ending by closing the skin with continuous Sarnoff stitches. The patient was discharged from the neurosurgery

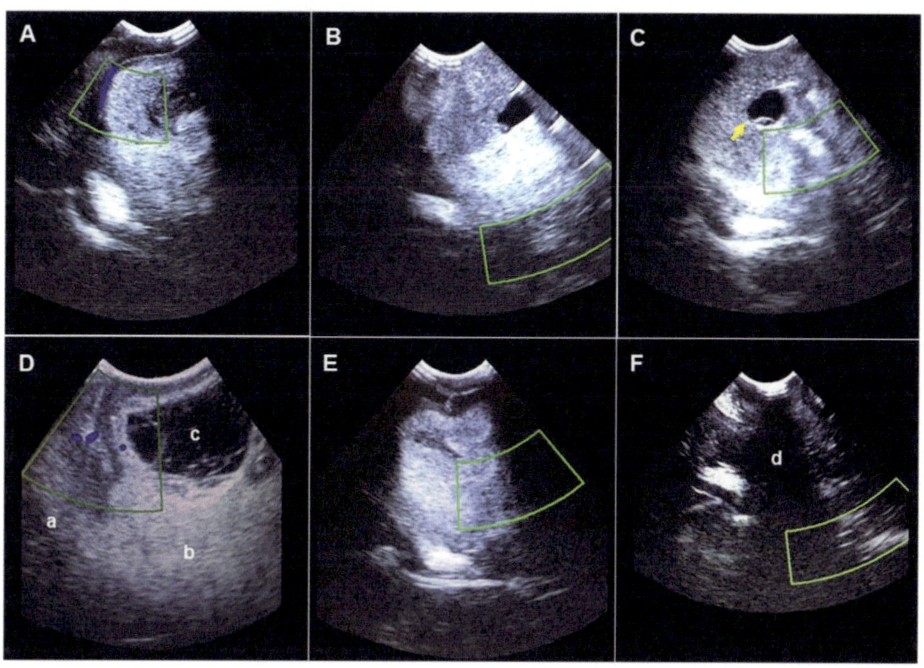

Figure 3.
Intraoperative 2D ultrasound (2D-US). A. One of the advantages of US is to show the perilesional vascular structures as shown in blue in the image. B. The tumoral lesion of the patient of shows a cystic component, also useful to define the characteristics of the tumor. C. The yellow arrow indicates an intratumorally cystic degeneration. D. In this image, it is possible to distinguish the echogenicity of different brain tissues: normal brain tissue (a), tumoral mass (b), and cystic component (c). E. 2D-US allows defining the limits of the tumor lesion, as shown in the differences of echogenicity. F. Secondary navigation after surgical resection allows to evaluate the complete tumor resection, and to avoid resection lodge artifact, it is suggested steering clear of putting hemostatic materials and the surgical field is filled with warm injectable solution to continue iUS mapping (d).

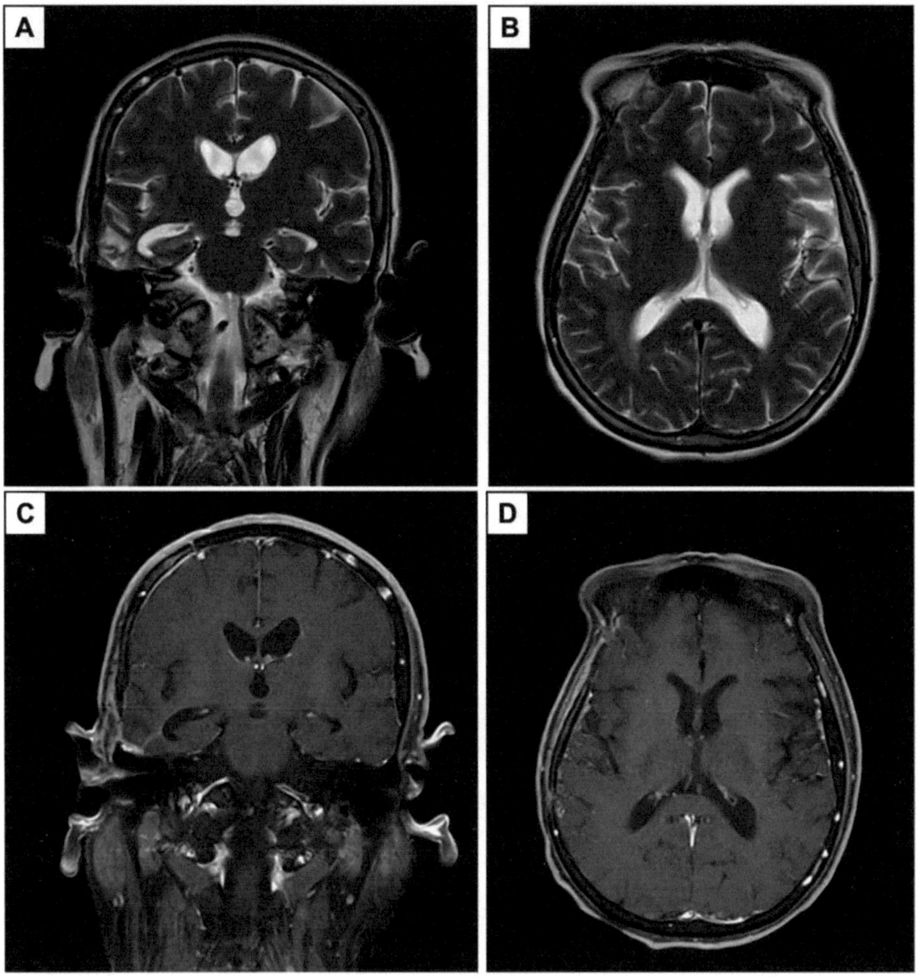

Figure 4.
Postoperative brain magnetic resonance imaging (MRI). T2-weighted MRI (A-B) A. Coronal view. B Axial view. T1. Contrast-enhanced T1-weighted MRI (C-D). C. Coronal view. D. Axial view. The images show a gross total resection of the lesion without recurrence.

service 3 days after the intervention without neurological alterations. MRI studies were obtained at 3, 6, and 10 months, where **Figure 4** shows the last imaging study at 10-month follow-up, showing a gross total resection of the lesion. The histopathological report confirmed the presence of glioblastoma, so it was decided to start adjuvant therapy (Stupp R. protocol) with radiotherapy (fractionated focal irradiation in daily fractions of 2 Gy given 5 days per week for 6 weeks, for a total of 60 Gy) plus continuous daily temozolomide (75 mg per square meter of body surface area per day, 7 days per week from the first to the last day of radiotherapy), followed by six cycles of adjuvant temozolomide (150 mg per square meter for 5 days during each 1 month cycle) [46]. Although recurrence is common in tumors such as glioblastoma, in this case at 10 months of follow-up no recurrence data were observed, due to the large resection of the tumor added to postoperative adjuvant management with chemotherapy and radiotherapy.

3.3 Case discussion

Most first-world countries have adequate technology to achieve complete resections in most of their cases, and it allows them to have better survival rates [47]. However, this requires a very high economic investment in terms of operating room equipment for neurological surgery. In contrast with developing countries, where health systems are limited to federal budgets, it is complicated to have all the tools to ensure maximum resection, so alternative methods to those commonly used (trans-operative MRI, neuronavigation, stereotaxic, or fluorescence through a special filter in the microscope) should be used in developed countries [48]. Our neurosurgery service has continued to use 2D-US as a routine tool in brain tumor surgery, because it is an available and accessible tool (low cost). The fact that it is not cutting-edge technology does not mean that it is less useful, and as the advantages shown in **Table 1**, this imaging tool has a series of modalities that offer great advantages during the evaluation of tumor resection during the intraoperative period.

Among the main disadvantages of the use of 2D-US for the resection of brain tumors is that it requires learning in its use and experience since it requires experience of the neurosurgeon. This means that whoever decides to use this method as a guide for maximum resections must prepare and learn ultrasonography prior to its use in the operating room, either with animal models or simulators. On the other hand, another disadvantage is the inability to plan before the intervention, a very clear advantage of neuronavigation and stereotaxic guided surgery. However, the main advantages of the US are as follows: the correct identification of the lesion after craniotomy and during the procedure (1), the identification of the tumor margins (2), the evaluation of the characteristics of the tumor (3), the evaluation of the vascular structures within the tumor and in its periphery (4), and the compensation phenomena in real time (avoid brain-shift) (5) [3].

In the case presented earlier, as neuronavigation and fluorescence were not available, it was decided to guide the resection with 2D-US, all with the aim of increasing the degree of resection with maximum safety for the patient and achieving adequate survival. As can be seen in the postoperative images, once the craniotomy was performed, an epidural recording of the lesion was started with the transducer (**Figure 2**), the durotomy was planned, and after it, the brain was repeatedly scanned to identify the edges of the lesion (**Figure 3D** and **E**), including some cystic portions and vessels at the periphery of the tumor (**Figure 3A–C**). Throughout the surgical procedure, the extension of the resection was verified with this method, until it was completed (**Figure 3F**), achieving the main objective (maximum resection) (**Figure 4**). Although in some places it is already considered an obsolete method, derived from advances in technology and the implementation of better imaging methods for intraoperative use. According to the literature search, and the results obtained in more than 50 patients (on published data) in which iUS was used for tumor resection including the illustrative case exposes in this book chapter, we consider that this method could be a great alternative due to the advantages mentioned earlier, since it is in real time and does not depend on planning and being very accessible compared to other methods. However, it is necessary to perform well-powered, well-designed, randomized prospective studies that compare the different trans-operative techniques such as MRI, neuronavigation, stereotaxic, fluorescence, and iUS, in terms of survival and cost-effectiveness.

4. Conclusion

During the resection of a brain tumor, efforts are aimed at minimizing the repercussion of the tumor on the neurological integrity of the patient, trying to preserve function with the highest degree of resection possible. Because the US can provide intraoperative (real-time) information, it is useful in guiding surgical resection. The background highlights the reliability of US in the management of tumor pathology, where despite the existence of multiple limitations compared to other methods of tumor resection such as artifacts that occur in the resection cavity and variability, it is necessary to carry out further studies that allow evaluating the efficacy of US in terms of survival, intraoperative tumor identification, and cost-effectiveness, compared with other alternatives.

Conflict of interest

The authors declare no conflict of interest.

Permissions

The permission to use the images/materials included in this study has been obtained.

Acronyms and abbreviations

CSF	Cerebrospinal fluid
CT	computed tomography
CE-US	contrast-enhanced ultrasound
D-US	Doppler ultrasound
HF-US	high-frequency ultrasound
iUS	intraoperative ultrasound
MRI	magnetic resonance imaging
3D-US	three-dimensional ultrasound
2D-US	two-dimensional ultrasound
US	ultrasound
US-E	ultrasound elastogy

DOI: http://dx.doi.org/10.5772/intechopen.106798

Author details

José Luis Navarro-Olvera[1,2], Armando Armas-Salazar[1,3], Jesús Q. Beltrán[1], Gustavo Aguado-Carrillo[1], Fiacro Jiménez-Ponce[1], Edgar Abarca-Rojano[3] and José Damián Carrillo-Ruiz[1,4,5]*

1 Unit of Functional and Stereotactic Neurosurgery and Radiosurgery, General Hospital of Mexico. "Dr. Eduardo Liceaga", Mexico City, Mexico

2 Faculty of Medicine, National Autonomous University of Mexico, Mexico City, Mexico

3 School of Higher Education in Medicine, National Polytechnic Institute, Mexico City, Mexico

4 Faculty of Health Sciences, Anahuac University, Mexico City, Mexico

5 General Hospital of Mexico. "Dr. Eduardo Liceaga", Mexico City, Mexico

*Address all correspondence to: josecarrilloruiz@yahoo.com

References

[1] Chandler WF, Knake JE, McGillicuddy JE, Lillehei KO, Silver TM. Intraoperative use of real-time ultrasonography in neurosurgery. Journal of Neurosurgery. 1982;**57**(2):157-163. DOI: 10.3171/jns.1982.57.2.0157

[2] Unsgaard G, Gronningsaeter A, Ommedal S, Nagelhus Hernes TA. Brain operations guided by real-time two-dimensional ultrasound: New possibilities as a result of improved image quality. Neurosurgery. 2002;**51**(2):402-412

[3] Sastry R, Bi WL, Pieper S, et al. Applications of ultrasound in the resection of brain tumors. Journal of Neuroimaging. 2017;**27**(1):5-15. DOI: 10.1111/jon.12382

[4] Serra C, Stauffer A, Actor B, et al. Intraoperative high frequency ultrasound in intracerebral high-grade tumors. Ultraschall Medizin. 2012;**33**(7):E306-E312. DOI: 10.1055/s-0032-1325369

[5] Moran CM, Pye SD, Ellis W, et al. A comparison of the imaging performance of high resolution ultrasound scanners for preclinical imaging. Ultrasound in Medicine & Biology. 2011;**37**(3):493-501. DOI: 10.1016/j.ultrasmedbio.2010.11.010

[6] Sos Sosna J, Barth MM, Kruskal JB, Kane RA. Intraoperative sonography for neurosurgery. Journal of Ultrasound in Medicine. 2005;**24**(12):1671-1682. DOI: 10.7863/jum.2005.24.12.1671

[7] Unsgaard G, Rygh OM, Selbekk T, et al. Intra-operative 3D ultrasound in neurosurgery. Acta Neurochirurgica. 2006;**148**(3):235-253. DOI: 10.1007/s00701-005-0688-y

[8] Selbekk T, Jakola AS, Solheim O, et al. Ultrasound imaging in neurosurgery: Approaches to minimize surgically induced image artefacts for improved resection control. Acta Neurochirurgica. 2013;**155**(6):973-980. DOI: 10.1007/s00701-013-1647-7

[9] Nelson TR, Pretorius DH, Hull A, Riccabona M, Sklansky MS, James G. Sources and impact of artifacts on clinical three-dimensional ultrasound imaging. Ultrasound in Obstetrics & Gynecology. 2000;**16**(4):374-383. DOI: 10.1046/j.1469-0705.2000.00180.x

[10] Riccabona M, Nelson TR, Weitzer C, Resch B, Pretorius DP. Potential of three-dimensional ultrasound in neonatal and paediatric neurosonography. European Radiology. 2003;**13**(9):2082-2093. DOI: 10.1007/s00330-003-1845-4

[11] Smith SW, Pavy HR, von Ramm OT. High-speed ultrasound volumetric imaging system. I. Transducer design and beam steering. IEEE Transactions on Ultrasonics, Ferroelectrics, and Frequency Control. 1991;**38**(2):100-108. DOI: 10.1109/58.68466

[12] Coburger J, Scheuerle A, Kapapa T, et al. Sensitivity and specificity of linear array intraoperative ultrasound in glioblastoma surgery: A comparative study with high field intraoperative MRI and conventional sector array ultrasound. Neurosurgical Review. 2015;**38**(3):499-509. DOI: 10.1007/s10143-015-0627-1

[13] Coburger J, Scheuerle A, Thal DR, et al. Linear array ultrasound in low-grade glioma surgery: Histology-based assessment of accuracy in comparison to conventional intraoperative ultrasound and intraoperative MRI. Acta

Neurochirurgica. 2015;**157**(2):195-206. DOI: 10.1007/s00701-014-2314-3

[14] Anderson T, McDicken WN. The difference between colour doppler velocity imaging and power doppler imaging. European Journal of Echocardiography. 2002;**3**(3):240-244. DOI: 10.1053/euje.2002.0150

[15] Rubin JM, Bude RO, Carson PL, Bree RL, Adler RS. Power Doppler US: A potentially useful alternative to mean frequency-based color Doppler US. Radiology. 1994;**190**(3):853-856. DOI: 10.1148/radiology.190.3.8115639

[16] Scholz M, Noack V, Pechlivanis I, et al. Vibrography during tumor neurosurgery. Journal of Ultrasound in Medicine. 2005;**24**(7):985-992. DOI: 10.7863/jum.2005.24.7.985

[17] Prada F, Perin A, Martegani A, et al. Intraoperative contrast-enhanced ultrasound for brain tumor surgery. Neurosurgery. 2014;**74**(5):542-552. DOI: 10.1227/NEU.0000000000000301

[18] Arlt F, Chalopin C, Müns A, Meixensberger J, Lindner D. Intraoperative 3D contrast-enhanced ultrasound (CEUS): A prospective study of 50 patients with brain tumours. Acta Neurochirurgica. 2016;**158**(4):685-694. DOI: 10.1007/s00701-016-2738-z

[19] Lekht I, Brauner N, Bakhsheshian J, et al. Versatile utilization of real-time intraoperative contrast-enhanced ultrasound in cranial neurosurgery: Technical note and retrospective case series. Neurosurgical Focus. 2016;**40**(3):E6. DOI: 10.3171/2015.11.FOCUS15570

[20] White T, Zavarella S, Jarchin L, Nardi D, Schaffer S, Schulder M. Combined brain mapping and compact intraoperative MRI for brain tumor resection. Stereotactic and Functional Neurosurgery. 2018;**96**(3):172-181. DOI: 10.1159/000488991

[21] Black PM, Moriarty T, Alexander E 3rd, et al. Development and implementation of intraoperative magnetic resonance imaging and its neurosurgical applications. Neurosurgery. 1997;**41**(4):831-845. DOI: 10.1097/00006123-199710000-00013

[22] Kanayama S, Hara T, Hamada Y, Matsumaru Y. Potential of 80-kV high-resolution cone-beam CT imaging combined with an optimized protocol for neurological surgery. Neuroradiology. 2015;**57**(2):155-162. DOI: 10.1007/s00234-014-1447-7

[23] Wittek A, Kikinis R, Warfield SK, Miller K. Brain shift computation using a fully nonlinear biomechanical model. Medical Image Computing and Computer-Assisted Intervention. 2005;**8**(Pt 2):583-590. DOI: 10.1007/11566489_72

[24] Hammoud MA, Ligon BL, el Souki R, Shi WM, Schomer DF, Sawaya R. Use of intraoperative ultrasound for localizing tumors and determining the extent of resection: A comparative study with magnetic resonance imaging. Journal of Neurosurgery. 1996;**84**(5):737-741. DOI: 10.3171/jns.1996.84.5.0737

[25] Solheim O, Selbekk T, Jakola AS, Unsgård G. Ultrasound-guided operations in unselected high-grade gliomas—Overall results, impact of image quality and patient selection. Acta Neurochirurgica. 2010;**152**(11):1873-1886. DOI: 10.1007/s00701-010-0731-5

[26] Yu SQ, Wang JS, Chen SY, et al. Diagnostic significance of intraoperative ultrasound contrast in evaluating the

resection degree of brain glioma by transmission electron microscopic examination. Chinese Medical Journal. 2015;**128**(2):186-190. DOI: 10.4103/0366-6999.149194

[27] Wang J, Liu X, Hou WH, et al. The relationship between intra-operative ultrasonography and pathological grade in cerebral glioma. The Journal of International Medical Research. 2008;**36**(6):1426-1434. DOI: 10.1177/147323000803600632

[28] LeRoux PD, Winter TC, Berger MS, Mack LA, Wang K, Elliott JP. A comparison between preoperative magnetic resonance and intraoperative ultrasound tumor volumes and margins. Journal of Clinical Ultrasound. 1994;**22**(1):29-36. DOI: 10.1002/jcu.1870220107

[29] Krekel NM, Zonderhuis BM, Schreurs HW, et al. Ultrasound-guided breast-sparing surgery to improve cosmetic outcomes and quality of life. A prospective multicentre randomised controlled clinical trial comparing ultrasound-guided surgery to traditional palpation-guided surgery (COBALT trial). BMC Surgery. 2011;**11**:8

[30] Un Unsgaard G, Selbekk T, Brostrup Müller T, et al. Ability of navigated 3D ultrasound to delineate gliomas and metastases—Comparison of image interpretations with histopathology. Acta Neurochirurgica. 2005;**147**(12):1259-1269. DOI: 10.1007/s00701-005-0624-1

[31] Sure U, Benes L, Bozinov O, Woydt M, Tirakotai W, Bertalanffy H. Intraoperative landmarking of vascular anatomy by integration of duplex and Doppler ultrasonography in image-guided surgery. Technical note. Surg Neurol. 2005;**63**(2):133-142. DOI: 10.1016/j.surneu.2004.08.040

[32] Šteňo A, Jezberová M, Hollý V, Timárová G, Šteňo J. Visualization of lenticulostriate arteries during insular low-grade glioma surgeries by navigated 3D ultrasound power Doppler: Technical note. Journal of Neurosurgery. 2016;**125**(4):1016-1023. DOI: 10.3171/2015.10.JNS151907

[33] Kanno H, Ozawa Y, Sakata K, et al. Intraoperative power Doppler ultrasonography with a contrast-enhancing agent for intracranial tumors. Journal of Neurosurgery. 2005;**102**(2):295-301. DOI: 10.3171/jns.2005.102.2.0295

[34] Engelhardt M, Hansen C, Eyding J, et al. Feasibility of contrast-enhanced sonography during resection of cerebral tumours: Initial results of a prospective study. Ultrasound in Medicine & Biology. 2007;**33**(4):571-575. DOI: 10.1016/j.ultrasmedbio.2006.10.007

[35] Bloch O, Han SJ, Cha S, et al. Impact of extent of resection for recurrent glioblastoma on overall survival: Clinical article. Journal of Neurosurgery. 2012;**117**(6):1032-1038. DOI: 10.3171/2012.9.JNS12504

[36] Aizer AA, Bi WL, Kandola MS, et al. Extent of resection and overall survival for patients with atypical and malignant meningioma. Cancer. 2015;**121**(24):4376-4381. DOI: 10.1002/cncr.29639

[37] Chacko AG, Kumar NK, Chacko G, et al. Intraoperative ultrasound in determining the extent of resection of parenchymal brain tumours—A comparative study with computed tomography and histopathology. Neurochir (Wien). 2003;**145**:743-748

[38] Woydt M, Krone A, Becker G, Schmidt K, Roggendorf W, Roosen K. Correlation of intra-operative ultrasound with histopathologic findings after

tumour resection in supratentorial gliomas. A method to improve gross total tumour resection. Acta Neurochirurgica. 1996;**138**(12):1391-1398. DOI: 10.1007/BF01411117

[39] Gerganov VM, Samii A, Akbarian A, Stieglitz L, Samii M, Fahlbusch R. Reliability of intraoperative high-resolution 2D ultrasound as an alternative to high-field strength MR imaging for tumor resection control: A prospective comparative study. Journal of Neurosurgery. 2009;**111**(3):512-519. DOI: 10.3171/2009.2.JNS08535

[40] Risholm P, Pieper S, Samset E, Wells WM 3rd. Summarizing and visualizing uncertainty in non-rigid registration. Medical Image Computing and Computer-Assisted Intervention. 2010;**13**(Pt 2):554-561. DOI: 10.1007/978-3-642-15745-5_68

[41] Coupé P, Hellier P, Morandi X, Barillot C. 3D rigid registration of intraoperative ultrasound and preoperative MR brain images based on hyperechogenic structures. International Journal of Biomedical Imaging. 2012;**2012**:531319. DOI: 10.1155/2012/531319

[42] Toews M, Wells WM 3rd. Bayesian registration via local image regions: Information, selection and marginalization. Information Processing in Medical Imaging. 2009;**21**:435-446. DOI: 10.1007/978-3-642-02498-6_36

[43] Mercier L, Fonov V, Haegelen C, Del Maestro RF, Petrecca K, Collins DL. Comparing two approaches to rigid registration of three-dimensional ultrasound and magnetic resonance images for neurosurgery. International Journal of Computer Assisted Radiology and Surgery. 2012;7(1):125-136. DOI: 10.1007/s11548-011-0620-2

[44] Reinertsen I, Lindseth F, Unsgaard G, Collins DL. Clinical validation of vessel-based registration for correction of brain-shift. Medical Image Analysis. 2007;**11**(6):673-684. DOI: 10.1016/j.media.2007.06.008

[45] Mercier L, Araujo D, Haegelen C, Del Maestro RF, Petrecca K, Collins DL. Registering pre- and postresection 3-dimensional ultrasound for improved visualization of residual brain tumor. Ultrasound in Medicine & Biology. 2013;**39**(1):16-29. DOI: 10.1016/j.ultrasmedbio.2012.08.004

[46] Stupp R, Mason WP, van den Bent MJ, et al. Radiotherapy plus concomitant and adjuvant temozolomide for glioblastoma. The New England Journal of Medicine. 2005;**352**(10):987-996. DOI: 10.1056/NEJMoa043330

[47] Allemani C, Matsuda T, Di Carlo V, et al. Global surveillance of trends in cancer survival 2000-14 (CONCORD-3): Analysis of individual records for 37 513 025 patients diagnosed with one of 18 cancers from 322 population-based registries in 71 countries. Lancet. 2018;**391**(10125):1023-1075. DOI: 10.1016/S0140-6736(17)33326-3

[48] Fatemi P, Zhang M, Miller KJ, Robe P, Li G. How intraoperative tools and techniques have changed the approach to brain tumor surgery. Current Oncology. 2018;**20**(11):89

Section 6

Experimental Therapeutics for the Brain Tumors

Chapter 10

Zika Virus for Brain Cancer Treatment?

Mateus Gonçalves de Sena Barbosa and Nicollas Nunes Rabelo

Abstract

Malignant brain tumors are among the most aggressive cancers with poor prognosis and no effective treatment despite all available therapies and technologies. The search for treatments for gliomas allowed the discovery that the Zika virus (ZIKV), a flavivirus, has a tropism for brain tumor cells and acts with an oncolytic effect, reaching brain tumors, in addition to stimulating the antitumor immunity of the host. Thus, it provides long-term immunity against cancer remission, reduces tumor burden, less metastasis and complete remission in some animals, consequently increases survival. There has been support that treatment with ZIKV against glioblastoma can be effective, suggesting a new future therapy that could revolutionize the prognosis of patients with brain tumors.

Keywords: Zika, neurotropism, glioblastoma, MSI1, AXL, oncolytic, brain cancer, brain tumor

1. Introduction

Central nervous system (CNS) tumors are pathologies that occur due to an exacerbated and disorganized cell proliferation. According to GLOBOCAN 2020, more than 300,000 new cases were recorded in 2020, with a mortality rate of 2.5%. The available treatments are neurosurgery, radiotherapy and chemotherapy [1, 2].

Glioblastomas (GBS) are considered the most aggressive and common primary brain tumor, with rapid progression and poor prognosis. Usual treatment includes neurosurgery, chemotherapy, radiation therapy, and alternative therapies that reduce neurological effects. In this case, there is no cure, so the treatment aims to increase survival with as much quality of life as possible [2–4].

Many recent studies present possible options for biochemical and intracellular pathways, therefore, the use of ZIKV is being suggested to reduce and/or inhibit the proliferation of tumor cells and induce apoptosis. Specific viral proteins and molecules have been observed in controlled and oriented studies to obtain stem cells, using attenuated vaccines, encapsulated viral fragments and viral therapy [2, 5, 6].

2. Methodology

A systematic and comprehensive literature review was performed from MEDLINE, EMBASE, Cochrane Central Register of Controlled Trials, Web of Science

IntechOpen

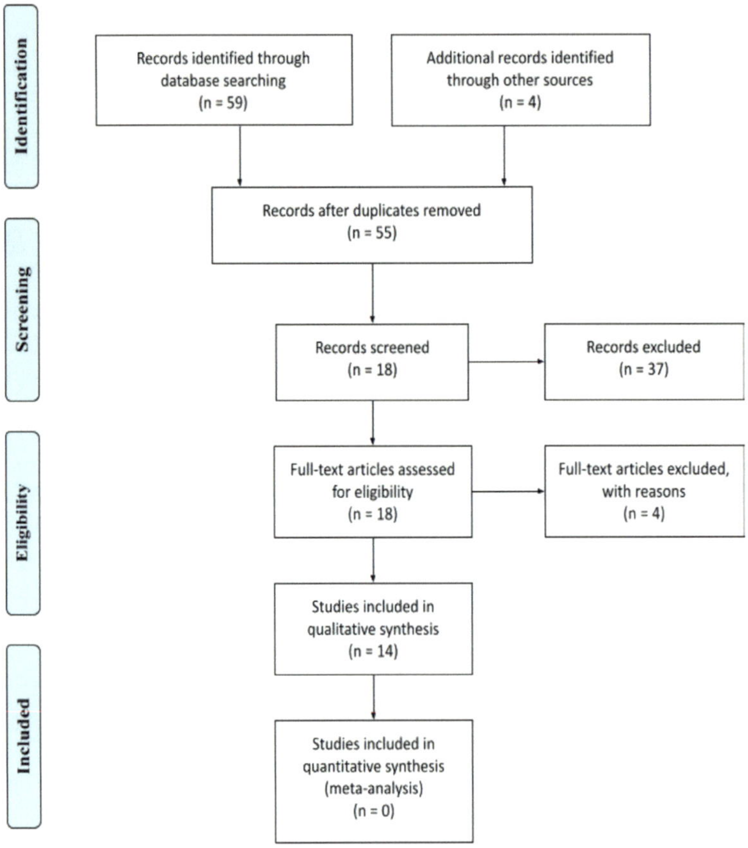

Figure 1.
Flowchart: Represent identification, screening, eligibility and Inclusion and exclusion criteria of this systematic review.

and SciELO, using the following keywords: "brain tumor", "brain cancer", "brain neoplasm", "glioma", "glioblastoma", "neuroblastoma", "stem cells", "oncology", "zika virus", "oncolytic", "oncolysis", "treatment", "therapy", "immunotherapy", "immunology" ", "approach", "outcome", "outcome", "vaccine" and "anticancer". These are in combination with the Boolean operators: "AND" and "OR". The keywords were searched in the "all fields" modality. Each article and its respective references were obtained in full and carefully analyzed.

The articles were included based on presenting scientific evidence from studies demonstrating the presence or absence of the oncolytic capacity of the zika virus against brain tumors and/or presenting the efficacy or inefficacy of this virus in the fight against brain tumors. Only articles in English, Spanish or Portuguese, without data restrictions (**Figure 1**).

3. Results/discussion

Table 1 contains the main objective aspects of each article selected for the qualitative synthesis. There are in vitro, in vivo and in vitro/in vivo studies. In the articles they have different signaling pathways and different biomarkers.

Reference	Title of the study	ZIKV strain	Cell lineage	Biomarker	Outcomes
Chen Qi, Wu Jin, Ye Qing, et al. 2018 [7]	Treatment of Human Glioblastoma with a Live Attenuated Zika Virus Vaccine Candidate	FSS 13025/ GZ01	GSCs specimens 387 and 4121		ZIKV-LAV was shown to be safe and significantly intracerebral tumor growth and reduced animal survival by selectively killing GSCs within the tumor
Crane AT, Chrostek MR, Krishna VD, et al. 2020 [8]	Zika virus-based immunotherapy enhances long-term survival of rodents with brain tumors through upregulation of memory T-cells	ZIKV H/ PF/2013	GL261 GBM cells; GS-9 L glioma cell line	—	ZIKV immunotherapy could be an adjuvant to tumor vaccines to intensify long-term survival, through enhanced T-cell response
Dabaja MZ, Lima EO, Oliveira DN, et al. 2018 [5]	Metabolic alterations induced by attenuated Zika virus in glioblastoma cells	$ZIKV^{BR}$	U-251 GBM cells	Phospholipids[1], chlorinated metabolite[2], phosphatidylinositol-3-phosphate	ZVp might be an alternative treatment for GBM, given the cytopathic effects and cell damage induced on neural tumor cells
Iannolo G, Sciuto MR, Cuscino N, et al. 2019 [9]	Zika virus infection induces MiR34c expression in glioblastoma stem cells: new perspectives for brain tumor treatments	ZIKV H/ PF/2013	GSCs U87MG and T98G	CD133, SOX-2, Musashi-1, and nestin	ZIKV infection induced miR34c expression and its overexpression reproduced an effect equivalent to that of infection. Mir34c can inhibit GSCs and reduce Bcl2, which could potentially enhance the effect of chemotherapy/radiotherapy.
Kaid C, Goulart E, Caires-Júnior LC, et al. 2018 [6]	Zika Virus Selectively Kills Aggressive Human Embryonal CNS Tumor Cells In Vitro and In Vivo	$ZIKV^{BR}$	Embryonal CNS tumor cell lines: DAOY, USP13-MED,USP7-ATRT	Wnt/β-catenin pathway	ZIKV has oncolytic properties and specifically targeted stem-like cancer cells from embryonal CNS tumors
Kaid C, Madi R, Astray R, et al. 2020 [2]	Safety, Tumor Reduction, and Clinical Impact of Zika Virus Injection in Dogs with Advanced-Stage Brain Tumors	$ZIKV^{BR}$	CNS primary tumor with neural origin, excluding meningioma and other non-neural tumors	anti-ZIKV NS2B antibody	Shown for the first time significant CNS tumor remission following ZIKVBR intrathecal injections in two dogs bearing spontaneous intracranial tumors with an absence of clinical side effects associated with ZIKV infection.

Reference	Title of the study	ZIKV strain	Cell lineage	Biomarker	Outcomes
Li H, Hu Y, Huang J, et al. 2019 [4]	Zika virus NS5 protein inhibits cell growth and invasion of glioma	PRVABC59	HEK293T, U87 and GL261 glioma cell lines	NS5	NS5 viral protein inhibited cell growth and proliferation and tumorsphere formation
Li M, Zhang D, Li C, et al. 2020 [10]	Characterization of Zika Virus Endocytic Pathways in Human Glioblastoma Cells	kv963796	Glioblastoma T98G cells	clathrin heavy chain	Viruses penetrate cells by various mechanisms, including fusion with the cell membrane or entering by receptor-mediated endocytosis. Clathrin-mediated endocytosis is the most frequently used pathway. ZIKV can enter T98G cells through not only clathrin-dependent but also clathrin-independent pathways
Lima E, Guerreiro T, Melo C, et al. 2017 [11]	MALDI-Imaging detects endogenous Digoxin in glioblastoma cells infected by Zika virus – would it be the oncolytic key?	$ZIKV^{BR}$	M059J GBM cells	Digoxin	ZIKV induced cytopathic effects, associated with endogenous digoxin synthesis, at GBM cells
Luplertlop N, Suwanmanee S, Muangkaew W, et al. 2017 [12]	The impact of Zika virus infection on human neuroblastoma (SH-SY5Y) cell line	SV0127/14 and SV0010/15	human neuroblastoma cell line (SH-SY5Y)	-	
Mazar J, Li Y, Rosado A, et al. 2018 [13]	Zika virus as an oncolytic treatment of human neuroblastomacells requires CD24	PRVABC59	Neuroblastoma MYCN and non-MYCN	NS1	ZIKV infection reduces cell viability. However, the permiveness to zika virus depends on CD24 expression. It occours mainly on high metabolic activity progenitors, not having this effect on differentiated cells

Reference	Title of the study	ZIKV strain	Cell lineage	Biomarker	Outcomes
Nair S, Mazzoccoli L, Jash A, et al. 2021 [3]	Zika virus oncolytic activity requires CD8+ T cells and is boosted by immune checkpoint blockade	ZIKV-Dakar	GL261 and CT2A GBM cells	CD8-depleting antibodies, isotype control IgG2b, antibodies against PD-1, IgG2a control	Histological analysis revealed comparable tumor sizes between the ZIKV and PBS groups at day 14 after tumor implantation (7 days after ZIKV treatment) but a decrease in tumor size 1 week later at day 21 after tumor implantation (14 days after ZIKV treatment) in response to ZIKV treatment. It was observed infiltration of immune cells in the tumor microenvironment at days 14 and 21 after tumor implantation in animals treated with ZIKV. ZIKV treatment also increased the tumor-associated myeloid cell response in the tumor bed, particularly the monocyte and microglia populations.
Trus I, Berube N, Jiang P, et al. 2020 [14]	Zika Virus with Increased CpG Dinucleotide Frequencies Shows Oncolytic Activity in Glioblastoma Stem Cells	PRVABC59	C6/36 cells		In vitro: reduced infection kinetics in nonmalignant brain cells but high infectivity and oncolytic activity in GSCs. In ovo: efficiently replicated with a significant reduction of tumor growth
Zhu Z, Mesci P, Bernatchez J, et al. 2020 [15]	Zika Virus Targets Glioblastoma Stem Cells through a SOX2-Integrin avb5 Axis	H/PAN/2016/ BEI-259634 and PRVABC59	293FT Cell Line, ENSA (ENS-tem-A), NSC11, NM53, NM55, NM177, NPC C4–7, hNP1 (STEMEZ hNP1) and H1 ESC		avb5 integrin was shown to be a functional marker of cancer stem cells essential for maintenance of GBM and ZIKV infection

Abbreviations: CNS (central nervous system), GBM (glioblastoma), MALDI (matrix laser desorption/ionization mass spectrometry imaging), ZVp (attenuated ZIKV prototype).
[1]*Lysophosphatidic acid, oxidized phosphatidylserine and simple phosphatidylserine.*
[2]*5-methyltetrahydropteroyltri-L-glutamate.*

Table 1.
Summary of the main in vitro/in vivo studies (2017–2021) investigating the oncolytic effects of Zika virus (ZIKV) in CNS tumors.

A research carried out with the aim of understanding how human embryonic CNS tumor stem cells behave in the face of ZIKV infection. Therefore, the study focused on analyzing three embryonic CNS tumor cell lines (DAOY, USP13-MED and USP7-ATRT), as well as three non-CNS tumor cell lines from breast, colorectal and prostate cancer. All six cell lines were infected with ZIKV to assess the in vitro oncolytic effects of ZIKV infection. Seventy two hours after infection, researchers observed cell death and/or reduced growth in all CNS tumor lineages, although DAOY infection was less pronounced when compared to USP13-MED and USP7-ATRT. Flow cytometry analysis was performed and showed an increase in the population of PI-positive CNS tumor lines as a consequence of ZIKV infection, suggesting cell death by rupture of the plasma membrane. It was also stated that ZIKV infection interfered with CNS tumor spheres, mainly in CNS embryonic tumor spheres. However, a slight or no effect on oncolytic properties and tumor sphere disruption was observed in non-CNS tumor cell lines. Based on these findings, the authors proposed a selective ZIKV infection and cell death of CNS tumor cells when compared to normal CNS stem cells and other tumor cell lines (prostate, breast, colorectal). Two years later, the same author showed for the first significant remission of the CNS tumor after intrathecal injections of ZIKV BR in two dogs bearing spontaneous intracranial tumors with no clinical side effects associated with ZIKV infection [2, 6].

Then, an in vivo study was performed with intracerebroventricular injection of ZIKV in BALB/c nude mice after a period of tumor establishment in the CNS (1 to 2 weeks for DAOY, USP13-MED and USP7-ATRT cell lines). In this study, ZIKV was shown to induce remission in 20 of the 29 animals in the experimental group, with complete remission in seven mice. When compared to the sham group, the OS of USP7-ATRT tumor-bearing mice treated with ZIKV infection was statistically increased ($P = 0.0046$) and 60% of the group had complete metastatic remission ($n = 3$). Reduction of tumor growth rate in USP7-ATRT and USP13-MED was also observed, although the DAOY cell line had a poor response to ZIKV infection, which fits the in vitro findings. In addition, the study suggests that the Wnt/β-catenin pathway may be involved in cell death associated with ZIKV infection, since USP7-ATRT, the cell line with the best results, showed hyperactivity of this specific pathway [7].

It was found that ZIKV interfered in cells infected with glioblastomas, through metabolic alterations. This happened, primarily, due to the non-structural protein of the virus (NS5), which considerably inhibits tumorigenicity due to the lesion of glioma stem cells, reducing their proliferation [4]. Moreover, cardiac glycoside molecules, such as digoxin, observed early in ZIKV infection, have already shown good results in patients with neuroblastoma, melanoma and breast cancer [11]. It has also been shown to increase p536 activity.

It was evidenced that the virus could act positively on other types of cancer, such as medulloblastoma, prostate, breast and rhabdoid teratoid tumor, however, they obtained good specific results for the central nervous system, especially the rhabdoid teratoid tumor, since they originate from cells -stem and neuroprogenitors, which are parts of greater tropism for the virus [6]. In another study, significant efficacy was observed for the treatment of neuroblastoma, in which the virus dominated most tumor cells in a few days [13].

Furthermore, tumor remission was observed in mice that survived glioblastoma by vaccination with cells previously infected with ZIKV and by intracranial injections of live attenuated virus or by previously infected cells. In this group, they obtained the possibility of long-term immunization from the generation of memory T cells, with significant survival. Therefore, ZIKV can contribute to the development of vaccines [8]. Another study showed that just one intracerebroventricular injection in mice was enough to reduce viral load, increase survival and reduce the incidence of remission and metastasis [6].

GBM has the characteristic of suppressing apoptosis pathways mediated by caspase activation, it was denoted that ZIKV infection induced the inhibition of the development of genes responsible for the maintenance and proliferation of tumor cells, such as NOTCH and NUMB. In addition, it decreased the expression of Bcl2, which may be responsible for the apoptotic response, with a reduction in NUMB, reducing AKT phosphorylation in glioblastoma cell lines. Down-modulation of NUMB induces p73 degradation in a proteasome-dependent manner. P73 has been found to confer an invasive phenotype on glioblastoma cells, and its deletion impairs invasion and chemoresistance in animal models and glioblastoma patients, with prolonged survival [9].

One study presented the analysis in GSCs and showed that there was an induction of miR34c production, consequently reducing the growth of these cells and regulating the expression of Bcl2 and NUMB, mimicking the same effect perceived in ZIKV infection. The answer obtained was that there is a reduction in tumor growth, promoting oncolytic activity in the treatment of GBM [9]. However, the ability of GBM to resist ZIKV activity in vivo still needs to be studied [14], it was noticed that some strains of GSC in vitro derived from CpG recoding in a ZIKV viral genome, using dinucleotide implementation technology CpG for candidate development may have different results for the oncolytic response. This dissonance of different recoded CpG variants demonstrates that the oncolytic activity of a virus can be modulated by adjusting the number of CpG dinucleotides introduced de novo into a viral genome. Thus, oncolytic therapy still needs to understand the behavior between the CpG-encoded viruses, the tumor, the tumor environment and the host responses for this oncolytic therapy to be more effective [9, 14].

4. Conclusion

ZIKV can be highly efficient and viable for brain cancer therapy, with safety, high T cell activity and can be used in conjunction with surgery/radiotherapy to improve survival. Despite the low number of studies and quality information to support the diligence and safety of ZIKV for the treatment of CNS studies, the results demonstrate efficacy and possibility of using this treatment in the future.

Funding

There is no financial support.

Conflict of interest

The authors declare that they have no conflict of interest.

Compliance with ethical standards

Nill.

Ethical approval

The local IRB waived the need for ethical approval due to the retrospective nature of the study.

Author details

Mateus Gonçalves de Sena Barbosa and Nicollas Nunes Rabelo*
Neurosurgery Department, Atenas University Center, Passos, Brazil

*Address all correspondence to: nicollasrabelo@hotmail.com

References

[1] Sung H, Ferlay J,Siegel RL, Laversanne M, Soerjomataram I, Jemal A, et al. Global cancer statistics 2020: GLOBOCAN estimates of incidence and mortality worldwide for 36 cancers in 185 countries. CA: A Cancer Journal for Clinicians. 2021;**71**(3):209-249

[2] Kaid C, dos Santos Madi RA, Astray R, Goulart E, Caires-Junior LC, Mitsugi TG, et al. Safety, tumor reduction, and clinical impact of zika virus injection in dogs with advanced-stage brain tumors. Molecular Therapy. 2020;**28**(5):1276-1286

[3] Nair S, Mazzoccoli L, Jash A, Govero J, Bais SS, Hu T, et al. Zika virus oncolytic activity requires CD8+ T cells and is boosted by immune checkpoint blockade. JCI Insight. 2021;**6**(1). DOI: 10.1172/jci.insight.144619

[4] Li H, Hu Y, Huang J, Feng Y, Zhang Z, Zhong K, et al. Zika virus NS5 protein inhibits cell growth and invasion of glioma. Biochemical and Biophysical Research Communications. 2019;**516**(2):515-520

[5] Dabaja MZ, Lima de OE, Oliveira de DN, Guerreiro TM, Melo CFOR, Morishita KN, et al. Metabolic alterations induced by attenuated Zika virus in glioblastoma cells. Cell & Bioscience 2018;**8**(1):1-9

[6] Kaid C, Goulart E, Caires-Júnior LC, Araujo BHS, Soares-Schanoski A, Bueno HMS, et al. Zika virus selectively kills aggressive human embryonal CNS tumor cells in vitro and in vivo. Cancer Research. 2018;**78**(12):3363-3374

[7] Chen Q, Wu J, Ye Q, Ma F, Zhu Q, Wu Y, et al. Treatment of human glioblastoma with a live attenuated zika virus vaccine candidate. MBio. 2018;**9**(5). DOI: 10.1128/mBio.01683-18

[8] Crane AT, Chrostek MR, Krishna VD, Shiao M, Toman NG, Pearce CM, et al. Zika virus-based immunotherapy enhances long-term survival of rodents with brain tumors through upregulation of memory T-cells. PLoS One. 2020;**15**(10):e0232858

[9] Iannolo G, Sciuto MR, Cuscino N, Pallini R, Douradinha B, Ricci Vitiani L, et al. Zika virus infection induces MiR34c expression in glioblastoma stem cells: New perspectives for brain tumor treatments. Cell Death & Disease. 2019;**10**(4):263

[10] Li M, Zhang D, Li C, Zheng Z, Fu M, Ni F, et al. Characterization of zika virus endocytic pathways in human glioblastoma cells. Frontiers in Microbiology. 2020;**11**:242

[11] Lima de E O, Guerreiro TM, Melo CFOR, de Oliveira DN, Machado D, Lancelloti M, et al. MALDI imaging detects endogenous digoxin in glioblastoma cells infected by Zika virus—Would it be the oncolytic key? Journal of Mass Spectrometry 2018;**53**(3):257-263

[12] Luplertlop N, Suwanmanee S, Muangkaew W, Ampawong S, Kitisin T, Poovorawan Y. The impact of Zika virus infection on human neuroblastoma (SH-SY5Y) cell line. Journal of Vector Borne Diseases. 2017;**54**(3):207

[13] Mazar J, Li Y, Rosado A, Phelan P, Kedarinath K, Parks GD, et al. Zika virus as an oncolytic treatment of human neuroblastoma cells requires CD24. PLoS One. 2018;**13**(7): e0200358

[14] Trus I, Berube N, Jiang P, Rak J, Gerdts V, Karniychuk U. Zika virus with increased CpG dinucleotide frequencies shows oncolytic activity in glioblastoma stem cells. Viruses. 2020;**12**(5):579

[15] Zhu Z, Mesci P, Bernatchez JA, Gimple RC, Wang X, Schafer ST, et al. Zika virus targets glioblastoma stem cells through a SOX2-integrin αvβ5 Axis. Cell Stem Cell. 2020;**26**(2):187-204.e10

Section 7

Spinal Central Nervous System Tumors

Chapter 11

Intramedullary Spinal Tumors

Gabriele Capo, Alberto Vandenbulcke and Cédric Yves Barrey

Abstract

Intramedullary spinal tumors are uncommon intra-axial lesions, which can be either primary or metastatic. Primary tumors arise from cell of spinal cord and account for 2–4% of all intrinsic tumors of the central nervous system, being much less common of brain tumors. They are slow-growing tumors, so symptoms precede diagnosis by an average of 2 years. Metastatic lesions usually originate from lung and breast tumors and are usually diagnosed within 1 month from symptom onset. Pain and weakness are the most common presenting symptoms. Magnetic resonance imaging represents the gold standard technique to study the spinal cord tumors, and first-line treatment is surgical resection, but it is not always curative. In selected situations, watchful waiting can be considered. Chemotherapy and radiation are considered, but controversy exists. Novel treatment options must be developed to supplement partial resection and recurrence.

Keywords: neurosurgery, spinal surgery, spinal cord, neurological outcome, neurological deficit, intramedullary tumors, ependymoma, astrocytoma, hemangioblastoma, vascular malformation

1. Introduction

Intramedullary tumors (ITs) refer to a group of heterogeneous neoplastic lesions, which arise from the cells of spinal cord, accounting approximately 2–4% of primary intra-axial tumors of the central nervous system (CNS) [1, 2], or from metastatic cells of extra-neural tumor. Primary tumors are most often derived of neuroepithelial cell origin, with ependymoma being the most common in adults, and astrocytoma the most common in children and adolescents. Metastatic lesions usually originate from lung and breast tumors.

ITs differ from the tumors of the adjacent structures of spinal canal as nerve roots and meninges, and they are so distributed [3]:

Children and adolescents, 65% ITs (36.3% neuroepithelial, 19.6% ependymal tumors), 17.2% nerve sheath tumors, 17.8 tumors of meninges.

Adults, 30.1% ITs (4.7% neuroepithelial tumors, 17% ependymal tumors), 30.4% nerve sheath tumors, 30.5% tumors of meninges.

We can classify the ITs related to the cell of origin:

Neuroepithelial (90–95% of all ITs)

- **Ependymal tumors** 60%, e.g., ependymoma, myxopapillary ependymoma.

- **Astrocytic tumors** 33%, e.g., pilocytic astrocytoma, diffuse astrocytoma, glioblastoma.
- Neuronal 1%, e.g., **ganglioglioma**.
- Embryonal tumors, e.g., primitive neuroectodermal tumors (PNET), atypical teratoid/rhabdoid tumor (AT/RT)

Non-neuroepithelial

- Mesenchymal tumors, e.g., **hemangioblastoma**
- Lymphocytic tumors, e.g., **primary lymphoma**
- Melanocytic tumors, e.g., **melanocytoma**
- **Metastatic tumors**

Intramedullary benign masses as vascular malformation or congenital/developmental lesions can be encountered, and they should be considered in differential diagnosis. They can be ectodermal inclusion as epidermoid and dermoid cyst, mesodermal inclusion as lipoma, and endodermal inclusion as neurenteric cyst.

Genetic factors correlate with ITs. The syndromes associated with these tumors are neurofibromatosis 1 (NF1, 19% of patients), 2 (NF2, 33–53% of patients), and Von Hippel Lindau disease (VHL) [4, 5]. These patients develop mostly astrocytoma in case of NF1, ependymoma in NF2, and hemangioblastoma in VHL.

Approximately 70% of intramedullary tumors are associated with cysts [6]. Two types of cysts are recognized: the *tumoral cyst* and the *reactive cyst/syringomyelia* (non-tumoral). The *tumoral cyst* contained within the tumor itself typically demonstrates peripheral enhancement and may result from necrosis, fluid secretion, or degeneration of the neoplasm. It normally needs to be resected along with the solid portion of the tumor because there is a high likelihood of neoplastic cells within the wall. It occurs in association with the following tumors: 46% for ganglioglioma, 22% for ependymoma, 21% for astrocytoma, and 2–4% for spinal hemangioblastoma [7–9].

The *reactive cyst or syringomyelia* (**Figure 1**) generally occurs rostral or caudal to the solid portion of the tumor. It is a cystic collection of the central canal, it does not enhance, and it is present in 25–58% of all ITs, most frequently associated with hemangioblastomas [6]. It may resolve once the neoplasm is resected.

1.1 Clinical presentation

The clinical features of ITs depends on their location, grow rate, and longitudinal extension. They can potentially lead to severe neurologic deterioration, decreased function, and poor quality of life. Diagnosis is often delayed, as symptoms are slowly progressive and nonspecific. An exception is intramedullary metastases, which are diagnosed within 1 month from symptom onset in up to 75% of cases [8].

The most common presenting symptom includes back or neck axial pain. It can be associated with irradiated radicular pain, weakness, sensory disturbance, spasticity, gait disturbance, and bowel or bladder dysfunction. The neurological symptoms do

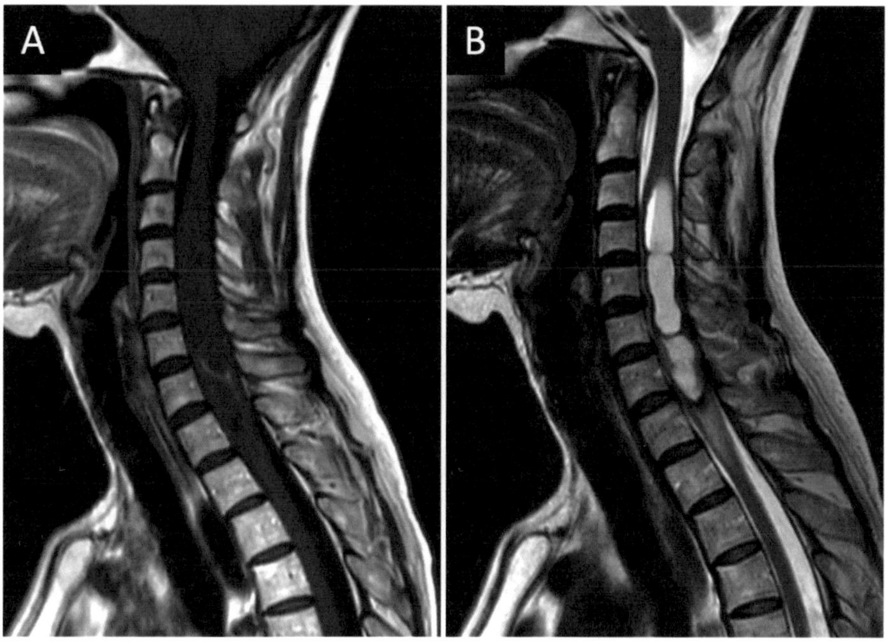

Figure 1.
Cervical ependymoma. Contrast-enhanced sagittal T1-weighted image (A) shows an enlarged spinal cord with an intramedullary lesion. It is a cervical ependymoma with light heterogeneous enhancement. Syringomyelia and caudal spinal cord edema are evident in sagittal T2-weighted image (B).

not involve head and face. Incomplete spinal cord syndrome as central, anterior, or Brown-Sequard may occur.

In children, progressive scoliosis may be seen in one-third of patients [10]. Motor regression and frequent falls may be the presenting features in young children [11].

1.2 Radiographic features

Radiographic evaluation can determine the location and extension of tumor. On plain radiograph and computerized tomography (CT), widening of the interpedicular distance, bony erosions, or scoliosis may be seen.

Myelography has been used in the past to evaluate the cord shape, but it is supplanted by MRI.

MRI is the preferred modality and helps to differentiate between lesions. General characteristics and T-1 and T-2 pattern of ITs are usually recognized, even if accurate diagnosis may be challenging. Focal spinal cord expansion and at least light contrast enhancement are seen. In contrast to intracranial neoplasms, even low-grade intramedullary tumors enhance to some degree.

Spinal angiography is mandatory to differentiate vascular lesions and for confirmed suspected diagnosis of hemangioblastoma.

Ependymomas are centrally located within the cord and display symmetric expansion with diffuse heterogeneous enhancement. Astrocytomas can be eccentrically positioned and non-enhancing. Hemangioblastomas are richly vascularized tumors with significant surrounding edema. Embolization can be useful in cases of hemangioblastoma. Metastatic lesions are well encapsulated, with no cystic change or hemorrhage. They are associated with cancer history.

1.3 Treatment and prognosis

The standard of care for most ITs is the surgical resection, which has improved with the modern operating microsurgery and intraoperative neuromonitoring.

Radiotherapy and chemotherapy are often reserved for high grade and infiltrative tumors and for recurrence. They are limited by adverse effects and blood-spinal cord barrier.

The best predictive factors of outcome are preoperative neurological status and tumor histology [12].

1.4 Differential diagnosis

Various expansile lesions non-neoplastic may mimic ITs. The differential diagnosis includes inflammatory disease, congenital-developmental lesions, and vascular malformation.

The inflammatory lesions can be:

- demyelination (e.g., multiple sclerosis), which usually presents no spinal cord enlargement, but diffuse plaque enhancement in brain and spinal cord correlated with acute lesion activity.

- transverse myelitis, which shows acute clinical course and typically occupy greater than two-thirds of the cross-sectional area of the cord.

- spinal cord abscess, with rim enhancement and restricted diffusion.

Among vascular lesion we find:

- Cavernous malformation, a low flow capillary malformation, which appears as rounded region of heterogeneous hyperintensity at T1 and T2-weighted images and peripheral hypointensity due to blood products of varying ages and hemosiderin deposition (“popcorn appearance”).

- Glomus arteriovenous malformation (AVM), a high-flow compact intramedullary nidus with AV shunting characterized by flow voids at spin-echo MRI.

- Spinal cord infarction appears hyperintense on T2-weighted images and DWI, without enhancement after contrast.

Congenital-developmental (ecto, meso, endoderm) no-enhancing lesions are:

- Epidermoid and dermoid cysts lined by squamous epithelium and skin appendages, whose signal at CT and MRI appear like cerebrospinal fluid (CSF), excepted for restricted diffusion and DWI.

- Lipoma, mature adipose tissue, characterized by homogeneous fat attenuation at CT and MRI.

- Neuroenteric cyst, usually ventral, which can manifest with varying signal intensity at T1 and T2-weighted imaging due to mucin content.

Spinal cord contusion is usually associated with other spinal injuries (osseous, ligament), and it is correlated with specific medical history (trauma, acute symptoms onset).

2. Spinal ependymoma

2.1 Epidemiology

Ependymomas are uncommon neuroepithelial tumors and represent 1.8% of all primary CNS tumors and 50–60% of all ITs. The annual incidence is reported between 0.14 and 0.21 per 100.000 person [13, 14]. They are classified in the WHO 2021 CNS tumor classification by anatomic site, (supratentorial, posterior fossa, spinal), histology (ependymoma, subependymoma, myxopapillary ependymoma), and molecular alterations.

Spinal ependymomas are now classified according to amplification status of MYCN, which regulates genes involved in cell growth. Spinal ependymomas are more common in adults than children, with a peak of incidence between the third and the fifth decade. They showed a slight male preponderance (male:female = 1.6:1), except for spinal subependymoma (SSE). Gender and age distribution showed slight variation according to different molecular types, while distribution along the spinal cord is extremely variable. SSE is predominantly in the cervical segment, followed by the thoracic. Conversely, spinal myxopapillary ependymomas (SMPEs) arise in the distal spinal cord (**Figure 2**) [15].

Extra-neural metastases from ependymomas are possible but uncommon.

2.2 Histopathology

Ependymomas are tumors of neuroectodermal origin. They are well-circumscribed lesions of ependymal differentiated cells and typically present eosinophilic cells with round nuclei and scant cytoplasm, organized in *rosette* around a central vessel.

Historically, they were supposed to origin from periventricular ependymal layer. Recent gene expression analysis suggested to origin from embryonic radial glial cells (RGCs) in the subventricular zone. RGCs in the supratentorial, infratentorial, and spinal canal have different chromosomal abnormalities and gene expression and consequently, morphologically similar ependymomas have different molecular profile [16].

Emerging evidence showed that despite histologic similarities, ependymomas arising in different localization widely differ for prognosis, molecular and genetic alteration.

The WHO 2021 CNS tumors classification introduced the anatomical and molecular pattern in the tumors type definition. The new classification defined 10 different CNS ependymal tumors. Types are defined based on the localization in one of the three neuroanatomical compartments, supratentorial, infratentorial and spinal cord, the molecular pattern, and the immunohistochemical analysis. Subependymoma and myxopapillary ependymoma are the only two types not restricted to a specific localization and may occur in the three different compartments.

Discordance between histological grade and clinical behavior cause controversy about grading system. Moreover, grading system showed to have high interobserver variability. For these reasons, treatment should not be based only on the histopathological grading system.

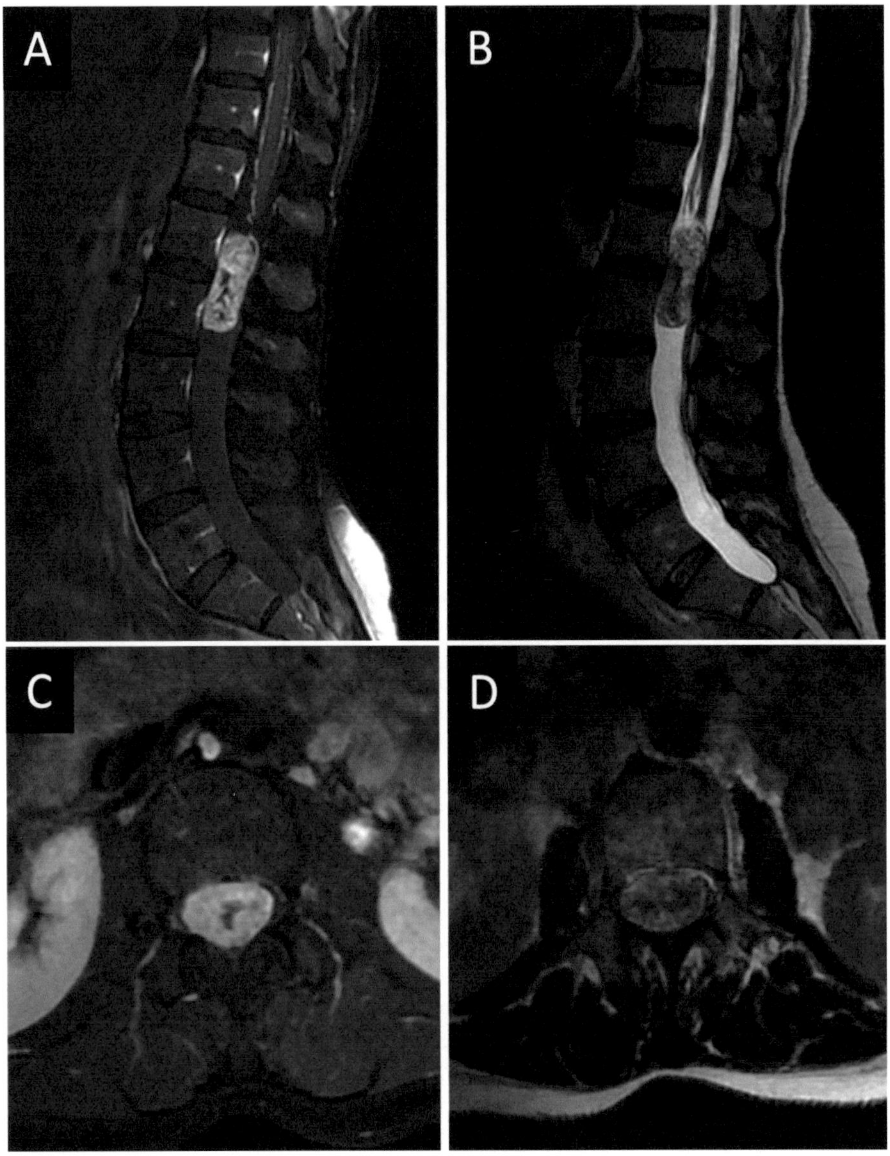

Figure 2.
Spinal myxopapillary ependymoma. Contrast-enhanced sagittal T1-weighted image (A) and non-enhanced sagittal T2-weighted image (B) show intradural lesion at distal part of spinal cord (lumbar region). The lesion presents heterogeneous contrast enhancement (A, C). In the axial plane (C, D), the myxopapillary ependymoma occupies the entire spinal canal, displacing and compressing cauda equina nerve roots.

Four different ependymomas types may involve the spinal cord: spinal ependymoma w/o MYCN amplification (SP-EPN), spinal ependymoma with MYNC amplification (SP-MYCN), SSE, and SMPE. Except for the spinal ependymoma with MYNC amplification, which shows aggressive characteristics, all of them are mostly benign.

SP-EPN is an ependymoma occurring in the spine without the morphological characteristics of SSE and SMPE. Most SP-EPNs have chromosome 22q losses that harbor the NF2 gene. The role of NF2 loss in ependymomas is still unclear, but SP-EPN is observed in 33–53% of NF2 patients [17]. Histologically, it shows a solid and circumscribed mass, composed of regular cells organized in perivascular pseudorosette and papillary organization. SP-EPN is classified as grade 2 or 3 according to general WHO grading system for CNS tumor.

SP-MYCN is a spinal ependymoma with MYNC amplification, and only a few cases have been described. This tumor occurs as large lesion with early leptomeningeal dissemination, high recurrence rate, rapid progression following recurrence, and poor responses to medical treatment. Aggressive histopathological features such as microvascular proliferation, high mitotic rate, and necrosis are described.

SSE arises in all neuroanatomical compartments. It is circumscribed glioma composed of cluster of cells with low mitotic rate and no nuclear atypia, embedded in a fibrillary matrix with microcystic changes and dystrophic calcification. It was classified as CNS WHO tumor grade I.

SMPE is characterized by myxoid changes, occurring along the neuroaxis but predominantly in the conus medullaris. It is mostly benign, but intradural dissemination and recurrence may occur. Histologically, the papillary organization around a fibrovascular core with perivascular myxoid changes and GFAP immunoreactivity are pathognomonic of this tumor. It was graded II in the WHO 2021 tumor classification.

2.3 Clinical presentation

Spinal ependymomas are centrally located lesion presenting with progressive signs and symptoms of spinal cord lesion. They depend on tumor size, location, and syrinx extension. Axial pain is primary initial symptom, predominant in supine position, and probably caused by dural distension. Radicular pain is uncommon. Then progressive neurological symptoms appear. Due to the not specific onset, diagnosis is often delayed, and symptoms last for 3–4 years before diagnosis.

Dysesthesia and paresthesia are common. Dissociated sensory loss with sacral sparing for somatotopic distribution of spinothalamic tract and bowel and bladder dysfunction occur early.

Posterior cord signs such as ataxia and giant instability occur later.

Para or tetraparesis appears with progressive growth, depending on the tumor site. Motor pattern is spastic in 50% of cases and frequently associated with muscle atrophy.

Pyramidal signs, irritations as hyper-reflexia, Babinski, Hoffman signs, clonus of the ankles are usually seen.

SMPE is predominant in the conus medullaris and presents with conus syndrome: autonomous bladder, fecal incontinence, impotence, saddle hypo or anesthesia, and distal legs weakness without pyramidal sings.

Preoperative paraclinical evaluation includes motor-evoked potentials (MEPs) and sensory evoked potentials (SEPs). They may identify subclinical deficit and show to have a functional prognostic value [18]. Urodynamic exam is routinely performed to explore bladder function.

2.4 Radiographic features

MRI with contrast enhancement is the gold standard for radiologic evaluation. Plain radiography and CT scan may identify nonspecific signs of bony remodeling (see above general overview) from intracanal lesions. Bony anomalies occurred tardively when neurological symptoms already justify an MRI evaluation.

Classic MRI appearance is well circumscribed, centered, enhancing masses causing spinal cord widening. Signal can be heterogeneous, especially for the SMPE type, for the presence of cysts (65% of case) and hemorrhagic components. But commonly, spinal ependymomas are described as hypointense to isointense from spinal cord signal at T1-weighted images and isointense to hyperintense at T2-weighted images.

More aggressive lesions with increased cellularity show lower signal.

The hemosiderin cap sign (hypointense T2) at rostral and caudal extremities is reported in up to one-third of cases and is highly suggestive.

Perilesional edema and syringomyelia are seen in more than 50% of cases.

SSE has different MRI features. It usually appears as expansile lobulated masses with hyperintense T2-weighted signal, without significant enhancement. Moreover, they are more eccentric compared to classic one and the steep spinal cord swelling causes a fusiform dilatation known as “bamboo leaf sign” [17].

Because of the risk of CSF dissemination, full craniospinal MRI is recommended especially for patients with NF2 at risk of multiple spinal ependymomas and schwannomas [19].

2.5 Treatment and prognosis

Complete microsurgical resection is the gold standard of treatment for these unencapsulated, well-circumscribed lesions. *En bloc* gross total resection (GTR) is preferred to avoid perioperative CSF dissemination, and it is now possible with good functional outcome in most of cases thanks to advances in modern microsurgery.

Since small tumor size and good preoperative status are associated with good functional outcome, early treatment is recommended. Due to the rarity of these lesions, referral center is preferred to improve GTR and functional outcome.

Intraoperative MEPs and SEPs are recommended. MEPs decline of 50% or more seem to be predictive of postoperative motor deficit [20]. An epidural electrode, the D-wave, may be placed on the caudal spinal cord to directly record the impulse on the corticospinal tract avoiding peripheric nerve conductance. The D-wave is considered the most specific monitoring for the corticospinal tract and is consequently the strongest predictor of postoperative motor deficit [21]. SEPs decrease or disappear following midline myelotomy, which is less predictive for functional outcome.

Standard posterior midline approach with multilevel facet sparing laminectomy is usually performed. Laminectomy should include one level above and below the lesion extension. Multilevel laminectomies at the cervical and cervico-thoracic junction level are associated with long-term kyphotic deformity. Arthrodesis is suggested if more than three-level laminectomy is performed. Alternatively, laminoplasty or transtubular approaches may be used [22].

Intraoperative ultrasound may be used to identify the tumors’ boundaries before dural opening.

Midline durotomy and dural suspension are performed. The arachnoid is opened separately. A standard midline myelotomy through the posterior medial septum is performed. Spinal ependymomas have a smooth, reddish gray glistening tumor surface. Operative microscope allows to easily identify and develop the dissection plane. Tumoral cysts must be distinguished from reactive/non-tumoral cysts and removed accurately, especially in case of SMPE.

At the end, the arachnoid is grossly closed to avoid spinal cord tethering at the surgical site. A tight water suture of dura is mandatory to avoid postoperative CSF fistula. Postoperative bed rest of 36–48 hours is suggested to minimize CSF pressure and prevent fistula. A symptomatic CSF fistula with CSF leak is at risk of meningitis and should be treated aggressively with revision surgery. Small asymptomatic pseudo meningocele may be treated nonoperatively with close observation.

The second most frequent complication is surgical site hematoma and should be evacuated whenever is compressive.

Majority of patients experience sensory deterioration immediately after surgery as the results of the posterior myelotomy and posterior cord manipulation. Slight motor deterioration may also occur because of intraoperative manipulation. Corticoids are frequently used to reduce postoperative edema.

Long-term functional outcome is related to preoperative status. Patients with major chronic neurological impairment rarely recovered significantly. On the other hand, minor and recent deficit frequently improves. Preservation rather than restoration of the functional outcome should be the goal.

In SP-EPN GTR increases overall survival (OS) and progression-free survival (PFS). Reported OS at 5 years following GTR is between 90 and 100% [23]. Whereas GTR resection is not achievable, radiotherapy increases PFS from 48 to 96 months. In lesions showing histopathologic signs of aggressivity and classified as CNS WHO tumor grade III postoperative, radiotherapy is recommended independently of the extent of resection. The suggested recommended dose is 45–54 Gy.

SP-MYNCs are more aggressive, with a recurrence rate of 75–100% and a median OS and PFS of 87 and 17 months, respectively, Radiotherapy is generally used for these rare and aggressive ependymomas [24].

SSEs are benign lesions with excellent prognosis, recurrence is extremely rare, even in case of subtotal resection (STR).

SMPEs are recognized to be at high risk of local recurrence and intradural spreading. The reported 10-year OS is of 92.4% and the PFS of 69.5 and 61.2% at 5 and 10 years, respectively. Local recurrence, increased by capsular violation, occurs in 84% of cases while CSF spreading is reported in 9.3% of patients. The irregular shape, the adherence to the cauda equine, and the myxoid matrix make GTR challenging. Postoperative radiotherapy increases PFS from 40–70% in patients with STR. While adjuvant postoperative radiotherapy following GTR showed increased local control compared to GTR alone in a small series. Larger prospective studies are needed to confirm these results.

A few data are available regarding chemotherapy, the topoisomerase-2 inhibitor showed partial responses in 20% of cases with good tolerance in recurrent tumors. Bevacizumab can provide clinical benefits, but no extensive data are available.

Because of the risk of CSF spreading, lumbar puncture for CSF cytology is recommended 3 weeks after surgery. Immediate postoperative MRI should be performed to evaluate the grade of resection and repeated regularly to identify relapse.

In case of relapse, reoperation should be considered.

3. Spinal astrocytoma

3.1 Epidemiology

Gliomas are primary tumors of the CNS of neuroepithelial origins. Spinal astrocytomas (SAs) correspond to 3% of CNS gliomas. They represent approximately 30% of all ITs, with an incidence of 0.07–0.1 per 100.000 person per year. They are the most common ITs in children representing the 60% of all tumors and 90% of tumors in patients younger than 10 years. SAs are rarely observed in patients older than 60 years old. Up to 60% of SAs occur in the cervical and cervicothoracic region. A slight male predilection is reported. SAs may be associated with NF1.

3.2 Histopathology

SAs are classified according to the 2021 WHO CNS classification and grading system, ranging from 1 to 4. Genetic markers have been incorporated to histopathological characteristics into the WHO grading system.

Histopathologic features are equivalent to the corresponding intracranial astrocytoma.

The new 2021 WHO CNS classification distinguishes the adult and pediatric gliomas. The pediatric subgroups include low-grade pilocytic astrocytoma and diffuse astrocytoma while adult type includes astrocytoma IDH-mutant (possible grade 2, 3, and 4) and astrocytoma IDH-wild type (glioblastoma-like tumor).

Pilocytic astrocytoma is characterized by biphasic cell population, Rosenthal fibers, and eosinophilic granular bodies. Distinction with a grade II astrocytoma may be not easy on morphological criteria. Molecular findings, as BRAF fusion is usually reported in pilocytic astrocytoma.

Astrocytoma (grade 2, 3, 4) is an infiltrating tumor. WHO grading is based on the presence of histological signs of malignity. They appear as hypercellular areas with tumor cells mixed with normal cellular elements. Tumor cells have elongated nuclei and eosinophilic fibrillary cytoplasm. Tumor cells clustering around the vessels are frequently founded. Necrosis and microvascular proliferation are observed in grade 4. Nuclear atypia, pleomorphism, increased mitotic count, and Ki-67/MIB-1 proliferative index increase with tumor grade. Moreover, the presence of CDK2A/B homozygous deletion in IDH-mutant astrocytoma is a negative prognostic factor, classifying tumor as grade 4, independently from necrosis and microvascular proliferation. Astrocytoma IDH-wild type with intermediate behavior is very rare, so it is now classified as glioblastoma IDH-wild type, independently from the histopathologic grade [25].

Diffuse and pilocytic astrocytomas are the most frequent ITs and account for 75% of all intramedullary SAs. Pilocytic astrocytoma is more common in the pediatric population while high-grade (grade 3 and 4) astrocytoma occurs mostly in adults.

3.3 Clinical presentation

Clinical presentation is like the other ITs (see above section "Spinal Ependymoma"). Axial pain is still the most frequent symptom. Slow progressive signs of spinal cord injury vary on form depending on the spinal location and tumoral extension. SAs tend to occur more eccentrically with signs and symptoms of unilateral spinal cord sufferance or incomplete Brown-Sequard syndrome (ipsilateral upper motor neuron paralysis and loss of proprioception, as well as contralateral loss of pain and temperature sensation). A zone of partial preservation or segmental ipsilateral lower motor neuron weakness and analgesia may be noted. Symptoms often appear from distal to proximal at the unilateral extremities before affecting the opposite site. Upper cervical lesion may involve lower cranial nerve [2].

3.4 Radiographic features

SAs appear as intramedullary fusiform multilevel intramedullary lesions on spinal cord MRI. Compared to spinal ependymomas, they are eccentric, and exophytic component can be observed. Moreover, they tend to be less defined and separate from normal spinal cord. Syringomyelia is less frequent compared to the other ITs and occurs in 20% of cases. SAs are hypo to iso-intense on T1-weighted images and hyper-intense on T2-weighted images. Contrast enhancement may be uniform, minimal, or patchy. In high-grade lesion, it is usually heterogeneous for necrosis and cysts. Peritumoral edema is observed in up to 40% of cases. Intra-tumoral and reactive (perilesional/non-tumoral) cysts occur in 20 and 15% of cases, respectively, while hemorrhage is rare [2, 26].

Diffuse tensor imaging (DTI) tractography, which shows white matter tracts, has been proposed as a diagnostic tool. It may help to distinguish tumor lesion, which displaces or destroys fibers of spinal cord, from acute inflammatory lesions, which are crossed by [27]. DTI can predict the presence of a dissecting plane between tumor and lesion or identify a "safe" entry zone [28].

Pilocytic astrocytomas are well circumscribed showing displacement of the spinal cord lesion and contrast enhancement. Cystic and syringomyelia are more frequent compared to other SAs.

Grade II SAs are infiltrating tumors, with no clear boundaries and dissection plane. Contrast enhancement varies from absent, heterogeneous, or homogeneous.

Glioblastomas show constant enhancement. Necrotic areas can be seen at MRI. Perilesional edema is more frequent due to the infiltrative and aggressive pattern [2, 26].

Plain RX and CT scan may be useful in case of extended bony erosion.

3.5 Treatment and prognosis

Treatment modalities for SAs are derived from brain glioma experience. Specific guidelines are still lacking, especially for diffuse and extensive cases. Surgical resection is generally proposed in patients experiencing neurological deficits, while it is still debated for asymptomatic patients.

The surgical management of SA should achieve the maximal degree of resection without major neurological deterioration. The surgeon should balance the functional and oncological outcomes. Finally, the extent of resection depends on histopathological diagnosis, clinical presentation, tumor extension, and modifications at intraoperative monitoring.

Resection of well-circumscribed lesions with benign behavior results in good functional and oncological outcome. Aggressive GTR without severe neurological deterioration can be achieved in these cases.

For high-grade infiltrative tumors, multimodal treatment is preferred. Biopsy or partial resection followed by adjuvant therapy as radiotherapy and chemotherapy is suggested. In these patients, GTR is usually unachievable without severe functional impairment and a high risk of recurrence is still present.

Standard midline approach as described above is performed. Midline myelotomy is usually performed, the dorsal root entry zone may be used for more lateralized lesions. Operating microscope is used to identify lesion borders whenever is possible. The lesion is resected alternating debulking and dissection from normal spinal cord to obtain vascular deafferentation. Debulking allows dynamic retraction and lesion mobilization, limiting spinal cord traction.

Intraoperative neuromonitoring is mandatory. PEM registration has a high sensitivity (84%) and specificity (83%) in detecting motor impairment, but it has a delay of several seconds from the injury to recognition. It is also influenced by heart rate, blood pressure, and anesthetic drugs. Conversely, the D-wave shows immediate changes and increased reliability. In highly infiltrative lesions, resection should be stopped if significant PEM and PES amplitude reduction are observed.

Watertight dural closure and hemostasis are crucial to avoid postoperative complications. Perioperative biopsy may be performed. Partial removal should be considered if malignancy is detected in extemporaneous examination of samples.

Early postoperative enhanced MRI is recommended to evaluate the extent of resection.

As for spinal ependymomas, patients usually experience a transient worsening of preoperative status, caused by posterior myelotomy and manipulation of the spinal cord. An improvement of the preoperative status is rare.

In a recent meta-analysis, surgical resection and low histopathologic grade show to improve local control and survival [29]. GTR increases 10-year OS from 45–71% and mean OS from 50 to 67 months for low-grade SAs. The 5-year OS results of 100% in WHO grade II lesions, and 67–83% in mixed series. The range PFS in all SAs is 7–138.8 months.

Radiotherapy and chemotherapy are used in high-grade lesions or in case of progression following surgical resection. There are no randomized trials to guide recommendations for adjuvant treatment, so institutional practice varies. Some authors suggest fractionated radiotherapy for low-grade tumors partial resected and for all high-grade.

Radiotherapy improves OS in high-grade SAs, but no benefits are reported for low-grade lesions.

The potential benefits of radiotherapy should be balanced with the high risk of radiotoxicity. The spinal cord has a limited radiosensitivity, and these lesions occur mostly in children, who are at higher risk of adverse effect.

Limited data are available for chemotherapy too. It is reserved for high-grade SAs, which progress following resection and radiotherapy. It is also proposed to children younger than 3 years old, in whom radiotherapy is not performed. Chemotherapy regimens are based on the Stupp protocol for brain glioblastomas and Temozolomide is mostly used. Some small series reported promising results for recurrent or unresectable lesion, but controversies still exist [30].

4. Spinal hemangioblastoma

4.1 Epidemiology

The spinal hemangioblastoma (SH) is a benign lesion of mesenchymal origin, arising from the vascular system. It is the third most frequent intramedullary lesion and accounts for 3–4%. The annual incidence is approximately 0.01 per 100.000 persons. 30% of patients with SH present VHL syndrome, which is characterized by mutation of VHL gene causing increased expression of the vascular endothelial growth factor (VEGF), responsible for the development of these vascular tumors. Patients affected by VHL syndrome usually present multiples CNS hemangioblastomas and concomitant retinal hemangioblastomas, pheochromocytoma, renal cell carcinoma, and pancreatic cysts [31].

SH occurs more commonly in men and during the fourth decade, but they may remain asymptomatic for years. In half of the cases, they are located in the cervical spinal cord while thoracic and lumbar spines are involved in 37 and 12% of cases, respectively [32].

4.2 Histopathology

SH is a highly vascularized lesion, well demarcated but not capsulated. It usually has a pial attachment and arises from the dorsal or dorsolateral region of spinal cord. A solid nodule is normally found, and it is frequently associated with cysts. The liquid cysts are similar to blood plasma, and it is probably a vascular exudate of the hyper-vascularized nodule.

SH is composed of a rich vascular network of capillary containing endothelial cells, pericytes, and lipid-laden stromal cells. The cell of origin is unknown but genetic analysis of sporadic and syndromic hemangioblastomas suggests VEGF-secreting undifferentiated mesenchymal cell. The most common staining proteins are S100 and vimentin.

According to histopathological morphology, two forms of SH exist. The reticular form, composed of irregular nuclei and prominent vessels, and the cellular form, which has minor vascular component and increasing stromal cells. The latter one may be histologically similar to astrocytomas.

The two forms are classified as WHO tumor grade I [32].

4.3 Clinical presentation

Medical history is like the other intramedullary lesion, with a combination of axial-radicular pain and spinal cord compression signs. Posterior cord signs and symptoms may be predominant while motor impairment is more delayed because of the posterior location [32]. Unilateral spinal cord compression with dissociate sensory impairment may occur.

Despite the high vascularity, hemorrhage is rare. The hemorrhage is subarachnoid in 73% of cases and intramedullary in 27%. Subarachnoid hemorrhage generally manifests with acute headache and/or axial pain. Intramedullary bleeding causes acute neurological signs.

4.4 Radiographic features

SH is a well-circumscribed lesion typically founded in the posterior and posterolateral spinal cord.

MRI allows differentiation from other ITs in most of the cases. SH appears as hypervascular highly enhancing nodule arising from the pial surface (**Figure 3**). In T1-weighted images, the nodule is usually iso to hypointense compared to spinal cord and identification is difficult. T2-weighted images show an iso- to hyperintense nodule associated with flow voids, vascular anomalies, and vasogenic edema. Cysts formation is observed in 50–70% of cases and syrinx in more than 50% of cases. Spinal cord widening is commonly observed and is mainly related to vascular congestion and consequent edema.

Spinal angiography is usually performed preoperatively, and it clearly identifies the main arterial feeders and draining veins. It allows a better comprehension of the vascular anatomy to confirm diagnosis and aiding surgical planning. Embolization may be performed in selected cases [33].

4.5 Treatment and prognosis

Surgery is recommended for all symptomatic SHs, otherwise observation is recommended for asymptomatic lesions. Surgical resection is extremely favorable

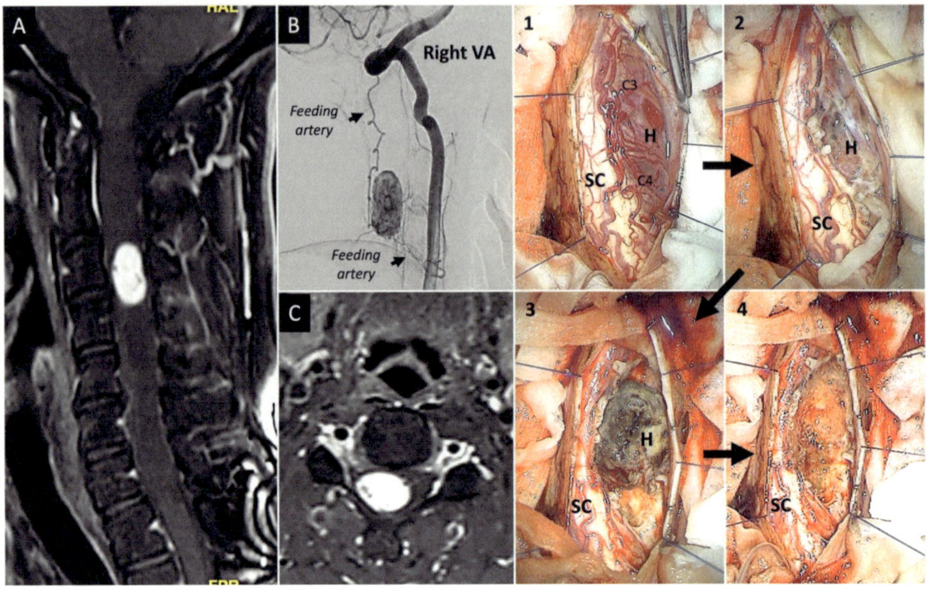

Figure 3.
Spinal hemangioblastoma. Preoperative MRI (A, C) shows a highly enhancing lesion. Angiography (B) confirms the hypervascularity with multiple feeders from the right vertebral artery. Intraoperative sequences are reported: exposition [1], partial deafferentation [2, 3], and complete resection [4] of the hemangioblastoma. VA vertebral artery, SC spinal cord, H hemangioblastoma, C3-C4 third and fourth cervical nerve root.

due to the posterior localization, the limited size, and the well-demarcated margins. Commonly more than 95% of patients are addressed for surgical resection, and GTR is obtained in approximately 83.5% of cases [32]. Preoperative spinal angiography allows an extensive comprehension of the vascular anatomy. It may help to distinguish the arterial feeder and the draining veins from the normal vasculature. The understanding of the vascular anatomy simplifies the surgical resection decreasing the risk of erroneous artery sacrifice and spinal cord ischemia.

Preoperative embolization significantly reduces the risk of intraoperative bleeding. It is technically challenging and can be performed in selected cases. It is reported in around 8% of cases [32]. The superselective catheterization of the small tortuous feeders is frequently not possible. A more proximal embolization is at risk of spinal cord ischemia and may develop collateral revascularization of the tumor. A subtotal embolization is usually preferred to avoid vascular rupture and ischemia.

Surgical approach depends on localization of the lesion. Most of the SHs are posterior and surgical resection is then performed through a standard posterior midline approach. More lateral lesions may be exposed thanks to dentate ligament opening, mobilization, and gentle spinal cord rotation. Transtubular resection is possible depending on nodule size. Anterior approach is described for anterior locate lesions. Intraoperative monitoring is mandatory with PEM and PES registration. Epidural D-was is preferable.

After durotomy, SH is usually easily identified. It appears as a well-delimitated bright red lesion with pial attachment associated with adjacent vascular anomalies. The feeding arteries should be rapidly identified and coagulated, to obtain a complete devascularization. The draining veins should be coagulated at the final stage to avoid vascular surcharge and rupture. Sometimes it is not easy to discriminate the arterial feeders from the vessels supplying the normal spinal cord. The Indocyanine green video-angiography (ICG-VA) is a useful tool to distinguish arterial feeders and draining veins intraoperatively. Temporary clipping of the arterial feeders associated with intraoperative neuromonitoring may provide additional information to avoid spinal cord injury [34, 35]. Operative microscope is used to identify and dissect the tumors' margins from the pia. Complete *en bloc* resection is preferable. There is no evidence that syrinx or cysts opening may improve functional outcome, and they usually disappear following the resection of SH [36].

The most common postoperative complication is CSF leak, up to 30%, followed by surgical site hematoma and infection, reported in 20 and 16.6% of cases, respectively.

The outcome is generally good with a mortality rate lower than 2%. Compared to neuroepithelial lesions (ependymomas and astrocytoma), functional recovery is observed in most cases, because of the superficial and non-infiltrative features. Sensory symptoms and pain have shown to improve in 72 and 90% of cases in a recent systematic review [32].

Early postoperative enhanced spinal MRI to verify the extent of resection is usually performed. Follow-up is conducted with repeated MRI. The frequency depends on the estimated risk of recurrence.

Recurrence is reported in 8% of sporadic SH and in 22% of patients affected by VHL syndrome and is more frequent following STR.

Radiotherapy is reserved for recurrent or inoperable lesions. The advancement in radiosurgery improved the accuracy, reducing spinal cord irradiation.

5. Other intramedullary tumors

5.1 Spinal gangliogliomas

Gangliogliomas are benign tumors (WHO grade I and II) of neuronal and glial origins. Intramedullary gangliogliomas occur mostly in the pediatric populations. They are composed of ganglions and glial cells. The glial cells are at risk of malignant transformation. Two histologic subtypes are described: the classic ganglioglioma, which is reported in 59% of cases, and the pilocytic-like ganglioglioma (41% of cases) where ganglion cells are combined with histological features of pilocytic astrocytoma. Ganglioglioma is typically associated with scoliosis and at MRI, it is not easily differentiated from neuroepithelial spinal cord tumors.

Among treatment, surgery is the first option, with GTR generally obtained in about 80% of cases. Radiotherapy is reported for recurrence. The oncological outcome is favorable with a 10-year survival rate of 83% [37, 38].

5.2 Spinal lymphoma

Lymphoma in spinal cord is usually secondary. Primary intramedullary lymphoma accounts for 1% of all primary CNS lymphomas. Primary lymphoma is usually non-Hodgkin diffuse B-cell lymphoma. It occurs mostly in adults or elderly [2] and appears as a heterogeneously enhancing, diffuse lesion with hyperintensity in T2-weighted and ADC signal. It may be misdiagnosed with demyelinating lesions [26]. Chemotherapy is the recommended therapy. Treatment regimen is based on methotrexate and temozolomide. Surgery and radiotherapy are not suitable for the systemic nature and diffuse localization. Outcome is generally poor, and recurrence occurs in 2 months despite treatment [38].

5.3 Spinal melanoma

Primary intramedullary melanomas arise from the melanocytes normally present in the two inner meningeal layers (leptomeninges), the arachnoid and the pia. They are pigmented tumors of the spinal cord, without any evidence of systemic melanoma and account for 1% of all melanomas. They present a rapid growth and consequently symptoms of spinal cord compression progress promptly compared to other primary lesion of the spinal cord [2, 38]. At MRI they appear as lesion with homogeneous contrast enhancement. The presence of melanin gives hyperintense signal on T1-weighted images and causes susceptibility artifact in gradient recalled echo T2-weighted.

The protocol of treatment is based on anecdotal evidence in individual cases. Surgical resection seems to be the best treatment option, but GTR is rarely obtained, and radiotherapy is usually performed postoperatively. Intrathecal chemotherapy has been reported to improve OS and PFS [38].

5.4 Spinal metastases

Spinal metastases represent the 1–3% of ITs. They occur in 0.4% of patients with cancer and usually originate from lung and breast tumors [2]. Spinal metastases appear as circumscribed enhancing lesions with peripheric edema. They present typically two signs, which help to differentiate from primary spinal lesion, the rim, and the flame signs. The rim sign is a more intense peripheric enhancement compared to the central portion. The flame sign is a flame-shaped enhancement at the cranial and/or caudal portion [26]. Due to the rarity, few reports are available about treatment options. The outcome is poor, with a mean survival time of 4 months. Surgical resection may be attempted, but GTR is limited by the absence of clear margins. Long-course multifractionated radiotherapy is rarely an option for these patients with poor functional and oncological outcome. Chemotherapy shows controversial results [38].

6. Conclusions

ITs are rare tumors of CNS, potentially devastating. They represent a clinical and surgical challenge, although advances in the management were made. It is imperative to reduce delay in diagnosis and to develop novel treatments for aggressive and infiltrating type.

Clinical and radiological manifestations are quite homogeneous and preoperative diagnosis is rarely conclusive. Surgical resection is the primary treatment option in most cases and can be curative in benign lesions. Conversely, total resection avoiding major neurological impairment is demanding. Radiotherapy and chemotherapy are generally used for incomplete resection, recurrence, or inoperable lesions. No definitive guidelines exist for adjuvant treatments due to the rarity of these lesions. Functional improvement is rarely obtained, and neurological stability should be considered the goal. Oncological outcome is variable and depends on the histological grade.

Conflict of interest

The authors declare no conflict of interest.

Acronyms and abbreviations

ITs	intramedullary tumors
GTR	gross total resection
CNS	central nervous system
PNET	primitive neuroectodermal tumors
AT/RT	atypical teratoid/rhabdoid tumor
NF1	neurofibromatosis 1
NF2	neurofibromatosis
VHL	Von Hippel Lindau disease
AVM	arteriovenous malformation
CSF	cerebrospinal fluid
RGCs	radial glial cells
SP-EPN	spinal ependymoma
SP-MYCN	spinal ependymoma with MYNC amplification
SSE	subependymoma
SMPE	spinal myxopapillary ependymoma
MEPs	motor evoked potentials
SEPs	sensory evoked potentials
GTR	gross total resection
STR	subtotal resection
WHO	world health organization
SAs	spinal astrocytomas
DTI	diffuse tensor imaging
SH	spinal hemangioblastoma
VEGF	vascular endothelial growth factor
ICG-VA	Indocyanine green video-angiography.

Author details

Gabriele Capo[1,2]*, Alberto Vandenbulcke[1,3] and Cédric Yves Barrey[1,4]

1 Hôpital Pierre Wertheimer, Hospices Civils de Lyon, Claude Bernard University of Lyon 1, Lyon-Bron, France

2 IRCCS Humanitas Research Hospital, Rozzano, Milan, Italy

3 University Hospital of Lausanne, Lausanne, Switzerland

4 Laboratory of Biomechanics, ENSAM, Arts et Metiers ParisTech, Paris, France

*Address all correspondence to: gabriele.capo@gmail.com

References

[1] Ostrom QT, Cioffi G, Gittleman H, Patil N, Waite K, Kruchko C, et al. CBTRUS statistical report: Primary brain and other central nervous system tumors diagnosed in the United States in 2012-2016. Neuro-Oncology. 2019;**21**(Suppl. 5):V1-V100

[2] Samartzis D, Gillis CC, Shih P, O'Toole JE, Fessler RG. Intramedullary spinal cord tumors: Part I—epidemiology, pathophysiology, and diagnosis. Global Spine Journal. 31 Oct 2015;**5**(5):425-435

[3] Ostrom Q. University hospitals health system. Neuro Oncology [Internet. 2020;**22**(S1):1-96 Available from: https://academic.oup.com/neuro-oncology/article/22/Supplement_1/iv1/5943281

[4] Yagi T, Ohata K, Haque M, Hakuba A. Intramedullary spinal cord tumour associated with neurofibromatosis type 1. Acta Neurochirurgica. 1997;**139**(11):1055-1060

[5] Kushel' YV, Belova YD, Tekoev AR. Intramedullary spinal cord tumors and neurofibromatosis. Zh Vopr Neirokhir Im N N Burdenko. **81**(1):70-73

[6] Adam A, Dixon AK, Gillard JH, Schaefer-Prokop C, Grainger RG, Allison DJ. Grainger & Allison's diagnostic radiology: A textbook of medical imaging. 4th ed, 3 vols [book review]. Radiology. Mar 2003;**226**(3):706

[7] Wolfgang D. Radiology Review Manual. Brain Disorders: Von Hippellindau Disease. 2007. pp. 335-343

[8] Koeller KK, Rosenblum RS, Morrison AL. From the archives of the AFIP neoplasms of the spinal cord and filum terminale: Radiologie-pathologie correlation. Radiographics. 2000;**20**(6):1721-1749

[9] Seo HS, Kim JH, Lee DH, Lee YH, Suh SI, Kim SY, et al. Nonenhancing intramedullary astrocytomas and other MR imaging features: A retrospective study and systematic review. Available from: www.ajnr.org

[10] Jallo GI, Freed D, Epstein F. Intramedullary spinal cord tumors in children. Child's Nervous System. 2003;**19**(9):641-649

[11] Smith AB, Soderlund KA, Rushing EJ, SmirniotopolousJG. Radiologic-pathologic correlation of pediatric and adolescent spinal neoplasms: Part 1, intramedullary spinal neoplasms. American Journal of Roentgenology. 2012;**198**(1):34-43

[12] Karikari IO, Nimjee SM, Hodges TR, Cutrell E, Hughes BD, Powers CJ, et al. Impact of tumor histology on resectability and neurological outcome in primary intramedullary spinal cord tumors: A single-center experience with 102 patients. Neurosurgery. 2015;76(Supplement 1):S4-13. [cited 2022 Oct 7]; Available from: https://pubmed.ncbi.nlm.nih.gov/25692367/

[13] Ostrom QT, Gittleman H, Truitt G, Boscia A, Kruchko C, Barnholtz-Sloan JS. CBTRUS statistical report: Primary brain and other central nervous system tumors diagnosed in the United States in 2011-2015. Neuro-Oncology. 2018;**20**:iv1-i86

[14] Schellinger KA, Propp JM, Villano JL, McCarthy BJ. Descriptive epidemiology of primary spinal cord tumors. Journal of Neuro-Oncology. 2008;**87**(2):173-179

[15] Kresbach C, Neyazi S, Schüller U. Updates in the classification

of ependymal neoplasms: The 2021 WHO Classification and beyond. Brain Pathology. 1 Jul 2022;**32**(4)

[16] Taylor MD, Poppleton H, Fuller C, Su X, Liu Y, Jensen P, et al. Radial glia cells are candidate stem cells of ependymoma. Cancer Cell. 2005;**8**(4):323-335

[17] Patronas NJ, Courcoutsakis N, Bromley CM, Katzman GL, MacCollin M, Parry DM. Intramedullary and spinal canal tumors in patients with neurofibromatosis 2: MR imaging findings and correlation with genotype. Radiology. 2001;**218**(2):434-442

[18] Dauleac C, Boulogne S, Barrey CY, Guyotat J, Jouanneau E, Mertens P, et al. Predictors of functional outcome after spinal cord surgery: Relevance of intraoperative neurophysiological monitoring combined with preoperative neurophysiological and MRI assessments. Neurophysiologie Clinique. 2022;**52**(3):242-251

[19] Rudà R, Reifenberger G, Frappaz D, Pfister SM, Laprie A, Santarius T, et al. EANO guidelines for the diagnosis and treatment of ependymal tumors. Neuro-Oncology. 27 Mar 2018;**20**(4):445-456

[20] Chatain GP, Kortz MW, Serva S, Shrestha K, Hosokawa P, Ung TH, et al. Long-term neurologic outcome after spinal ependymoma resection with multimodal intraoperative electrophysiological recording: Cohort study and review of the literature. Neurospine. 2022;**19**(1):118-132

[21] Skrap B, Tramontano V, Faccioli F, Meglio M, Pinna G, Sala F. Surgery for intramedullary spinal cord ependymomas in the neuromonitoring era: Results from a consecutive series of 100 patients. Journal of Neurosurgery. Spine. 2022;**36**(5):858-868

[22] Duff JM, Omoumi P, Bobinski L, Belouaer A, Wuthrich SP, Zanchi F, et al. Transtubular image-guided surgery for spinal intradural lesions: Techniques, results, and complications in a consecutive series of 60 patients. Journal of Neurosurgery: Spine. 1 Jul 2022;**37**(1):121-129

[23] Khalid SI, Adogwa O, Kelly R, Metha A, Bagley C, Cheng J, et al. Adult spinal ependymomas: An epidemiologic study. World Neurosurgery. 2018;**111**:e53-e61

[24] Ghasemi DR, Sill M, Okonechnikov K, Korshunov A, Yip S, Schutz PW, et al. MYCN amplification drives an aggressive form of spinal ependymoma. Acta Neuropathologica. 2019;**138**(6):1075-1089

[25] Torp SH, Solheim O, Skjulsvik AJ. The WHO 2021 classification of central nervous system tumours: A practical update on what neurosurgeons need to know — A minireview. Acta Neurochirurgica. 2022:2453-2464

[26] Shih RY, Koeller KK. Intramedullary masses of the spinal cord: Radiologic-pathologic correlation. Radiographics. 2020:1125-1145

[27] Egger K, Hohenhaus M, Van Velthoven V, Heil S, Urbach H. Spinal diffusion tensor tractography for differentiation of intramedullary tumor-suspected lesions. European Journal of Radiology. 2016;**85**(12):2275-2280

[28] Setzer M, Murtagh RD, Murtagh FR, Eleraky M, Jain S, Marquardt G, et al. Diffusion tensor imaging tractography in patients with intramedullary tumors: Comparison with intraoperative findings and value for prediction of tumor resectability. Journal of Neurosurgery. Spine. 2010;**13**(3):371-380

[29] Golpayegani M, Edalatfar M, Ahmadi A, Sadeghi-Naini M, Salari F, Hanaei S, et al. Complete versus incomplete surgical resection in

intramedullary astrocytoma: Systematic review with individual patient data meta-analysis. Global Spine Journal. 2022;**2022**:1-15

[30] Hernández-Durán S, Bregy A, Shah AH, Hanft S, Komotar RJ, Manzano GR. Primary spinal cord glioblastoma multiforme treated with temozolomide. Journal of Clinical Neuroscience. 2015;**22**(12):1877-1882

[31] Dornbos D, Kim HJ, Butman JA, Lonser RR. Review of the neurological implications of von Hippel-Lindau disease. JAMA Neurology. 1 May 2018;**75**(5):620-627

[32] Jankovic D, Hanissian A, Rotim K, Splavski B, Arnautovic KI. Novel clinical insights into spinal hemangioblastoma in adults: A systematic review. World Neurosurgery. 2022;**158**:1-10

[33] Saliou G, Giammattei L, Ozanne A, Messerer M. Role of preoperative embolization of intramedullary hemangioblastoma. Neuro-Chirurgie. 2017;**63**(5):372-375

[34] Clark AJ, Lu DC, Richardson RM, Tihan T, Parsa AT, Chou D, et al. Surgical technique of temporary arterial occlusion in the operative management of spinal hemangioblastomas. World Neurosurgery. 2010;**74**(1):200-205

[35] Barrey CY, Baassiri W, Vandenbulcke A. Clipping test of a radiculomedullary artery during resection of a dorsal spinal meningioma. World Neurosurgery. 2022;**164**:159

[36] Oppenlander ME, Spetzler RF. Advances in spinal hemangioblastoma surgery. World Neurosurgery. 2010;**74**(1):116-117

[37] Dudley RWR, Torok MR, Gallegos DR, Mulcahy-Levy JM, Hoffman LM, Liu AK, et al. Pediatric low-grade ganglioglioma: Epidemiology, treatments, and outcome analysis on 348 children from the surveillance, epidemiology, and end results database. Neurosurgery. 2015;**76**(3):313-320

[38] Tobin MK, Geraghty JR, Engelhard HH, Linninger AA, Mehta AI. Intramedullary spinal cord tumors: A review of current and future treatment strategies and future treatment strategies. Neurosurgical Focus. 2015;**39**:1-10

Chapter 12

Surgical Principles for Spinal Meningiomas

Feyzi Birol Sarica

Abstract

Spinal meningiomas, which are usually benign character, rarely show an invasive course. Since they grow slowly in the intradural extramedullary space, clinical symptoms also progress slowly. It is usually diagnosed in the later periods, when the tumor reaches to large size. They most commonly show location in the thoracic region. Although it does not have a real capsule, they can be removed completely or close to total by microsurgical methods, since they are well-demarcated solitary tumors. The most important factor in the complete and safe removal of spinal meningioma is the selection of the surgical approach suitable for the size, localization, and topography of the tumor. In the postoperative period, improvement in neurological functions is observed generally and their prognosis is good. In this study, the natural history of the tumor is explained in detail, by examining the pathogenesis and predisposing factors and clinical symptomatology in the spinal meningiomas. Moreover, it has been also focused on describing the surgical approaches and operative techniques to be used in the complete and safe removal of the spinal meningioma, according to the localization and topography of the tumor.

Keywords: cervical spine, dorsal and dorsolateral region, lumbar spine, spinal meningioma, surgical approaches, thoracic spine, treatment modalities, ventral and ventrolateral region

1. Introduction

The spinal meningiomas (SMs), which originate from the cap cells of the arachnoid membrane, are generally benign character and tumors of which prognosis is positive [1]. While SMs constitute 25–46% of all intradural spinal tumors, and they constitute 12% of all meningiomas [2, 3]. Its incidence is 0.5–2/100,000 per year [4]. It progresses to the subarachnoid space by growing slowly in the intradural extramedullary distance. When they reach to large sizes, they first cause stretching of the surrounding arachnoid and then they press on the spinal cord and nerve roots. In these cases, the diagnosis is usually made late due to the slowly progressive character of clinical symptoms. Different clinical symptoms can be observed in patients with the SMs, depending on the localization, topographic structure, and size of the tumor. The tumors can mostly dissect from the spinal cord and nerve roots, because of their solitary structure and the presence of arachnoid and good surgical cleavage between the spinal cord and them. It is possible to remove total or near-total with microsurgical methods. They rarely exhibit invasive character [5]. In the postoperative period, a rapid improvement is observed in the neurological functions of the patients [6, 7].

2. Spinal meningioma

2.1 Epidemiology and predisposing factors

The SMs are more common in women than men and the female, male ratio was 4:1. It is frequently observed in middle-aged women and the mean age was 57.6 years [2, 6]. It has been thought that the reason why it is more common seen in women may be due to the response of the tissues to sex hormones [8]. However, the effects of hormones on SM development are still controversial [9]. Although no definite predisposing factor has been identified, it has been stated that steroid, aminergic, and growth factor receptors will be able to play a role in SM development pathogenesis [10]. However, neurofibromatosis type 2 accompanies 12% of the SM cases under 50 years of age. It has been also stated that the 22nd chromosome deletion and inactivation were frequently observed in the sporadic meningiomas accompanying neurofibromatosis type 2 in the genetic studies conducted [11]. It has been stated that SM was observed in the patients who received radiotherapy to the spinal region and also in the patients with a history of intraventricular ependymoma and breast adenocarcinoma in the literature [12].

2.2 Rare tumor forms

The intramedullary-located SMs, which are seen as rare, are frequently observed in the cervical region, especially in the C2–C4 localization. In fewer cases, the thoracic region localization has also been stated. There are varying degrees of neurological deficits in the clinic of these cases, which are frequently observed in the fifth decade. No specific tumor subtype has been stated for the intramedullary SMs [13–15]. Other rare extradurally located SMs show location in the thoracic region with a rate of 53% and in the cervical region with a rate of 42%. They are observed in women and before the third decade. It has also been stated in the literature that they could be removed totally; therefore, the recurrence rate was higher in these cases, due to their invasion of neighboring important anatomical structures in some cases of the extradural SM [16]. Rare cases of SM have also been stated in the literature, as a result of an intracranial meningioma reaching the spinal region via cerebrospinal fluid (CSF). Similarly, it has been stated in rare cases that SM was observed in another spinal region in the patient with a diagnosis of SM during the follow-up [17–19].

2.3 Localization and topography

In a systematic review conducted by Pereira et al. regarding the SMs, it was most commonly localized in the thoracic region with a rate of 64.6%, and this was followed by the cervical region with 22.7% and other region localizations with 12.7%, respectively [20]. In the literature, the thoracic region localization rates have been stated as 83% by Solero et al., as 79% by Voldrich et al., as 76% by Gottfried et al. and as 72% by Gezen et al. [7, 21–23]. On the other hand, in the analysis conducted by Ozkan et al. in the patients with the ventral and ventrolateral SM, the localization was observed in the thoracic region (between T1 and T9 levels) in the rate of 52.7%, in the cervical region in the rate of 27.3% (between C0 and C7 levels), and the thoracolumbar region (between T10 and L2 levels) in the rate of 20% [24].

In the literature, although there is no specific topographic classification for the SMs, it has been stated that the tumors were frequently located on the dorsal and dorsolateral of the spinal cord [2]. The ventral and ventrolateral localization rates have been stated as 39% by Roux et al., 33.5% by Ozkan et al., 13% by Yoon et al., and 15% by Solero et al. [7, 24–26]. On the other hand, in the topographic examination of the SMs, it has been stated lateral localization in 45–71%, dorsal localization in 10–31%, and ventral localization in 15–27% [7, 23, 27]. Generally, while the tumors localized in the thoracic region are observed in the dorsal spine of the spinal cord, the tumors localized in the cervical region are observed in the ventral part of the spinal cord [2, 7, 28]. Ozkan et al. have stated that only ventral-located cases were seen in 21.8% of the ventral and ventrolateral SMs and ventrolateral-located cases were seen in 78.2% of them [24].

Although they mostly show intradural extramedullary localization, approximately 10% of SMs are located extradurally or extra-intradurally. It is found as 5.4% by King et al., 14% by Gezen et al., and 17% by Cohen-Gadol et al. [5, 21, 23, 29].

2.4 Histopathological analysis and tumor subtypes

The World Health Organization (WHO) has classified SMs into three grades, according to the degree of malignancy. The WHO grade-I SMs constitute more than 90% of the tumors [30]. In a recent systematic review of the SMs, the histopathology of 1415 tumors has been analyzed and it has been stated that the WHO grade-I meningiomas were the most common with a rate of 94.8%. On the other hand, when the subtypes of the WHO grade-I meningiomas were examined, it has been stated that the psammomatous meningioma, which was found at a rate of 27.8%, and meningothelial meningioma, which was found at a rate of 25.2%, were the most common tumor subtypes. This was followed by the WHO grade-II meningiomas (clear cell, choroidal, and atypical) with a rate of 4.4% and the WHO grade-III meningiomas (anaplastic and papillary) with a rate of 0.8%, respectively [20]. There are spinal invasion, aggressive course, and high recurrence rates in the WHO grade-II and WHO grade-III SMs with high mitotic activity [31–34]. Similarly, in other studies stated in the literature; the transitional, fibrous, chordoid, and metaplastic meningioma subtypes have been observed to be less common. Moreover, it has also been stated that there was no correlation between the age of the patients and the histopathological subtypes of the tumor [12].

2.5 Clinical presentations

Different clinical symptoms are observed, depending on the location and topography of the tumor, its growth pattern, and size. The SMs cause misdiagnosis and/ or late diagnosis because of their different symptoms and slow growth potential. It is observed that the average diagnosis time is usually around 1 year [12, 29]. The most common symptom is pain. While localized pains are observed more, the pains in the radicular nature are less common [21]. Although it varies according to the growth pattern of the tumor in the extramedullary region, the spinal cord compression findings come to the fore, especially in large-dimensioned tumors. In these cases, various degrees of muscle weakness (spastic paresis or plegia), sensory deficit (hypoesthesia, anesthesia, or paresthesia), and corticospinal tract findings, such as sphincter dysfunctions and Brown-sequard syndrome, can develop [2, 6, 7, 23, 25, 35, 36]. In the study conducted by Voldrich et al., movement disorders depending on muscle weakness have been stated in 79%, sensory disorders in 70%, and sphincter dysfunction in 10%. In this study, the rate of asymptomatic cases was 11% [21]. On the other hand, Ozkan et al. have stated that the nonspecific symptoms, such as sensory impairment, were observed more frequently at a rate of 94.5%;therefore, the diagnosis was made later in these cases, especially in the ventral and ventral localized SMs [24]. While the most common symptom was radiculopathic pain in the study in which Han et al. analyzed the patients with high-grade SM, this was followed by motor weakness, sensory deficit, and sphincter disorders, respectively. In this study by Han et al.; it has been emphasized that the asymptomatic period observed in the patients with high-grade SMs was much shorter than in the WHO grade-I SMs [37].

2.6 Neurodiagnostic techniques

Spinal magnetic resonance imaging (MRI) is currently the best diagnostic tool for SMs. In earlier periods, when the spinal MRI technique was not used, these cases were often misdiagnosed [2, 23]. Klekamp and Samii have stated that early diagnosis can be made in these cases by means of the spinal MRI and they also affected the neurological outcome after surgery [27]. Ozkan et al. have stated that the time between the symptom duration and diagnosis was around 6 months by means of the spinal MRI [24]. In the spinal MRI T1- and T2-sequences, the tumors are usually observed isointense with the spinal cord. On the other hand, in the MRI images made after the intravenous injection of Gadolinium-DTPA, the SMs show intense homogeneous contrast enhancement. By means of the spinal MRI, the localization of the tumor, its size, the invasive behavior, and its relationship with neighboring tissues can also be examined in detail [25, 38]. The intratumoral calcifications can be shown by computed tomography (CT) [39]. Ono et al. have stated that the tumor stiffness developed due to calcifications would be able to be defined by the Spinal MRI T1-sequences and CT [40]. On the other hand, the tumors with ossification and infiltration of the adjacent structures with a broad tumor base have been radiologically defined as the "en plaque meningiomas" [35, 41, 42].

3. Surgical treatment

3.1 General surgical principles

The majority of SMs are benign, and the first choice in their treatment is surgery. The first successful surgical treatment of SM was performed by Sir Victor Horsley in 1887 [6]. The surgical timing is performed under emergency or elective conditions, by taking into account the patient's neurological picture. The gold standard in surgical treatment is total resection of the tumor by the microsurgical method [43, 44]. In the preoperative period, the tumor localization and size should be examined in detail with the contrast-enhanced spinal MRI, and the tumor level should be determined with the intraoperative C-arm scopy. The most important issue in surgical planning is to determine the appropriate surgical approach, according to the location and spread of the tumor in the spinal axis. Especially, in surgical approaches requiring a laminectomy, the laminectomies should be performed from the cranial to the caudal and the spinal cord should be rotated with appropriate techniques [43, 45, 46]. The aim of the surgery is to completely remove the SM without damaging the neural elements, such as the adjacent spinal cord and nerve roots, which are exposed to tumor compression. After the microsurgical tumor resection, the resection and/or coagulation of the tumor-infiltrated dural base should also be planned. It is very useful to use intraoperative neuromonitoring techniques (with somatosensory-evoked potential (SSEP) and motor-evoked potential (MEP) recordings) to increase surgical safety. On the other hand, intraoperative ultrasonography (USG) can be used in the internal debulking phase to reduce the volume of the tumor in large tumors [47].

3.2 Surgical approaches, principles, and operative techniques

3.2.1 Upper cervical spinal meningioma

Almost 27% of all cervical meningiomas have been stated in the upper cervical spine and only 3% in the foramen magnum area [48, 49]. Topographically, in approximately 50% of patients, the tumor is located ventral or ventrolateral to the spinal cord [50]. The gold standard in the surgery of upper cervical SMs is complete removal. The dorsal and dorsolaterally located upper cervical SMs can be safely and effectively removed with the standard posterior midline approach [51, 52].

3.2.1.1 Lateral and far-lateral approaches

The posterior midline approach is insufficient for surgical access to the ventral and ventrolateral of the upper cervical region. Because of this difficulty in surgical exposure, the tumors are often incompletely removed. Similarly, because of the posterior midline approach, which requires significant spinal cord and brainstem retraction, the tumors in this region have a high risk of postsurgical morbidity [51, 52].

The lateral and far-lateral approaches have been developed to avoid the disadvantages of the posterior midline approach and to access the foramen magnum and the upper cervical region ventral [53–60]. With the lateral transcondylar approach, which provides a more comprehensive surgical perspective from the lateral to the foramen magnum, the tumors located ventrally in the foramen magnum can now be successfully removed in many clinics [61–63]. George et al. expressed the borders of the foramen magnum as the region between the lower 1/3 of the clivus and the upper corner of the C2 vertebra corpus in the anterior, between the occipital squamous anterior edge and the C2 spinous process in the posterior, and between the jugular tubercles and the upper edges of the C2 laminae laterally [64]. The far-lateral approach was first described by George et al. in 1988 to reach the lesions in front of the foramen magnum. The lesions located in the ventral/ventrolateral of the foramen magnum and upper cervical region can be safely removed by means of the far-lateral approach and its modified subtypes developed in the following years.

The critical issue in the far-lateral approach is the manipulation of the vertebral artery [51]. The extreme-lateral craniocervical approach has been developed by modifying the far-lateral approach by Salas et al. in 1999. In later years, the extreme-lateral craniocervical approach has been modified and new approaches, such as transfacet and retrofacet approaches, have been developed for the removal of the intradural lesions located ventral to the upper cervical region. After all, the tumors located in the foramen magnum and upper cervical region ventrals are removed and are now used as a standard approach by many surgeons, by means of the far-lateral approach and its modified subtypes [54].

3.2.2 Subaxial cervical spinal meningioma

The SMs below the C2 level can be removed with both anterior and posterior approaches. On the other hand, in the removal of dorsal and dorsolateral subaxial SMs, the standard posterior approaches performed with the laminectomy or laminotomy are usually sufficient [43, 46]. The cervical SMs located ventrolaterally are operated with the modified posterior approaches by using laterally extended laminectomy techniques [2, 7, 23, 25, 27]. On the other hand, the standard anterior cervical approach is preferred for the removal of ventrally located subaxial cervical tumors [46].

3.2.2.1 Modified posterior approach with lateral extension

There are difficulties in the surgical removal of the SMs that are completely ventral and located with their dural base [2, 7, 23, 25]. Levy et al. stated that the prognosis was worse in ventrally located cervical SMs they operated [2]. To overcome these surgical difficulties, laterally extended modified posterior approaches have been developed. Klekamp et al. have operated on 130 patients with the SMs (27% ventrally located) for the laminectomy, by using the modified posterior approach with facetectomy added as needed [27]. On the other hand, Roux et al. have operated on 54 patients with SM (39% ventral and ventrolateral localization), by using a modified posterior midline approach with articular process resection added as needed [25]. After all, the lateral extension laminectomy techniques have been the most commonly used approach for the removal of the ventral cervical SMs. However, a modified posterior approach using the bilateral extended laminectomy has also been described to be able to minimize spinal cord manipulation. As an advantage of this technique, it has been emphasized that the tumor in front of the spinal cord could be approached bilaterally [7, 23, 28].

Solero et al. stated that all ventrally located cervical SMs were successfully removed with the modified posterior approach in which bilaterally extended laminectomy was used. In this study, they have stated that the dura was opened in a T-shaped and the dentate ligaments were also cut, in addition to bilaterally extended laminectomy to minimize spinal cord manipulation and to provide a better surgical perspective [7]. Similarly, Gezen et al. have stated that the postoperative results were good with bilaterally extended laminectomies in operated ventrally located SMs, as a result of the compilation that they perform an analysis for 36 patients [23]. After all, it has been stated that the prognosis was good in the patients operated with the modified posterior approaches by using a laterally extended laminectomy in the patient series stated in the literature all with ventrally located tumors [7, 23, 25].

3.2.2.2 Anterior cervical approach with corpectomy

Payer et al. stated that the most important advantages of the anterior cervical approach were the opening of a large bone window with corpectomy and reaching a direct ventral cervical SM without the need for spinal cord manipulation, as a result of the systematic review they made and other studies stated in the literature. In ventrally located SMs, extradural coagulation of pathological vascular structures, which are the tumor feeder observed in the anterior dura, can also be easily performed before the dura is opened [65–69].

In the literature, it has been stated the anterior cervical approach was used successfully in the removal of ventrally located cervical SMs. Giroux et al. have stated that the complete tumor resection was performed, without making spinal cord manipulation, after the C5 corpectomy and opening dura with a midline vertical incision with the anterior cervical approach. Better control of bleeding has also been stated [66]. Lenelle et al. have stated that the tumor was completely removed along with the tumor-infiltrated dural base, after opening the dura in an ellipsoid shaped in the cranial and caudal vertical axis with the tumor centered with the corpectomy involving the C4 corpus inferior, C5 corpus, and C6 corpus superior. Duraplasty has been performed by using fascia taken from the iliac region. Moreover, they have emphasized that the surgery was more comfortable by means of the coagulation of pathological dural vascular structures, which are tumor feeders, with this approach [67]. Sava et al. have stated that the tumor was completely removed with the dural base in the cranio-caudal direction, by making multiple corpectomy from C3 to T1 of intradural SM extending between foramen magnum and T2 vertebra levels with this approach. The lumbar CSF drainage has been also applied to prevent CSF leakage in the patient who underwent duraplasty by using fascia [68]. Payer et al. have stated that the intradural ventrally located broad-based SM extending between C5 and C7 levels were completely removed by performing C5, C6, and C7 corpectomy with the anterior cervical approach. The dura has been opened with a midline vertical incision, and the tumor has been dissected from the spinal cord nerve roots and dural base. It has been also emphasized that the tumor-infiltrated dural base was coagulated intradurally and the inner layer of the dura was extensively coagulated by separating it with a microdissector, after the tumor removal [65].

3.2.3 Thoracic and lumbar spinal meningioma

The standard posterior midline approach with laminectomy or laminotomy is usually sufficient in the removal of dorsal, lateral, and ventrolateral thoracic SMs. Nowadays, laminectomies can be extended laterally with the techniques of adding articular process resection to the hemilaminectomy or adding unilateral facetectomy to the laminectomy. On the other hand, in tumors that are completely or mostly ventrally located, the laminectomies can be also extended laterally bilaterally to provide bilateral exposure. In these cases, laminoplasty techniques with miniplates are also used in the same session to avoid spinal instability. While the hemilaminectomy or laminoplasty techniques are preferred more in the cervical localized cases, the laminectomy techniques are generally preferred in the thoracic and thoracolumbar localized cases. In tumors in which the ventrolateral component is larger, hemilaminectomy or laminoplasty techniques are preferred [24].

Moreover, the modified posterior approaches with the lateral extension improved by adding techniques, such as unilateral total facetectomy, pedicle resection, costotransversectomy, and partial vertebrectomy to laminectomy or laminotomy have also been developed to reach ventrally located thoracic tumors [43, 46, 70]. The anterior transthoracic approach is no longer used today since serious vascular injuries have been stated with severe lung retraction in ventrally located thoracic tumor resections [46, 71]. The posterior and modified posterior approaches are sufficient in most cases in the removal of dorsal, lateral, ventrolateral and ventral lumbar SMs. On the other hand, another advantage of using the posterior approaches used in tumor resections at the lumbar level is that the spinal cord and nerve root retraction, which is necessary for revealing the tumor, can be performed more safely by the surgeon. Despite these approaches, the anterior transabdominal approach and the lateral retroperitoneal approach, which are rarely used nowadays, can be preferred in very few cases where the tumor cannot be removed [46, 72].

3.2.3.1 Posterior midline approach and operative technique

The posterior approaches with the laminectomy or laminotomy are usually sufficient in the surgical resection of dorsal and dorsolateral SMs [43]. Considering the extent of tumoral dural involvement, compression, and displacement levels in the spinal cord that is proportional to the size of the tumor, and findings, such as CSF blockage and laminectomy or laminotomy, should be planned. Generally, the laminectomy or laminotomy is performed at a lower and an upper level together with the tumor level in a way it will cover the cranial and caudal poles of the tumor, which is revealed under the guidance of fluoroscopy [45, 46, 61]. In order to prevent spinal instability that will be able to develop in the long-term postoperatively in the posterior approaches, the laminoplasty techniques are now preferred by using laminotomies or microplates performed with pneumatic cutters instead of the laminectomy [24]. The laminectomy and/or laminotomy are performed starting from the cranial in order to prevent postoperative neurological losses that will be able to develop due to spinal cord herniation. If possible, it would also be helpful at this stage to check the localization and extent of the tumor by intraoperative ultrasonographic examination. The dura is opened by making a linear incision in the dorsal small SMs [45, 46]. The dura is ellipsoid-shaped and opened in the cases of large dorsal SM with a wide base and severe adhesion to the dura in order to perform a total resection of the dural base, where the tumor is attached, together with the tumor [46]. The dural leaves are suspended with the sutures. In the arachnoid dissection stage, the patient is placed in the slight trandelenburg position and cotonoids are placed in the cranial and caudal regions of the surgical field in order to reduce CSF leakage and blood flow to the subarachnoid space [45]. Although they do not have a true capsule, the SMs can be separated from the normal tissue by a good surgical cleavage through the arachnoid [47]. The microsurgical tumor resection should be performed with intraoperative neuromonitoring techniques in order not to damage the spinal cord and nerve roots. With these surgical procedures, the tumor volume is reduced by the internal debulking first, and then a total resection of the tumor is performed with the tumor-infiltrated dural base (according to Simpson grade-I resection). The cavitron ultrasonic aspirators (CUSA) can be used for the internal debulking of large tumors with a wide dural base. However, during the use of CUSA, utmost care should be taken not to damage the spinal cord [45, 61, 73, 74]. In the surgeries, where only the tumor is removed and the tumor-infiltrated dural base is coagulated (according to Simpson's grade-II resection), the dura is closed by primary suturing in a water-tight manner. However, in the surgeries in which the tumor is completely removed with the tumor-infiltrated dural base (according to Simpson's grade-I resection), the dural opening is usually closed by duraplasty (using autografts and allografts) and fibrin tissue adhesives are placed on it [45]. The total resection (according to Simpson's grade-I resection) and gross-total resection (according to Simpson's grade-II resection) can be successfully performed in most dorsal SM cases with the posterior midline approach following the above surgical procedures.

3.2.3.2 Modified posterior approach and operative technique

The modified posterior approaches have been developed in the removal of ventrally located thoracic SMs since more lateral exposure is required in surgery. In this approach, the laminectomy or laminotomy can be extended more laterally, depending on the location and topography of the tumor, by means of the techniques described above. For ventrally located tumors, the dura can be opened with a straight, curve-linear, or T-shaped incision and arachnoid dissection is performed. The dentate ligament is tractioned with a silk suture placed on one side. The spinal cord is then rotated slightly to provide a better surgical perspective of the ventral spinal cord. A much wider surgical exposure can be achieved by cutting the dentate ligaments after the dura is opened [24]. With the increase in the size of the ventrally located tumor, the spinal cord compression increases, and the spinal cord is displaced. For this reason, in order to minimize spinal cord injury in ventrally located large tumors, an incision is made on the side of the dural attachment and away from the spinal cord. Then, the tumor volume is reduced by internal debulking accompanied by intraoperative neuromonitoring. Thus, the spinal cord is decompressed and tumor borders can be observed better. While internal debulking is performed in large tumors, and can be used in the CUSA. However, extreme care should be taken to avoid serious spinal cord injuries due to the size of the CUSA probes [50]. During the complete removal of the SMs, the sensory nerves attached to the tumor can be cut [24]. Thus, the completely free tumor is mobilized by placing a traction suture, and the SM is completely removed (according to Simpson's grade-II resection) [61, 73, 74].

However, in large-sized thoracic tumors that are completely ventrally located, the total resection of the tumor cannot always be performed with the modified posterior approach described above. In this situation, there is a need for the modified posterior approaches (with the classical laminectomy or laminotomy with unilateral total facetectomy, pedicle resection, costotrasversectomy, and/or partial vertebrectomy added) that provide more lateral surgical exposure. The dural resection is almost impossible in ventrally located tumors with a wide base and severe adhesion to the dura; therefore, the tumor-infiltrated dural base is coagulated, by leaving it in place (according to Simpson's grade-II resection) [46, 61]. In addition, in the microsurgery of the SMs located in the thoracic and thoracolumbar regions, maximum care should be taken not to injury the Adamkiewicks artery (arteria radicularis magna; 90% observed between T7 and L1 levels and on the left side), which is a serious feeder of the spinal cord [45].

3.2.3.3 Illustrative case

A 68-year-old female patient having localized back pain for the last 3 months applied to our outpatient clinic. Her neurological examination was normal. In the contrast-enhanced spinal MRI of the patient, at T12 vertebral level, a mass lesion, which as intradural extramedullary located, smooth-contoured, in 18x14 mm size, showed a location in the spinal cord ventral, and was compatible with spinal meningioma, was detected. Moreover, it was also observed that the tumor located in the ventral of the spinal cord displaced the conus medullaris posteriorly (**Figure 1**). The patient was operated with a modified posterior midline approach with the bilateral extended laminectomy. First, T11 and then T12 bilateral extended laminectomy was made from the cranial to the caudal, and then right unilateral median facetectomy was performed. The dura was opened with a slight curve-linear vertical incision. The tumor was completely removed, by leaving the tumor-infiltrated dural base in place with the neuromonitoring and microsurgical technique. The tumor-infiltrated dural base was coagulated with the bipolar. Thus, the tumor was completely removed according to Simpson's grade-II tumor resection. The neurological examination of the patient in the postoperative period revealed that the left leg muscle strength was grade 4+/5. After a 10-day physical therapy and rehabilitation program, the patient's

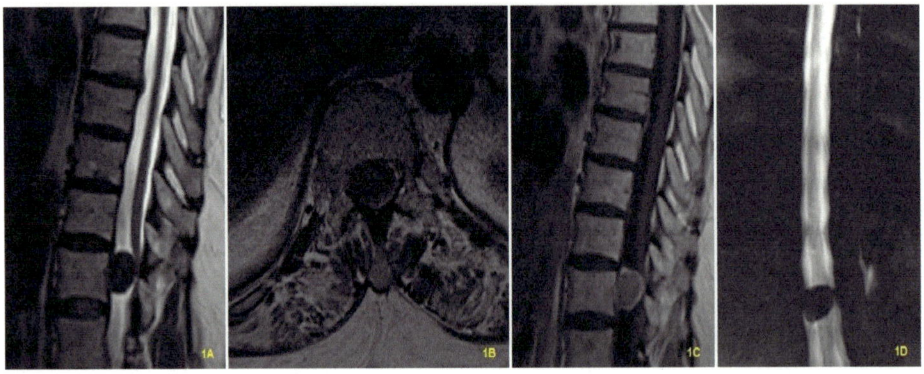

Figure 1.
In the preoperative period spinal magnetic resonance imaging; at T12 vertebral level, a mass lesion, which was intradural-extramedullary localized, displaced the conus medullaris posteriorly in the ventral of the spinal cord, was 18 x 14 mm in size, and was a hypointense and well-contoured in the unenhanced sagittal T2- (A) and axial T2- (B) sequences, was observed. In the contrast-enhanced sagittal T1- sequence (C), homogeneous contrast enhancement is observed in the lesion. In the spinal MRI-myelography (D), the CSF blockade is observed at the level of the relevant spinal cord.

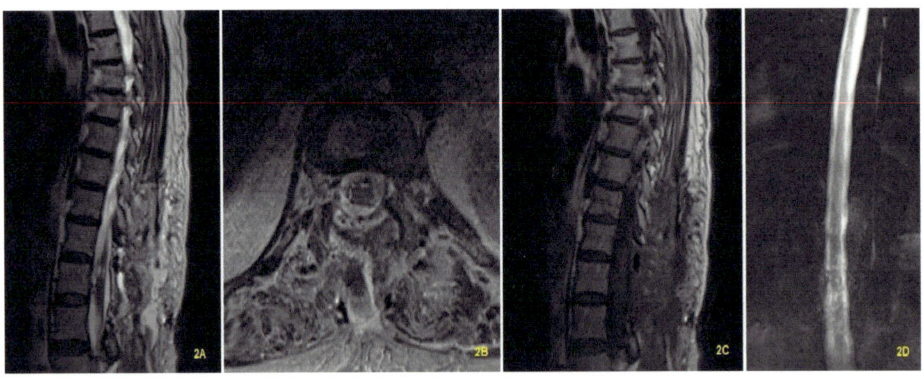

Figure 2.
In the contrast-enhanced spinal magnetic resonance imaging performed on the 7th postoperative day, in the unenhanced sagittal T2- (A) and axial T2- (B) sequences, the mass lesion observed in the preoperative period was removed, and contrast enhancement in favor of residual tumor was not detected in the contrast-enhanced sagittal T1- sequence (C). The spinal MRI-myelography (D) shows that CSF flow is normal.

left leg muscle strength improved to grade 5/5. The pathology result came as psammomatous meningiomas (WHO grade-I). In the contrast-enhanced spinal MRI performed on the 7th postoperative day, the contrast enhancement was not detected in favor of the residual tumor (**Figure 2**).

3.3 Types of surgical tumor removal

The grading system defined by Simpson for intracranial meningiomas is used to evaluate the scope of surgical resection in SMs [75]. The tumor-infiltrated dural base can be resected more radically in the microsurgery of the intracranial meningiomas compared to the SMs. Therefore, the use of Simpson's grading system in SM surgery is limited. While the term complete is used for Simpson's grade-I and grade-II resections in some clinics, in some clinics, gross-total resection terms are used for Simpson's grade-I and grade-II resections, and subtotal resection terms are used for grade-III and higher resections. The complete tumor removal rates of the SMs observed in all localizations range from 82 to 98% [2, 7, 8, 22, 23, 27, 50]. In a systematic review conducted by Pereira et al., it has been stated that 94.5% of the SMs were extracted according to Simpson grade-I and grade-II resection, and 5.5% of them, the extraction was performed according to Simpson grade-III or higher resection [20].

Abou-Madawi et al. have stated the results of 23 patients (Foramen magnum in 10 patients, C1–C2 levels in 7 patients, C2–C3 levels in 4 patients, and C3–C4 levels in 2 patients) with the ventral (7 patients) and ventrolateral (16 patients) foramen magnum and upper cervical meningiomas operated with the retrofacet approach, which was a subtype of the far-lateral approach. In this study, it has been stated that the tumor was removed completely in 91.3% of the patients, and subtotal removal was performed in 8.7% of the patients because the tumor has adhered to the intradural vertebral artery. As a result of this study, it has been emphasized that the far-lateral approach was a safe surgical corridor [76]. On the other hand, it has been stated by Slin'ko et al. that the total tumor resection was performed in only 74% of the ventral/ventrolaterally located patients operated with the standard posterior midline approach and its modified forms [77].

The subaxial cervical SMs located intradurally ventrally are excised with the anterior cervical approach performed with the uni- or multi-segmental corpectomies. Giroux et al. and Banczerowski et al. stated that the intradural ventral SMs at the C5 level were completely removed with the anterior cervical approach [66, 69]. A ventrally located SM at the level of the C5 vertebra has been removed by Lenelle et al. with the anterior approach, along with the tumor-infiltrating dural base, and the tumor was completely excised [67]. Payer et al. have completely removed an intradural broad-based ventrally located SM extending between C5 and C7 levels with an anterior approach accompanied by the multi-segmental corpectomy [65]. On the other hand, the tumor has been completely removed by Sawa et al. with the tumor-infiltrating dural base with the multi-segmental corpectomy anterior cervical approach of the intradural SM extending between the foramen magnum and T2 vertebrae from C3 to T1.

Ozkan et al. have stated the surgical results of the patients (29 patients (52.7%) with the SMs with only ventral and ventrolateral localization between T1–T9 and surgical results in 11 patients (20%) they operated with a modified posterior approach by using the technique of lengthening laminectomies to the laterals. It has been stated that 53 (96.4%) of a total of 55 SMs were successfully removed with this approach (according to Simpsons grade-II resection) [24].

3.3.1 Surgical difficulty in tumor removal: en plaque, calcified, and recurrent tumors

Although complete tumor resection is the gold standard in SM surgery, the complete removal of en plaque and recurrent tumors with arachnoid infiltration is very difficult [34, 43, 44]. The ossified SMs are observed from0.7% to 5.5% of all SMs. The complete removal of the ossified SMs is difficult due to their hard consistency and strong adhesion to the spinal cord [44, 78, 79]. Therefore, the surgical approaches that offer a narrower surgical perspective make the removal of ossified tumors more difficult and increase the postoperative morbidity in these cases. Therefore, the microsurgical dissection of the tumor and pia-mater is recommended in the ossified SMs. It has been stated that the tumor could be removed as a block with this method [78]. The ventral location of the tumor is another factor that complicates the complete resection. In the study conducted by Ozkan et al. on 55 patients with the SM located ventrally and ventrolaterally have stated the total removal of the SM, according to Simpson's grade-II resection in 53 patients (96.4%), and the subtotal removal of the SM because of intratumoral calcification in 2 patients (3.6%) [24]. Similarly, Levy et al. have emphasized that the total excision of the tumors should not be performed in the calcified meningiomas located close to the spinal cord due to the high risk of postoperative morbidity [2]. It has been stated that the complete removal of the tumor together with the tumor-infiltrated dural base, if possible, in the SM surgery, and coagulation of the dura in cases where removal was not possible, reduced the tumor recurrence. Moreover, the surgical technique in which the inner and outer dura layers of the dura are separated and the inner dura layer is removed with the tumor, and the intact outer dura layer is sutured has been described in the literature. By means of this technique, there will be no need for the duraplasty using the fascia or synthetic dura grafts [24, 47, 80]. The arachnoid scar formation also complicates the total removal of recurrent tumors [20].

4. Surgical outcomes

4.1 Improvement in neurological functions

A specific classification developed for the SMs has not been stated in the evaluation of the neurological functions of patients in the preoperative and postoperative period. However, it has been observed that the McCormick classification was used in the spinal ependiomas in some clinics, and other functional neurological classifications, such as modified McCormick (MMC), Frankel, and Japanese Orthopedic Association (JOA) classifications, were used in some clinics [24, 37, 70, 76]. In the patients having whole SMs, functional and neurologic recovery rates after surgery range from 61 to 98% [2, 7, 23, 25, 27, 48, 81]. In the patients with the SMs, recovery of neurological functions is observed with rapid recovery in the postoperative period [73, 74]. Klekamp and Samii have stated that 80% of the patients with the SMs were able to walk 1 year after surgery [27]. Riad et al. have stated some improvement in sphincter dysfunction in 67% of the cases [82]. Specifically, in the study involving the ventral and ventrolateral SMs, while the rate of independent walking in the preoperative period was 72.7% in the preoperative period, it increased to 90.9% with a significant improvement in the postoperative period [24]. After all, it is understood that the postoperative functional and neurologic recovery rates in the ventral and ventrolateral SMs are compatible with all SMs. In the studies published in recent years, the postoperative permanent neurological deterioration rates have been stated in the range from 0 to 10% [2, 22, 26, 29, 50, 83, 84]. Many potential risk factors that will be able to cause permanent postoperative neurological deterioration have been stated in the literature [7, 24, 25, 48, 85].

4.2 Incomplete removal of calcified tumor and surgical outcome

It is observed that the neurologic deterioration rates are higher in the postoperative period in patients with especially SM with massive calcification, in which the complete removal of the tumor by microsurgery is difficult [2, 24, 44, 86, 87]. Levy et al. have stated poor postoperative clinical outcomes in three (75%) of four patients with the calcified SMs. As a result of this study, it has been emphasized that the total resection of tumors should not be performed in calcified meningiomas located close to the spinal cord [2]. Ozkan et al. have stated a total of seven patients (12.7%) with the calcified SMs in their series of 55 patients with ventrally located SMs. In this study, they have stated total the removal of SM (according to Simpson's grade-II resection) in five patients with ventrally located calcified tumors and the subtotal removal of meningioma in two patients. In this study, it has been stated that postoperative neurological deterioration was detected in five patients (9.1%), and four of these patients recovered in the early postoperative period [24]. When this study and other studies in the literature are evaluated together, it is understood that the calcified SMs should be evaluated separately as a specific issue.

4.3 Histopathological subtypes of the tumor and surgical outcome

Schaller et al. stated in their series that the neurological deficits of 33 patients (8 dorsal, 6 ventral, and 19 ventrolateral tumors) improved in 79% of the patients in the postoperative period, and neurological functions worsened in 21% [48]. In this study, the histopathology of the tumor has been observed to be psammomatous meningioma in all cases whose neurological functions worsened in the postoperative period [48]. On the other hand, Ozkan et al. stated in their study on the ventral SMs that they did not find any relationship between the psammomatous meningioma subtype and the negative clinical outcomes of the patients [24]. Han et al. analyzed the results of 20 operated patients with high-grade SMs. In this study, the SMs have been removed according to Simpson's grade-II resection in 80% of the patients and resection has been performed in 20% of the patients according to Simpson's grad-III. As a result of this study in which the surgical results were evaluated with the MMC grading, it has been stated that 73.7% of the patients improved in their neurological functions and no change occurred in the neurological functions of 15.7%.

4.4 Tumor localization and surgical outcome

4.4.1 Upper cervical spinal meningioma and surgical outcome

4.4.1.1 Lateral and far-lateral approaches

Abou-Madawi et al. evaluated the postoperative results of the patients with ventrally located foramen magnum and upper cervical region meningioma, which they operated with the far-lateral retrofacet approach, according to the JOA score, and they have stated that 70% of the patients had completed recovery and 30% of the patients had a reduction in preoperative symptoms. It has been also stated that there was no worsening of the neurological functions in the postoperative period in any of the patients [76]. On the other hand, Slin'ko et al. have analyzed the results of a total of 140 patients with the SMs, which were topographically located at 24% ventrally and 76% ventrolaterally, they operated with different approaches, such as posterior approach, laterally extended modified posterior approach, and anterolateral approach. In the postoperative period, it has been stated that 50% of the patients recovered completely, 38% improved, 7% did not change their neurological functions compared to the preoperative period, and 5% worsened [77]. After all, in many studies stated in the literature, it has been stated that the postoperative results in the ventral/ventrolateral SMs operated with the lateral approach were better than those operated with the posterior midline approach and its modified forms [44, 49, 77, 88, 89].

4.4.2 Subaxial cervical spinal meningioma and surgical outcome

4.4.2.1 Modified posterior midline approach with lateral extension

Slin'ko et al. have stated that the postoperative clinical outcomes were worse in the patients with ventral tumor, who were operated with different approaches, such as posterior approach, laterally extended modified posterior approach, and anterolateral approach, according to tumor topography, compared to the patients with ventrolateral tumor [77]. Joachim et al. have recommended cutting the dentate ligaments to prevent postoperative neurological deterioration in the tumors located ventrally. It has been stated with this technique that the stretch of the spinal cord released from the dentate ligaments was reduced and it could be mobilized more easily [88]. On the other hand, Ozkan et al. have stated the surgical results of 55 patients (27.3% localized between C0–C7 levels) with ventral and ventrolateral SMs localized in all spinal regions they operated with a modified posterior approach by using the technique of lengthening laminectomies to the laterals. They have stated successful complete removal of the SM (according to Simpsons grade-II resection) in 53 patients (96.4%) with this approach. They have stated that they were removed incompletely due to calcification of the tumor in two cases located close to the spinal cord. With this approach, the rate of independent walking, which was observed at a rate of 72.7% in the preoperative period for all patients according to Frankel grading, improved significantly in the postoperative period and increased to 90.9% [24].

4.4.2.2 Anterior cervical approach with corpectomy

In most of the studies reported in the literature, it has been stated that the neurologic functions mostly improved in the postoperative period in cases where the intradural ventrally located subaxial SMs were completely removed by the operation with an anterior cervical approach with uni- or multi-segmental corpectomy [65–67, 69]. In a case with the intradural SM extending between the foramen magnum and T2 vertebra level, the tumor has been completely removed by Sawa et al. with the tumor-infiltrated dural base by the anterior approach. Multi-segmental corpectomy has been performed from C3 to T1. It has been observed that the quadriparesis observed in this patient first deteriorated in the postoperative period, but improved significantly within months [68].

4.4.3 Thoracic and Lumbar spinal meningioma and surgical outcome

4.4.3.1 Modified posterior approach with lateral extension

Goel et al. have stated that the postoperative clinical results of 17 patients with the SM located ventral and ventrolateral and operated with the posterior midline approach (82.3% gross-total resection) were bad [90]. On the other hand, Ozkan et al. have stated the surgical results of 55 patients (52.7% localized between T1–T9 levels and 20% between T10–L2 levels) with the ventral and ventrolateral SMs localized in all spinal regions they operated with the modified posterior approach by using the technique of lengthening laminectomies to the laterals. They have stated successful complete removal of the SM (according to Simpsons grade-II resection) in 53 patients (96.4%) with this approach. They have stated that they removed the tumor incompletely due to calcification located close to the spinal cord in two cases.

With this approach, the rate of independent walking, which was observed at a rate of 72.7% in the preoperative period for all patients according to Frankel grading, improved significantly in the postoperative period and increased to 90.9%. As a result of this study, it has been stated that the technique of extending laminectomies to the laterals (modified posterior approach) could be applied bilaterally when necessary by providing a wider and more reliable surgical perspective bilaterally for the ventral-located tumor. In addition, it has been emphasized that spinal cord manipulation could be performed more reliably without excessive traction by means of the technique of bilateral lengthening of the laminectomy [24].

4.4.3.2 Anterior approach

D'Aliberti et al. have evaluated the results of 145 patients with lesions located in the thoracic and lumbar spinal regions that were operated with the anterior approach and suggested that the ventral approach should be used for the removal of extradural lesions [91].

5. Management of the postoperative complications

5.1 Overview of postoperative complications

The postoperative complication rates vary depending on the localization and topographic structure of the tumor and the surgical approach in SMs. Sandalcioglu et al. have stated that postoperative complications developed in 3.3% of the patients in their series of 131 patients with the SMs, who were operated with the standard posterior midline approach [50]. On the other hand, Ozkan et al. have stated the postoperative complication rate was 13.5% in a series of 55 patients with the ventral and ventrolateral SMs. They operated with the modified posterior approach extended laterally [24]. When the postoperative complications are examined, the CSF leakage draws attention, especially. In addition, the complications, such as venous thrombosis, epidural hematoma, and myocardial infarction, delayed wound healing and bifrontal intracranial air trapping have been reported in the literature [21, 24, 50, 66–69, 76, 92].

5.2 Cerebrospinal fluid leakage and management

The rate of CSF leakages observed in the postoperative period in the SMs has been stated between 0 and 4% [4, 22]. It is most commonly observed after the surgery for the SMs located in the upper thoracic region due to the stretch in the interscapular region [45]. Sandalcioglu et al. have stated the postoperative CSF leakage rate of 0.8% in a series of 131 patients with the SMs that they operated with the standard posterior midline approach [50]. On the other hand, Ozkan et al. have stated the postoperative CSF leakage rate as 5.5% in a series of 55 patients with the ventral and ventrolateral SMs that they operated with the modified posterior approach extended laterally [24]. The CSF leakage observed in the postoperative period in the lateral and far-lateral approaches used for the removal of ventrally located cervical SMs is particularly noteworthy. The postoperative CSF leakage was detected in 4 (17.3%) of 23 patients with the ventral/ventrolateral SM in the upper cervical region who were operated with the far-lateral retrofacet approach, and all of these patients recovered with CSF drainage [76]. Sen et al. have stated that CSF leakage was detected in the postoperative period in 2 (33.3%) of 6 patients with the foramen magnum and cervical intradural lesions, who were operated with the extreme-lateral approach. It has been emphasized that the CSF leakage developed due to excessive dural coagulation [92]. Similarly, CSF leakage has also been stated in the postoperative period in the anterior cervical approach used for the removal of ventrally located cervical SMs [66–69]. Therefore, in the majority of the studies reported in the literature, it has been recommended that excessive coagulation of dura should be avoided in order to prevent CSF leakage [66–69, 76, 92].

In the majority of cases, the CSF leakages developed from the small dural openings. To prevent CSF leakage, the dura leaves should be closed with primary suturing, especially in a water-tight manner. However, if the dural opening is too large to be closed with the primary suturing, the duraplasty should be performed by using autografts (with fascia) or allografts (with dural synthetic grafts). Then, the fibrin tissue adhesives are placed on the sutured dura area in the necessary cases. In the cases with CSF leakage that cannot be prevented by these surgical strategies, the autogenous blood injection into the epidural space and the lumbar CSF drainage can be performed, respectively. If there is no improvement in the CSF leakage within 3 days in the postoperative period, the surgical field should be reopened and dura repair should be performed [45].

5.3 Spinal instability and fusion requirement

In the posterior midline approaches used for the removal of SMs observed in the cervical and cervico-thoracic junction, the kyphotic deformity will be able to develop in the long-term postoperatively when the multilevel laminectomy is performed. Therefore, arthrodesis is recommended in cases with more than three levels of laminectomy. In these cases, laminoplasty techniques can be used as an alternative [93]. Moreover, spinal instability also develops in the modified posterior approaches, where the total facetectomy is performed with the laminectomy in the cervical and lumbar regions [45]. To prevent spinal instability, posterior stabilization with instrumentation should be performed with lateral mass screwing for the cervical region and transpedicular screwing for the lumbar region, in the same session [45, 46, 94]. In the thoracic region, spinal instability due to the laminectomy is observed very rarely, even in patients who have undergone facetectomy [24]. Menku et al. have recommended that the lamina provided a safe mechanical barrier; therefore, the laminoplasty should be performed in posterior approaches, where laminectomy is used [95]. Therefore, the laminoplasty techniques performed by placing the mini-plates on the laminotomy sites with the pneumatic cutters are preferred in patients who need multi-segmental laminectomy [45, 95]. Even if the laminotomy is performed to reduce the risk of postoperative spinal instability, in all cases, where posterior approaches are used in surgery, all anatomical structures in the surgical area, especially interspinous ligaments should be closed by suturing regularly and tightly. In the anterior transabdominal approaches, where the extensive vertebrectomy is performed, which is now very rarely preferred, the instrumented fusion with the corpectomy cage should be performed in the same session to prevent postoperative instability [46, 94].

One of the most important disadvantages of the anterior cervical approach with the corpectomy used for the removal of ventrally located cervical SMs is spinal instability. It has been stated that placing an autogenous bone graft or cage in the corpectomy area and fusion with the anterior cervical plate-screw system was sufficient in patients who have undergone one- or two-level corpectomies. On the other hand, in cases with three or more corpectomies, the risk of pseudoarthrosis increases after the anterior cervical fusion described above. Therefore, posterior cervical stabilization is recommended to prevent spinal instability that will be able to develop in these cases [96, 97]. Ozkan et al. have stated that 53 of 55 ventrally located SMs were completely removed with the modified posterior approach, in which the laminectomies were extended laterally, and that the secondary stabilization was not performed in any of these cases due to the potential instability due to laminectomy [24].

5.4 Postoperative pain

The somatic pain observed in the preoperative period in the SMs mostly resolves in the postoperative period. On the other hand, analgesic drugs are used together with psychotherapy in the postoperative period, especially in the sub-observed prolonged central pain. The dorsal colon stimulation and morphine pumps can also be used in resistant cases [45].

6. Recurrence

6.1 Extent of surgical tumor removal

The surgical resection coverage is very important in terms of the postoperative tumor recurrence and thus prognosis in the SMs [21]. In the systematic review conducted by Pereira et al., it has been stated that Simpson grade-I and grade-II resection was performed in 94.5% of the SMs, and Simpson grade III or higher resection was performed in 5.5% of them. In this study, the tumor recurrence rate was reported as 4.3% in the SM cases [20]. As a result of another study, it has been stated that the tumor recurrence rate range from 1.3 to 6.4%, and tumor recurrences developed within 1 to 17 years [6].

When other series in the literature were examined, the rates of complete tumor removal in SMs have been reported between 82% and 98% [2, 7, 8, 22, 23, 27]. Similarly, the tumor recurrence rates reported in retrospective studies range from 1 to 15% [5, 22, 23, 27]. While the local tumor recurrence was observed in the majority of SM cases, the tumor recurrence has also been reported in a spinal region other than the region where the tumor was first removed [2].

Voldrich et al. have emphasized that the patient follow-up periods after surgery were also important in determining the frequency of tumor recurrence in Simpson's grade-II resection cases [21, 98]. In the retrospective study conducted by Mirimanoff et al., the tumor recurrence rates were reported as 7%, 10%, and 12% in 5, 10, and 15-year follow-up periods of all meningiomas (intracranial and spinal meningioma) who underwent total resection. However, it has been also stated that 8% of the cases included in this study had SM [85]. On the other hand, Naito et al. have performed a retrospective analysis of 35 patients with the WHO grade-I SMs and stated that no local recurrence was observed in 31 patients (88.6%), who underwent Simpson's grade-I and grade-II resections during 2 years of follow-up [99].

In the study conducted by Klekamp and Samii, they stated that tumor recurrence was observed at a rate of 29.5% in the cases with complete resection, and at a rate of 100% in the cases with partial resection [27]. As a result of many studies reported in the literature, it has been stated that there was no relationship between the treatment modalities (dural resection or dural coagulation) applied to the tumor-infiltrated dural base and tumor recurrence in SMs, unlike intracranial meningiomas [5, 7, 23, 27]. In the systematic study conducted by Pereira et al., although it has been emphasized that partial tumor resection was a risk factor for tumor recurrence [100], it has not been shown that the subtotal tumor resection could definitely lead to the recurrence [5].

6.2 Histopathological tumor subtype and recurrence

In addition to the scope of surgical resection in the SMs, the histological WHO grade of the tumor plays a very important role in tumor recurrence [101]. Most of the SMs are WHO grade-I meningiomas with psammomatous, meningothelial, and other subtypes. The WHO grade-II atypical meningiomas with clear-cell and chordoid subtypes and the WHO grade-III malignant meningiomas are observed less frequently. In particular, the risk of local recurrence is higher in the WHO grade-III malignant meningiomas [102]. The tumor recurrences can be observed rarely in the WHO grade-II atypical meningiomas and very rarely in the WHO grade-I meningiomas [12]. In conclusion, it has been observed in the literature that the risk of tumor recurrence was higher in the WHO grade-II and WHO grade-III SMs and their subtypes, in proportion to the increase in the degree of malignancy [13, 18, 23]. Setzer et al. have stated that the tumor recurrence rates observed in the WHO grade-I, WHO grade-II, and WHO grade-III SMs were 1.4%, 50%, and 100%, respectively. Zorludemir et al. stated that the recurrence rate in the clear cell SMs was 61%. Han et al. analyzed 20 patients with high-grade SMs who were operated on. In this study, it has been stated that the SM was removed according to Simpson's grade-II resection in 16 (80%) patients and it has been removed according to Simpson's grade-III resection in 4 patients (20%), and the tumor recurrence has been observed in a total of 3 patients (15%) [37]. Mauri et al. have stated that the arachnoid invasion in the SMs and the high Ki-67 proliferative index of the tumor were risk factors for tumor recurrence. On the other hand, it has been stated in the same study that the microsurgical dural resection grade, tumor size, and progesterone receptor expression were not risk factors for tumor recurrence [103].

6.3 Reoperation during relapse

Nakamura et al. stated that the WHO grade-I SMs were completely removed with the tumor-infiltrated dural base (according to Simpson's grade-I resection) and reported that the tumor recurrence was lower than in the cases in which the tumor-infiltrated dural base was coagulated and left in place and only the tumor was completely removed (according to Simpson's grade-II resection). However, Sandalcioglu and King have stated that the tumor recurrence was low in the WHO grade-I SMs, even if the tumor-infiltrated dural base was not removed [5, 50, 104]. The total removal of recurrent tumors is difficult due to the arachnoid scar formation. For this reason, the tumor recurrence will be able to be seen in the reoperated cases. Therefore, the aim of surgery should be the total removal of the SM in the first operation [20]. The total removal of recurrent high-grade SMs is difficult because they adhere tightly to the surrounding tissues, spinal cord, and nerve roots. Han et al. stated the results of four patients with recurrent high-grade SM. In this study, they have stated that the SM was incompletely removed (according to Simpson's grade-III resection) in three cases with the ventral location and tightly adhered to the spinal cord, and complete removal of the SM in one case with the challenging surgery (according to Simpson's grade-II resection) [37].

7. Adjuvant therapies

7.1 Adjuvant radiotherapy and stereotactic radiosurgery

Adjuvant radiotherapy is still a controversial issue because of radiation-induced spinal cord damage (radiation myelopathy) [23]. The radiation myelopathy develops, especially as a result of the radiotherapy applications to a 10 cm part of the spinal cord at a dose of more than 1400 cGy [45]. Therefore, the opinion that adjuvant radiotherapy should be used in multiple recurrent tumors or SMs with atypical (WHO grade-II) or malignant (WHO grade-III) histopathology has gained weight [50, 105]. In addition, it has been stated that the adjuvant stereotactic radiosurgery was beneficial in cases with a radiological increase in tumor size [106, 107]. Flores et al. stated in their review that successful local tumor control was achieved with the fractionated stereotactic radiosurgery in one patient with ventrally located foramen magnum meningioma who was operated with the far-lateral approach [52].

7.2 Medical and physical therapy

The physical therapy applied in the postoperative period has a great role in improving the neurological functions of patients. Therefore, physical therapy and rehabilitation programs should be started as soon as possible in patients with SM, who have neurological dysfunction in the postoperative period [61]. Moreover, it will be beneficial to use the peroperative methyl-prednisolone treatment in patients with SM pressing on the spinal cord [108].

8. Prognosis

The prognosis is good in most of the patients with the SMs, and significant improvement in neurological functions is observed in the postoperative period. The rates of improvement in neurological functions in the postoperative period have been stated in the range from 61 to 98%. The permanent postoperative worsening rates have been observed in the literature between 0% and 10% [24, 82]. In a systematic review, the mortality rate has been stated to be 3%. In the literature, it has been stated that aspiration pneumonia, stroke, and myocardial infarction caused more postoperative mortality, especially in pulmonary embolism [5, 27]. It has been observed that the prognosis was better in the SMs localized below the C4 level and topographically located dorsally and dorsolaterally. Moreover, it has been observed that the prognosis was better in patients under 60 years of age and in patients with short duration of clinical symptoms [48]. On the other hand, it has been stated that the prognosis was worse in the SM cases with intratumoral calcifications due to the difficulties experienced in the surgery [2].

Moreover, by means of the developments in the imaging techniques, such as spinal MRI and digital subtraction angiography, the SMs could be diagnosed early and endovascular embolization could be performed in the preoperative period of vascular structures that were tumor feeders. Performing the microsurgical procedures with intraoperative neuromonitoring, ultrasonography, and cavitron ultrasonic aspirator facilitate safe complete removal of the tumor. The use of these preoperative techniques contributes to the significant reduction in the postoperative morbidity and mortality rates in patients with the SMs, and ultimately to a better prognosis [5, 7, 22, 109].

9. Conclusions

The SMs, which are usually benign and grow slowly, are usually diagnosed late. However, the presence of a good surgical cleavage between the spinal cord and the tumor enables the total or near-total removal of SMs by microsurgical methods. The most important factor in the complete and safe removal of the SM is the selection of the surgical approach suitable for the localization and topography of the tumor. In surgical approaches with a high risk of spinal instability, the instrumented fusion should also be performed in the same session. In the postoperative period, rapid improvement in neurological functions is observed in most of the patients. In order to prevent CSF leakage, which is the most common postoperative complication, the excessive coagulation of dura should be avoided. Adjuvant radiotherapy or stereotactic radiosurgery can be used in recurrent SMs with malignant histopathology.

Conflict of interest

The authors declare no conflict of interest.

Acronyms and abbreviations

CSF	cerebrospinal fluid
CT	computerized tomography
CUSA	cavitron ultrasonic surgical aspirator
JOA	Japanese orthopedic society
MEP	motor-evoked potentials
MMC	modified McCormick
MRI	magnetic resonance imaging
SSEP	somatosensory-evoked potentials
SM	spinal meningioma
USG	ultrasonography
WHO	World Health Organization

Author details

Feyzi Birol Sarica
Department of Neurosurgery, Giresun University Faculty of Medicine, Giresun Education and Research Hospital, Giresun, Turkey

*Address all correspondence to: saricafb@gmail.com

References

[1] Katz K, Reichenthal E, Israeli J. Surgical treatment of spinal meningiomas. Neurochirurgia (Stuttg). 1981;**24**(1):21-22. DOI: 10.1055/s-2008-1053837

[2] Levy WJ, Bay J, Dohn D. Spinal cord meningioma. Journal of Neurosurgery. 1982;**57**:804-812. DOI: 10.3171/jns.1982.57.6.0804

[3] Russell DS, Rubinstein LJ. Pathology of Tumours of the Nervous System. 5th ed. London: Edward Arnold; 1989. pp. 449-532

[4] Setzer M, Vatter H, Marquardt G, Seifert V, Vrionis FD. Management of spinal meningiomas: Surgical results and a review of the literature. Neurosurgical Focus. 2007;**23**(4):E14. DOI: 10.3171/FOC-07/10/E14

[5] King AT, Sharr MM, Gullan RW, Bartlett JR. Spinal meningiomas: A 20-year review. British Journal of Neurosurgery. 1988;**12**(6):521-526. DOI: 10.1080/02688699844367

[6] Namer IJ, Pamir MN, Benli K, Saglam S, Erbengi A. Spinal meningiomas. Neurochirurgia (Stuttg). 1987;**30**(1):11-15. DOI: 10.1055/s-2008-1053647

[7] Solero CL, Fornari M, Giombini S, Lasio G, Oliveri G, Cimino C, et al. Spinal meningiomas: Review of 174 operated cases. Neurosurgery. 1989;**25**(2):153-160

[8] Morandi X, Haegelen C, Riffaud L, Amlashi S, Adn M, Brassier G. Results in the operative treatment of elderly patients with spinal meningiomas. Spine (Phila Pa 1976). 2004;**29**(19):2191-2194. DOI: 10.1097/01.brs.0000141173.79572.40

[9] Nelson JS, Parisi JE, Schochet SS. Principles and practice of neuropathology. In: Parisi JE, Mena H, editors. Non-Glial Tumors. St. Louis, MO: Mosby-Year Book, Inc.; 1993. pp. 203-213

[10] Wang XQ, Zeng XW, Zhang BY, Dou YF, Wu JS, Jiang CC, et al. Spinal meningioma in childhood: Clinical features and treatment. Child's Nervous System. 2012;**28**(1):129-136. DOI: 10.1007/s00381-011-1570-2

[11] Shen Y, Nunes F, Stemmer-Rachaminov A, James M, Mohapatra G, Plotkin S, et al. Genomic profiling distinguishes familial multiple and sporadic multiple meningiomas. BMC Medical Genomics. 2009;**2**:42. DOI: 10.1186/1755-8794-2-42

[12] Parry DM, Eldridge R, Kaiser-Kupfer MI, Bouzas EA, Pikus A, Patronas N. Neurofibromatosis 2 (NF2): Clinical characteristics of 63 affected individuals and clinical evidence for heterogeneity. American Journal of Medical Genetics. 1994;**52**(4):450-461. DOI: 10.1002/ajgm.1320520411

[13] Moriuchi S, Nakagawa H, Yamada M, Kadota T. Intramedullary spinal cord meningioma—Case report. Neurologia Medico-Chirurgica. 1996;**36**:888-892. DOI: 10.2176/nmc.36.888

[14] Park SH, Hwang SK, Park YM. Intramedullary clear cell meningioma. Acta Neurochirurgica. 2006;**148**(4):463-466. DOI: 10.1007/s00701-005-0695-z

[15] Salvati M, Artico M, Lunardi P, Gagliardi FM. Intramedullary meningioma: Case report and review of the literature. Surgical Neurology. 1992;**37**(1):42-45. DOI: 10.1016/0090-3019(92)90064-t

[16] Frank BL, Harrop JS, Hanna A, Ratliff J. Cervical extradural meningioma: Case report and literature review. The Journal of Spinal Cord Medicine. 2008;**31**(3):302-305. DOI: 10.1080/10790268.2008.11760727

[17] Erkutlu I, Buyukhatipoglu H, Alptekin M, Berkyurek E, Tutar E, Gok A. Spinal drop metastases from a papillary meningioma: A case report and review of the literature: Utility of CSF sampling. Medical Oncology. 2009;**26**(2):242-246

[18] Kamiya K, Inagawa T, Nagasako R. Malignant intraventricular meningioma with spinal metastasis through the cerebrospinal fluid. Surgical Neurology. 1989;**32**(3):213-218. DOI: 10.1016/0090-3019(89)90181-x

[19] Akbay A, Altundağ MK, Ozişik Y, Zorlu AF, Palaoğlu S. Reverse seeding of recurrent intraspinal malignant meningioma. Oncology. 2002;**62**(4):386-388. DOI: 10.1159/000065072

[20] Pereira BJA, de Almeida AN, Paiva WS, de Aguiar PHP, Teixeira MJ, Marie SKN. Neuro-oncological features of spinal meningiomas: Systematic review. Neuro-Chirurgie. 2020;**66**(1):41-44. DOI: 10.1016/j.neuchi.2019.09.027

[21] Voldrich R, Netuka D, Benes V. Spinal meningiomas—92 patients operated our department. Cesk Slov Neurol N. 2019;**115**(6):664-669. DOI: 10.14735/amcsnn2019664

[22] Gottfried ON, Gluf W, Quinones-Hinojosa A, Kan P, Schmidt MH. Spinal meningiomas: Surgical management and outcome. Neurosurgical Focus. 2003;**14**(6):e2. DOI: 10.3171/foc.2003.14.6.2

[23] Gezen F, Kahraman S, Canakci Z, Bedük A. Review of 36 cases of spinal cord meningioma. Spine (Phila Pa 1976). 2000;**25**(6):727-731. DOI: 10.1097/00007632-200003150-00013

[24] Ozkan N, Dammann P, Chen B, Schoemberg T, Schlamann M, Sandalcioglu IE, et al. Operative strategies in ventrally and ventrolaterally located spinal meningiomas and review of the literature. Neurosurgical Review. 2013;**36**(4):611-619. DOI: 10.1007/s10143-013-0462-1

[25] Roux FX, Nataf F, Pinaudeau M, Borne G, Devaux B, Meder JF. Intraspinal meningiomas: Review of 54 cases with discussion of poor prognosis factors and modern therapeutic management. Surgical Neurology. 1996;**46**:458-463. DOI: 10.1016/S0090-3019(96)00199-1

[26] Yoon SH, Chung CK, Jahng TA. Surgical outcome of spinal canal meningiomas. Journal of Korean Neurosurgical Association. 2007;**42**(4):300-304. DOI: 10.3340/jkns.2007.42.4.300

[27] Klekamp J, Samii M. Surgical results for spinal meningiomas. Surgical Neurology. 1999 Dec;**52**(6):552-562. DOI: 10.1016/s0090-3019(99)00153-6

[28] Sisti M, Stein B. Surgery of spinal meningiomas. In: Al-Mefty (ed.), editor. Meningiomas. New York: Raven Press; 1991. pp. 615-620

[29] Cohen-Gadol AA, Zikel OF, Koch CA, Scheithauer BW, Krauss WE. Spinal meningiomas in patients younger than 50 years of age: A 21-year experience. Journal of Neurosurgery. 2003;**98**(Suppl. 3):258-263. DOI: 10.3171/spi.2003.98.3.0258

[30] Kshettry VR, Hsieh JK, Ostrom QT, Kruchko C, Benzel EC, Barnholtz-Sloan JS. Descriptive epidemiology

of spinal meningiomas in the United States. Spine (Phila Pa 1976). 2015;**40**(15):E886-E889. DOI: 10.1097/BRS.0000000000000974

[31] Mawrin C, Perry A. Pathological classification and molecular genetics of meningiomas. Journal of Neuro-Oncology. 2010;**99**(33):379-391. DOI: 10.1007/s11060-010-0342-2

[32] Louis DN, Perry A, Reifenberger G, von Deimling A, Figarella-Branger D, Cavenee WK, et al. The 2016 World Health Organization classification of tumors of the central nervous system: A summary. Acta Neuropathologica. 2016;**131**(6):803-820. DOI: 10.1007/s00401-016-1545-1

[33] Jain D, Sharma MC, Sarkar C, Suri V, Garg A, Singh M, et al. Clear cell meningioma, an uncommon variant of meningioma: A clinicopathologic study of nine cases. Journal of Neuro-Oncology. 2007;**81**(3):315-321. DOI: 10.1007/s11060-9237-7

[34] Sun SQ, Cai C, Ravindra VM, Gamble P, Yarbrough CK, Dacey RG, et al. Simpson Grade I-III resection of spinal atypical (World Health Organization Grade II) meningiomas is associated with symptom resolution and low recurrence. Neurosurgery. 2015;**76**(6):739-746. DOI: 10.1227/NEU.0000000000000720

[35] Freidberg SR. Removal of an ossified ventral thoracic meningioma. Case report. Journal of Neurosurgery. 1972;**37**(6):728-730. DOI: 10.3171/jns.1972.37.6.0728

[36] Weinstein JN, McLain RF. Tumors of the Spine. In: Rothman RH, Simeone FA, editors. The Spine. 3rd ed. Philadelphia: WB Saunders Co.; 1992. pp. 1299-1300

[37] Han B, Zhang L, Jia W, Yang J. Clinical features and surgical outcomes of high-grade spinal meningiomas: Report of 19 cases and literature review. Journal of Clinical Neuroscience. 2020;**72**:264-269. DOI: 10.1016/j.jocn.2019.11.020

[38] Kaiser MC, Ramos L. MRI of the spine. In: Tumors. New York: Thieme Medical Publishers, Inc; 1990. pp. 67-68

[39] Lee JW, Lee IS, Choi KU, Lee YH, Yi JH, Song JW, et al. CT and MRI findings of calcified spinal meningiomas: Correlation with pathological findings. Skeletal Radiology. 2010;**39**(4):345-352. DOI: 10.1007/s00256-009-0771-1

[40] Ono K, Shimizu T, Fujibayashi S, Otsuki B, Murata K, Sakomoto A, et al. Predictive value of heterogeneously enhanced magnetic resonance imaging findings with computed tomography evidence of calcification for severe motor deficits in spinal meningioma. Neurospine. 2020;**18**(1):163-196. DOI: 10.14245/ns.2040494.247

[41] Gamache FW Jr, Wang JC, Deck M, Heise C. Unusual appearance of an en plaque meningioma of the cervical spinal canal. A case report and literature review. Spine. 2001;**26**(5):E87-E89

[42] Stechison MT, Tasker RR, Wortzman G. Spinal meningioma en plaque. Report of two cases. Journal of Neurosurgery. 1987;**67**(3):452-455. DOI: 10.3171/jns.1987.67.3.0452

[43] Arima H, Takami T, Yamagata T, Naito K, Abe J, Shimokawa N, et al. Surgical management of spinal meningiomas: A retrospective case analysis based on preoperative surgical grade. Surgical Neurology International. 2014;**5**(Suppl. 7):S333-S338. DOI: 10.4103/2152-7806.139642

[44] Kim CH, Chung CK, Lee SH, Jahng TA, Hyun SJ, Kim KJ, et al. Long-term recurrence rates after the removal of spinal meningiomas in relation to Simpson grades. European Spine Journal. 2016;**25**(12):4025-4032. DOI: 10.1007/s00586-015-4306-2

[45] Unal F. Spinal intradural ekstramedüller tümörler. In: Aksoy K, Palaoglu S, Pamir N, Tuncer R, editors. Temel Nörosirurji. Section 3, Chapter 122. Turkey: Turkish Neurosurgery Society Publications; 2005. pp. 1121-1128. ISBN: 975-96290-8-9

[46] Rasras S, Kiani A. Intradural extramedullary spinal tumors. In: Morgan LR, Sarica FB, editors. Brain and Spinal Tumors—Primary and Secondary. London, United Kingdom: InTechOpen Limited. pp. 43-53

[47] Bozkus H. Spinal meningiomlar. Turk Nörosirurji Dergisi. 2011;**21**(2):202-206

[48] Schaller B. Spinal meningioma: Relationship between histological subtypes and surgical outcome? Journal of Neuro-Oncology. 2005;**75**(2):157-161. DOI: 10.1007/s11060-005-1469-4

[49] Arnautovic KI, Al-Mefty O, Husain M. Ventral foramen magnum meningiomas. Journal of Neurosurgery. 2000;**92**(1 Suppl):71-80. DOI: 10.3171/spi.2000.92.1.0071

[50] Sandalcioglu IE, Hunold A, Müller O, Bassiouni H, Stolke D, Asgari S. Spinal meningiomas: Critical review of 131 surgically treated patients. European Spine Journal. 2008;**17**(8):1035-1041. DOI: 10.1007/s00586-008-0685-y

[51] George B, Dematons C, Cophignon J. Lateral approach to the anterior portion of the foramen magnum: Application to surgical removal of 14 benign tumors: Technical note. Surgical Neurology. 1988;**29**(6):484-490. DOI: 10.1016/0090-3019(88)90145-0

[52] Flores BC, Boudreaux BP, Klinger DR, Mickey BE, Barnett SL. The far-lateral approach for foramen magnum meningiomas. Neurosurgical Focus. 2013;**35**(6):E12. DOI: 10.3171/2013.10.FOCUS13332

[53] Lanzino G, Paolini S, Spetzler RF. Far-lateral approach to the craniocervical junction. Neurosurgery. 2005;**57**(4 Suppl):367-371. DOI: 10.1227/01.neu.0000176848.05925.80

[54] Salas E, Sekhar LN, Ziyal IM, Caputy AJ, Wright DC. Variations of the extreme-lateral craniocervical approach: Anatomical study and clinical analysis of 69 patients. Journal of Neurosurgery. 1999;**90**(2 Suppl):206-219. DOI: 10.3171/spi.1999.90.2.0206

[55] Kratimenos GP, Crockard HA. The far lateral approach for ventrally placed foramen magnum and upper cervical spine tumours. British Journal of Neurosurgery. 1993;**7**(2):129-140. DOI: 10.3109/02688699309103469

[56] Sen C, Shrivastava R, Anwar S, Triana A. Lateral transcondylar approach for tumors at the anterior aspect of the craniovertebral junction. Neurosurgery. 2010;**66**(3 Suppl):104-112. DOI: 10.1227/01.NEU.0000365930.95389.60

[57] Margalit NS, Lesser JB, Singer M, Sen C. Lateral approach to anterolateral tumors at the foramen magnum: Factors determining surgical procedure. Neurosurgery. 2005;**56**(2 Suppl):324-336. DOI: 10.1227/01.neu.0000156796.28536.6d

[58] Angevine PD, Kellner C, Haque RM, McCormick PC. Surgical management of ventral intradural spinal lesions. Journal of Neurosurgery. Spine. 2011;**15**(1):28-37. DOI: 10.3171/2011.3.SPINE1095

[59] Ayoub B. The far lateral approach for intra-dural anteriorly situated tumours at the craniovertebral junction. Turkish Neurosurgery. 2011;**21**(4):494-498

[60] Liu JK, Rao G, Schmidt MH, Couldwell WT. Far lateral transcondylar transtubercular approach to lesions of the ventral foramen magnum and craniovertebral junction. Contemp Neurosurg. 2007;**29**(10):1-7. DOI: 10.1097/01.CNE.0000268054.70330.62

[61] Keles E, Ozer AF. İntradural ekstramedüller omurilik tümörleri. In: Zileli M, Ozer AF, editors. Omurilik ve Omurga Cerrahisi. 2002. pp. 1113-1119

[62] Al-Mefty O. Meningioms. New York: Raven Press; 1991

[63] McDonnell DE. Anterolateral cervical approach to the craniovertebral junction. In: Rengachary SS, Wilkins RH, editors. Neurosurgical Operative Atlas. Baltimore.: Williams & Wilkins; 1991. pp. 147-164

[64] George B, Lot G, Boissonnet H. Meningioma of the foramen magnum: A series of 40 cases. Surgical Neurology. 1997;**47**(4):371-379. DOI: 10.1016/s0090-3019(96)00204-2

[65] Payer M. The anterior approach to anterior cervical meningiomas: Review illustrated by a case. Acta Neurochirurgica. 2005;**147**(5):555-560. DOI: 10.1007/s00701-005-0502-x

[66] Giroux JC, Nehra O. Anterior approach for removal of al cervical intradural tumor. Case report and technical note. Neurosurgery. 1978;**2**(2):128-130. DOI: 10.1227/00006123-197803000-00009

[67] Lenelle J, Born JD, Collignon J. Ablation by the anterior transcorporeal approach of an ante-spinal cord cervical meningioma. Apropos of a case. Neurochirurgie. 1986;**32**(3):262-265

[68] Sawa H, Tamaki N, Kurata H, Nagashima T. Complete resection of a spinal meningioma extending from the foramen magnum to the second thoracic vertebral body via the anterior approach: Case report. Neurosurgery. 1993;**33**:1095-1098. DOI: 10.1227/00006123-199312000-00019

[69] Banczerowski P, Lipoth L, Vajda J, Veres R. Surgery of ventral intradural midline cervical spinal pathologies via anterior cervical approach: Our experience. Ideggyógyászati Szemle. 2003;**56**:115-118

[70] McCormick PC. Surgical management of dumbbell and paraspinal tumors of the thoracic and lumbar spine. Neurosurgery. 1996;**38**(1):67-74. DOI: 10.1097/00006123-199601000-00017

[71] Bohlman HH, Zdeblick TA. Anterior excision of herniated thoracic discs. The Journal of Bone and Joint Surgery. 1988;**70**(7):1038-1047

[72] Ando K, Imagama S, Ito Z, Kobayashi K, Ukai J, Muramoto A, et al. Unilateral instrumented fixation for cervical dumbbell tumors. Journal of Orthopaedic Surgery and Research. 2014;**9**:2

[73] Meyer FB, Ebersold MJ, Reese DF. Benign tumors of the foramen magnum.

Journal of Neurosurgery. 1984;**61**(1):136-142. DOI: 10.3171/jns.1984.61.1.0136

[74] Stein BM, Leeds NE, Taveras JM, Pool JL. Meningiomas of the foramen magnum. Journal of Neurosurgery. 1963;**20**:740-751. DOI: 10.3171/jns.20.9.0740

[75] Simpson D. The recurrence of intracranial meningiomas after surgical treatment. Journal of Neurology, Neurosurgery, and Psychiatry. 1957;**20**(1):22-39. DOI: 10.1136/jnnp.20.1.22

[76] Abou-Madawi EK et al. Far-lateral approach for ventral and ventrolateral upper cervical meningiomas: A case series and literature reviewn. The Spine Journal. 2021;**15**(5):584-595. DOI: 10.31616/asj.2020.0270

[77] Slinko E, Al-Qashqish I. Intradural ventral and ventrolateral tumors of the spinal cord: Surgical treatment and results. Neurosurgical Focus. 2004;**17**(1):ECP2. DOI: 10.3171/foc.2004.17.1.9

[78] Taha MM, Alawamry A, Abdel-Aziz HR. Ossified spinal meningioma: A case report and a review of the literature. Surgery Journal. 2019;**5**(4):e137-e141. DOI: 10.1055/s-0039-1697634

[79] Tola S, De Angelis M, Bistazzoni S, Chiaramonte C, Esposito V, Paolini S. Hemilaminectomy for spinal meningioma: A case series of 20 patients with a focus on ventral- and ventrolateral lesions. Clinical Neurology and Neurosurgery. 2016;**148**:35-41. DOI: 10.1016/j.clineuro.2016.06.015

[80] Saito T, Arizono T, Maeda T, Terada K, Iwamoto Y. A novel technique for surgical resection of spinal meningioma. Spine (Phila Pa 1976). 2001;**26**(16):1805-1808. DOI: 10.1097/00007632-200108150-00017

[81] Postalci L, Tugcu B, Gungor A, Guclu G. Spinal meningiomas: Recurrence in ventrally located individuals on long-term follow-up; a review of 46 operated cases. Turkish Neurosurgery. 2011;**21**(4):449-453

[82] Riad H, Knafo D, Segnarbieux F, Lonjon N. Spinal meningiomas: Surgical outcome and literature review. Neuro-Chirurgie. 2013;**59**(1):30-34. DOI: 10.1016/j.neuchi.2012.10.137

[83] Aydin MD, Cesur M, Aydin N, Alici HA. Disappearance of phantom limb pain during cauda equina compression by spinal meningioma and gradual reactivation after decompression. Anesthesia and Analgesia. 2005;**101**(4):1123-1126. DOI: 10.1213/01.ANE.0000175768.11507.BC

[84] Haegelen C, Morandi X, Riffaud L, Amlashi SF, Leray E, Brassier G. Results of spinal meningioma surgery in patients with severe preoperative neurological deficits. European Spine Journal. 2005;**14**(5):440-444. DOI: 10.1007/s00586-004-0809-y

[85] Mirimanoff RO, Dosoretz DE, Linggood RM, Ojemann RG, Martuza RL. Meningioma: Analysis of recurrence and progression following neurosurgical resection. Journal of Neurosurgery. 1985;**62**(1):18-24. DOI: 10.3171/jns.1985.62.1.0018

[86] Maiti TK, Bir SC, Patra DP, Kalakoti P, Guthikonda B, Nanda A. Spinal meningiomas: Clinicoradiological factors predicting recurrence and functional outcome. Neurosurgical Focus. 2016;**41**(2):E6. DOI: 10.3171/2016.5.FOCUS16163

[87] Ruggeri AG, Fazzolari B, Colistra D, Cappelletti M, Marotta N, Delfini R. Calcified spinal meningiomas. World Neurosurgery. 2017;**102**:406-412. DOI: 10.1016/j.wneu.2017.03.045

[88] Joaquim AF, Almeida JP, Dos Santos MJ, Ghizoni E, de Oliveira E, Tedeschi H. Surgical management of intradural extramedullary tumors located anteriorly to the spinal cord. Journal of Clinical Neuroscience. 2012;**19**(8):1150-1153. DOI: 10.1015/j.jocn.2011.08.044

[89] Komotar RJ, Zacharia BE, McGovern RA, Sisti MB, Bruce JN, D'Ambrosio AL. Approaches to anterior and anterolateral foramen magnum lesions: A critical review. Journal of Craniovertebr Junction Spine. 2010;**1**(2):86-99. DOI: 10.4103/0974-8237.77672

[90] Goel A, Desai K, Muzumdar D. Surgery on anterior foramen magnum meningiomas using a conventional posterior suboccipital approach: A report on an experience with 17 cases. Neurosurgery. 2001;**49**(1):102-106. DOI: 10.1097/00006123-200107000-00016

[91] D'Aliberti G, Talamonti G, Villa F, Debernardi A, Sansalone CV, LaMaida A, et al. Anterior approach to thoracic and lumbar spine lesions: Results in 145 consecutive cases. Journal of Neurosurgery. 2008;**9**(5):466-482. DOI: 10.3171/SPI.2008.9.11.466

[92] Sen CN, Sekhar LN. An extreme lateral approach to intradural lesions of the cervical spine and foramen magnum. Neurosurgery. 1990;**27**(2):197-204. DOI: 10.1097/00006123-199008000-00004

[93] Duff JM, Omoumi P, Bobinski L, Belouaer A, Plaza Wuthrich S, Zanchi F, et al. Transtubular image-guided surgery for spinal intradural lesions: Techniques, results, and complications in a consecutive series of 60 patients. Journal of Neurosurgery. 2022;**2022**:1-9. DOI: 10.3171/2021.10.SPINE211168

[94] Abumi K, Panjabi M, Kramer K, Duranceau J, Oxland T, Crisco JJ. Biomechanical evaluation of lumbar spinal stability after graded facetectomies. Spine. 1990;**15**:1142-1147. DOI: 10.1097/00007632-199011010-00011

[95] Menku A, Koc RK, Oktem IS, Tucer B, Kurtsoy A. Laminoplasty with miniplates for posterior approach in thoracic and lumbar intraspinal surgery. Turkish Neurosurgery. 2010;**20**(1):27-32

[96] Sasso RC, Ruggiero RA Jr, Reilly TM, Hall PV. Early reconstruction failures after multilevel cervical corpectomy. Spine (Phila Pa 1976). 2003;**28**(2):140-142. DOI: 10.1097/00007632-200301150-00009

[97] Vaccaro AR, Falatyn SP, Scuderi GJ, Eismont FJ, McGuire RA, Singh K, et al. Early failure of long segment anterior cervical plate fixation. Journal of Spinal Disorders. 1998;**11**(5):410-415

[98] Voldrich R, Netuka D, Benes V. Spinal meningiomas: Is Simpson grade II resection radical enough? Acta Neurochirurgica. 2020;**162**(6):1401-1408. DOI: 10.1007/s00701-020-04280-2

[99] Naito K, Yamagata T, Arima H, Takami T. Low recurrence after Simpson grade II resection of spinal benign meningiomas in a single-institute 10-year retrospective study. Journal of Clinical Neuroscience. 2020;**77**:168-174. DOI: 10.1016/j.Jocn.2020.04.113

[100] Iacoangeli M, Gladi M, Di Rienzo A, Dobran M, Alvaro L, Nocchi N, et al. Minimally invasive surgery for benign

intradural extramedullary spinal meningiomas: Experience of a single institution in a cohort of elderly patients and review of the literature. Clinical Interventions in Aging. 2012;7:557-564. DOI: 10.2147/CIA.S38923

[101] Barresi V, Caffo M, Tuccari G. Classification of human meningiomas: Lights, shadows, and future perspectives. Journal of Neuroscience Research. 2016;**94**(12):1604-1612. DOI: 10.1002/jnr.23801

[102] Saraceni C, Harrop JS. Spinal meningioma: Chronicles of contemporary neurosurgical diagnosis and management. Clinical Neurology and Neurosurgery. 2009;**111**(3):221-226. DOI: 10.1016/jcklineuro.2008.10.018

[103] Mauri F, De Caro MDB, Divitiis O, Guadagno E, Mariniello G. Recurrence of spinal meningiomas: Analysis of the risk factors. British Journal of Neurosurgery. 2020;**34**(5):569-574. DOI: 10.1080/02688697.2019.1638886

[104] Nakamura M, Tsuji O, Fujiyoshi K, et al. Long-term surgical outcomes of spinal meningiomas. Spine. 2012;**37**:E617-E623

[105] Schiebe ME, Hoffmann W, Kortmann RD, Bamberg M. Radiotherapy in recurrent malignant meningiomas with multiple spinal manifestations. Acta Oncologica. 1997;**36**(1):88-90. DOI: 10.3109/02841869709100743

[106] Dodd RL, Ryu MR, Kamnerdsupaphon P, Gibbs IC, Chang SD Jr, Adler JR Jr. CyberKnife radiosurgery for benign intradural extramedullary spinal tumors. Neurosurgery. 2006;**58**(4):674-685. DOI: 10.1227/01.NEU.0000204128.84742.8F

[107] Gerszten PC, Burton SA, Ozhasoglu C, McCue KJ, Quinn AE. Radiosurgery for benign intradural spinal tumors. Neurosurgery. 2008;**62**(4):887-896. DOI: 10.1227/01.neu.0000318174.28461.fc

[108] Frati A, Pesce A, Toccaceli G, Fraschetti F, Caruso R, Raco A. Spinal Meningiomas Prognostic Evaluation Score (SPES): Predicting the neurological outcomes in spinal meningioma surgery. Neurosurgical Review. 2019;**42**(1):115-125. DOI: 10.1007/s10143-018-0961-1

[109] McCormick PC, Post KD, Stein BM. Intradural extramedullary tumors in adults. Neurosurgery Clinics of North America. 1990;**1**(3):591-608